Breastfeeding: Benefits to Infant and Mother

Breastfeeding: Benefits to Infant and Mother

Guest Editor
Robert D. Roghair

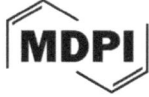 Basel • Beijing • Wuhan • Barcelona • Belgrade • Novi Sad • Cluj • Manchester

Guest Editor
Robert D. Roghair
Stead Family Department of
Pediatrics
University of Iowa
Iowa City
USA

Editorial Office
MDPI AG
Grosspeteranlage 5
4052 Basel, Switzerland

This is a reprint of the Special Issue, published open access by the journal *Nutrients* (ISSN 2072-6643), freely accessible at: https://www.mdpi.com/journal/nutrients/special_issues/35UH7CV876.

For citation purposes, cite each article independently as indicated on the article page online and as indicated below:

Lastname, A.A.; Lastname, B.B. Article Title. *Journal Name* **Year**, *Volume Number*, Page Range.

ISBN 978-3-7258-3523-2 (Hbk)
ISBN 978-3-7258-3524-9 (PDF)
https://doi.org/10.3390/books978-3-7258-3524-9

Cover image courtesy of Robert D. Roghair

© 2025 by the authors. Articles in this book are Open Access and distributed under the Creative Commons Attribution (CC BY) license. The book as a whole is distributed by MDPI under the terms and conditions of the Creative Commons Attribution-NonCommercial-NoDerivs (CC BY-NC-ND) license (https://creativecommons.org/licenses/by-nc-nd/4.0/).

Contents

About the Editor vii

Preface ix

Robert Roghair
Breastfeeding: Benefits to Infant and Mother
Reprinted from: *Nutrients* 2024, 16, 3251, https://doi.org/10.3390/nu16193251 1

Wafaa T. Elgzar, DaifAllah D. Al-Thubaity, Mohammed A. Alshahrani, Rasha M. Essa and Heba A. Ibrahim
The Relationship between Maternal Ideation and Exclusive Breastfeeding Practice among Saudi Nursing Mothers: A Cross-Sectional Study
Reprinted from: *Nutrients* 2023, 15, 1719, https://doi.org/10.3390/nu15071719 6

DaifAllah D. Al-Thubaity, Mohammed A. Alshahrani, Wafaa T. Elgzar and Heba A. Ibrahim
Determinants of High Breastfeeding Self-Efficacy among Nursing Mothers in Najran, Saudi Arabia
Reprinted from: *Nutrients* 2023, 15, 1919, https://doi.org/10.3390/nu15081919 22

M. Ascensión Olcina Simón, Rosita Rotella, Jose M. Soriano, Agustin Llopis-Gonzalez, Isabel Peraita-Costa and María Morales-Suarez-Varela
Breastfeeding-Related Practices in Rural Ethiopia: Colostrum Avoidance
Reprinted from: *Nutrients* 2023, 15, 2177, https://doi.org/10.3390/nu15092177 35

Lars Libuda, Birgit Filipiak-Pittroff, Marie Standl, Tamara Schikowski, Andrea von Berg, Sibylle Koletzko, et al.
Full Breastfeeding and Allergic Diseases—Long-Term Protection or Rebound Effects?
Reprinted from: *Nutrients* 2023, 15, 2780, https://doi.org/10.3390/nu15122780 48

Agnes Meire Branco Leria Bizon, Camila Giugliani and Elsa Regina Justo Giugliani
Women's Satisfaction with Breastfeeding and Risk of Exclusive Breastfeeding Interruption
Reprinted from: *Nutrients* 2023, 15, 5062, https://doi.org/10.3390/nu15245062 63

Sarah J. Melov, James Elhindi, Lisa White, Justin McNab, Vincent W. Lee, Kelly Donnolley, et al.
Previous High-Intensity Breastfeeding Lowers the Risk of an Abnormal Fasting Glucose in a Subsequent Pregnancy Oral Glucose Tolerance Test
Reprinted from: *Nutrients* 2024, 16, 28, https://doi.org/10.3390/nu16010028 73

Isabel Rodríguez-Gallego, Rafael Vila-Candel, Isabel Corrales-Gutierrez, Diego Gomez-Baya and Fatima Leon-Larios
Evaluation of the Impact of a Midwife-Led Breastfeeding Group Intervention on Prevention of Postpartum Depression: A Multicentre Randomised Clinical Trial
Reprinted from: *Nutrients* 2024, 16, 227, https://doi.org/10.3390/nu16020227 86

Rafael Vila-Candel, Francisco Javier Soriano-Vidal, Cristina Franco-Antonio, Oscar Garcia-Algar, Vicente Andreu-Esteve and Desirée Mena-Tudela
Factors Influencing Duration of Breastfeeding: Insights from a Prospective Study of Maternal Health Literacy and Obstetric Practices
Reprinted from: *Nutrients* 2024, 16, 690, https://doi.org/10.3390/nu16050690 101

Isabel Rodríguez-Gallego, Isabel Corrales-Gutierrez, Diego Gomez-Baya and Fatima Leon-Larios
Effectiveness of a Postpartum Breastfeeding Support Group Intervention in Promoting Exclusive Breastfeeding and Perceived Self-Efficacy: A Multicentre Randomized Clinical Trial
Reprinted from: *Nutrients* **2024**, *16*, 988, https://doi.org/10.3390/nu16070988 . . . . **116**

Cristina Verea-Nuñez, Nuria Novoa-Maciñeiras, Ana Suarez-Casal and Juan Manuel Vazquez-Lago
Factors Associated with Exclusive Breastfeeding during Admission to a Baby-Friendly Hospital Initiative Hospital: A Cross-Sectional Study in Spain
Reprinted from: *Nutrients* **2024**, *16*, 1679, https://doi.org/10.3390/nu16111679 . . . . **134**

Réka Anna Vass, Miaomiao Zhang, Livia Simon Sarkadi, Márta Üveges, Judit Tormási, Eszter L. Benes, et al.
Effect of Holder Pasteurization, Mode of Delivery, and Infant's Gender on Fatty Acid Composition of Donor Breast Milk
Reprinted from: *Nutrients* **2024**, *16*, 1689, https://doi.org/10.3390/nu16111689 . . . . **145**

Ebe D'Adamo, Chiara Peila, Mariachiara Strozzi, Roberta Barolo, Antonio Maconi, Arianna Nanni, et al.
Presepsin in Human Milk Is Delivery Mode and Gender Dependent
Reprinted from: *Nutrients* **2024**, *16*, 2554, https://doi.org/10.3390/nu16152554 . . . . **160**

About the Editor

Robert D. Roghair

Robert D. Roghair received his pharmacy degree and medical degree from the University of Iowa, and he has been a faculty neonatologist with the University of Iowa for nearly 20 years. He is now a full tenured Professor of Pediatrics, and he directs the Iowa Medical Student Research Program. For over 20 consecutive years, his laboratory has performed NIH-funded basic science and clinical research investigations into the roles of breast milk, leptin, and exercise in the developmental origins of disease. More recently, he has become a vocal advocate for increased inclusion of individuals with disabilities in healthcare and research careers, and he serves on the equity committee of multiple national and international organizations.

Preface

This Special Issue was created to support evidence-based recommendations regarding the initiation and maintenance of breastfeeding worldwide. The resulting compilation of articles significantly expands the depth of our understanding of the factors that facilitate breastfeeding initiation and continuation, in addition to the public health implications of breastfeeding success. Higher levels of knowledge and self-efficacy have consistently fostered maternal-defined breastfeeding satisfaction. While ongoing efforts are needed to increase breastfeeding rates, it is encouraging that many of the factors that contribute to a positive maternal attitude and experience are modifiable, as long as healthcare providers seek the identification of factors that could be interfering with breastfeeding success. There are important roles in this process for a multidisciplinary healthcare team as well as community stakeholders. In this Special Issue, that paradigm was demonstrated by the results of a randomized clinical trial that showed midwife-led postpartum support groups can lower maternal depression scores while simultaneously increasing self-efficacy and breastfeeding success. This Special Issue further clarifies the public health importance of breastfeeding with studies demonstrating a reduction in the odds of abnormal fasting glucose during subsequent pregnancies and protection of the breastfed infant from early eczema. This is a clear call for policymakers to increase resource allocation, including improved workplace and parental leave policies, to improve public health worldwide.

Robert D. Roghair
Guest Editor

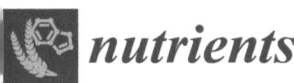

Editorial

Breastfeeding: Benefits to Infant and Mother

Robert Roghair

Stead Family Department of Pediatrics, Carver College of Medicine, University of Iowa, Iowa City, IA 52242, USA; robert-roghair@uiowa.edu

Citation: Roghair, R. Breastfeeding: Benefits to Infant and Mother. *Nutrients* **2024**, *16*, 3251. https://doi.org/10.3390/nu16193251

Received: 5 September 2024
Accepted: 20 September 2024
Published: 26 September 2024

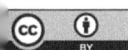

Copyright: © 2024 by the author. Licensee MDPI, Basel, Switzerland. This article is an open access article distributed under the terms and conditions of the Creative Commons Attribution (CC BY) license (https://creativecommons.org/licenses/by/4.0/).

1. Introduction

The provision of human milk to newborn infants is one of the most effective ways to reduce infant mortality. It has been estimated that nearly one million children's lives could be saved every year if all children were optimally breastfed [1]. Later in life, breastfed children perform better on intelligence tests, are less likely to be overweight or obese and less prone to diabetes [2]. Additional benefits are seen for birthing parents that provide their own milk for their infants, including a reduction in the rates of many types of cancer and decreased metabolic or cardiovascular disease [3,4]. Based on this evidence, the World Health Organization (WHO) and the United Nations International Children's Emergency Fund (UNICEF) recommend that children initiate breastfeeding within the first hour of birth and be exclusively breastfed for 6 months [5]. Unfortunately, more often than not, infants receive non-human milk feedings before 6 months, and the provision of breast milk often ends before the evidence-based target of at least 2 years. Beyond the global imperative, disparities in breastfeeding rates within countries are striking and the variable rate of breastfeeding across racial or ethnic groups and among individuals with different socioeconomic statuses is an under-appreciated public health crisis.

This Special Issue "Breastfeeding: Benefits to Infant and Mother" was created to develop evidence-based recommendations to increase the initiation and maintenance of breastfeeding worldwide and further expand upon the health benefits of human milk across diverse populations. This effort was successful with dozens of submissions subjected to rigorous peer review, resulting in twelve outstanding contributions to the medical literature in this important area. This editorial is intended to assist in the dissemination of this newfound knowledge and awareness. In turn, it is hoped that caregivers and care providers will be able to use this information to increase breastfeeding rates with positive impacts on child and adult health.

2. Overview of Published Articles

In the first contribution, Elgzar et al. utilized a retrospective, cross-sectional study to examine the correlation between specific components of maternal ideation on exclusive breastfeeding (EBF) practices in Saudi Arabia (contribution 1). The reported rate of EBF at 6 months within this cohort (41%) is consistent with global rates, supporting the widespread applicability of the inquiries. The investigation found that each construct of maternal ideation, including cognitive aspects (adequate knowledge and positive beliefs), psychological dimensions (self-efficacy) and social dimensions (social influence, descriptive and injective norms) were positive predictors of EBF, as were traditional factors, including maternal age, mode of delivery, occupation, and education.

Olcina Simón et al. added another layer to the investigations of Elgzar et al. by delving into the role of cognitive and social dimensions in the persistence of colostrum avoidance among a majority of women in rural Ethiopia (contribution 2). In their cross-sectional study, only 3% of birthing parents started breastfeeding within an hour of birth and 56% practiced colostrum avoidance. Maternal educational level, living conditions, beliefs about the dangers of colostrum, and attendance at delivery by relatives rather than healthcare providers predicted colostrum avoidance. Unfortunately, inaccessible health care contributed to limited or no prenatal care for most of the study participants, and this likely contributed to the persistence of the traditional feeding practices despite their association with increased infant mortality.

D'Adamo et al. published a related time-course investigation into the impact time since delivery on the breast milk content of presepsin, a truncated, soluble form of CD14 that has been used as a short-term biomarker for infection (contribution 3). Their prospective study demonstrated reductions in presepsin with advancing gestational age at delivery and elapsed time since delivery with relatively minor variation seen based on mode of delivery or infant gestation. Notably, presepsin levels are markedly higher in colostrum than transitional or mature milk, especially among preterm infants. While the impact of breast milk presepsin on gut health and innate immunity is an area of ongoing investigation, these data support the importance of colostrum feedings, especially in the context of preterm delivery.

Although it is certainly not available to all families, donor human milk can be used as a bridge towards the provision of maternal milk or as a substitute for maternal milk during prolonged neonatal hospitalizations. In those situations, it is important for donor milk to replicate the characteristics of maternal milk, and in this regard, the article by Vass et al. examined the impact of demographic parameters on the fatty acid composition of donor milk (contribution 4). While Holder pasteurization significantly reduced the content of multiple medium and long chain fatty acids, there were significantly increased levels of other fatty acids. Similar changes were seen, independent of pasteurization, based on mode of delivery with smaller effects identified in relation to the gender of the donor's infant. While the absolute differences in fatty acid content were relatively small, it is clear that further research is needed to define the effects of various pasteurization methods and donor selection strategies on the composition of donated human milk.

Returning to the investigation of the correlates of early EBF success, Verea-Nuñez et al. performed a cross-sectional study at a certified baby-friendly hospital in Spain with an EBF rate during admission of 73% (contribution 5). While there was an overall positive attitude towards breastfeeding, this was further enhanced by avoidance of pacifiers and the provision of proper breastfeeding information from healthcare providers. Beyond having a positive attitude, having a positive prior breastfeeding experience and an infant that did not require specialized care was associated with increased likelihood of EBF throughout the newborn admission. These results emphasize the importance of assisting initial breastfeeding efforts for benefits that extend beyond the current dyad to subsequent births.

A second cross-sectional contribution from Saudi Arabia by Al-Thubaity et al. focused on the determinants of maternal self-efficacy in the ability to breastfeed satisfactorily, a key component of EBF ideation, especially when extra effort or persistence are needed in the context of unexpected barriers or challenges (contribution 6). Reinforcing the findings of Elgzar et al. and Verea-Nuñez et al., maternal self-efficacy over the first 6 months following delivery was significantly influenced by a positive maternal attitude, as well as maternal occupation, education, and past EBF experiences. It is worth emphasizing the study's important, but perhaps not surprising, finding that housewives were nearly twice as likely to have a high EBF self-efficacy compared with working mothers, highlighting a need for improved workplace and parental leave policies.

The prospective cohort study performed in southern Brazil by Bizon et al. further emphasized the importance of a positive maternal attitude in the maintenance of EBF by directly correlating the level of maternal satisfaction at 1 month with ongoing EBF (contribution 7). In a multivariate model that corrected for maternal age, maternal education, cohabitation, and early breastfeeding difficulties, mothers with a higher level of satisfaction at 1 month were over four times as likely to be EBF at 6 months. While the results emphasize the importance of early interventions to achieve maternal satisfaction, the EBF rate at 6 months of only 24% among the cohort with high levels of early satisfaction emphasizes the need for additional and ongoing assessments and interventions.

In a complimentary investigation, Vila-Candel and colleagues explored the importance of health literacy in the prevention of breastfeeding abandonment (contribution 8). Their multicenter study across four regions of Spain prospectively assessed breastfeeding attrition over 6 months with rates gradually declining from 82% to 43%, consistent with global rates of breastfeeding abandonment. Health literacy, along with mobilization during labor and spontaneous labor were significantly associated with a reduced likelihood of breastfeeding abandonment, perhaps a reflection of improved feelings of maternal self-efficacy or control over the perinatal events. Interestingly, unlike the results of other studies within this Special Issue, maternal education level or economic status did not predict either health literacy or breastfeeding discontinuation, emphasizing the need for region-specific investigations.

With multiple studies demonstrating the importance of maternal support or education in the development of maternal self-efficacy, Rodríguez-Gallego led a remarkable randomized clinical trial that tested the effectiveness of a monthly midwife-led postpartum support group on breastfeeding outcomes at 4 months among 382 women from Andalusia (contribution 9). At 6 months, the rate of EBF was significantly higher in the intervention arm, and this appeared to be mediated by an increase in perceived self-efficacy. In a second contribution from the same interventional study, women in the postpartum support group also had significantly reduced Edinburgh Postnatal Depression Scale scores at 4 months (contribution 10). At both 2 months and 4 months, higher depression scores were significantly associated with reduced EBF rates. Beyond the correlation with EBF rates, the mitigation of maternal depression through enhanced support group participation has implications for the long-term health of both mother and child.

Continuing the shift towards long-term outcomes, Melov et al. investigated the association of prior breastfeeding with subsequent maternal health (contribution 11). In their retrospective cohort, an impressive 62% of multiparous women in Sydney, Australia, breastfed over 6 months in their prior pregnancy, although disparities were noted in association with maternal age, ethnicity, and economic status. Overall, high intensity breastfeeding for at least 3 months in the prior pregnancy was associated with nearly a 50% reduction in the odds of an abnormal fasting glucose in the subsequent pregnancy and a tendency towards a reduced likelihood of being diagnosed with gestational diabetes.

Finally, the long-term outcomes of breastfed infants were evaluated by Libuda and colleagues (contribution 12). Their observational study allayed concerns that breastfeeding could prevent early childhood eczema in higher-risk infants at the cost of a rebound increase in allergic diseases through young adulthood. Overall, beyond the known protection from early eczema, there was no association between breastfeeding and healthcare provider-diagnosed allergic diseases. There was, however, an interesting bidirectional interaction, based on the presence or absence of early eczema, between breastfeeding and long-term allergic rhinitis risk in those with no family history of allergic diseases.

3. Conclusions

This compilation of articles has significantly expanded the depth of our understanding of the factors that facilitate breastfeeding initiation and continuation, as well as the public health implications of those efforts. The role of maternal ideation, in particular self-efficacy, assumed a prominent role in this Special Issue, and for good reason, as multiple publications demonstrate the importance of maternal satisfaction in the decision to continue breastfeeding with implications for the health of the infant, the mother, and potential future pregnancies. Given the ongoing need to increase breastfeeding rates, it is encouraging that many of the factors that contribute to a positive maternal attitude can be modifiable.

Only when healthcare providers screen for and identify suboptimal levels of maternal knowledge or self-efficacy can discussions begin with families regarding factors that might be contributing. Those conversations can, in turn, open the door to possible interventions to promote a more positive experience for the mother–infant dyad and the prevention of premature breastfeeding abandonment. As the contributions in this Special Issue attest, there are important roles in this process for all members of the multidisciplinary healthcare team, including lactation consultants, midwives, and additional community-based allies that contribute towards our shared understanding of the benefits of human milk.

Beyond encouragement to implement expanded screenings and evidence-supported quality improvement projects, the contributions gathered for this Special Issue identify important areas for future research. These areas include the optimal design of breastfeeding education programs and/or interventions in developing as well as developed countries. While the public health importance of breastfeeding is a clear call for an overall increase in resource allocation by policy makers, in particular an improvement in parental leave policies and universal screenings, and because resources remain limited, there is a need to identify ways to risk-stratify individuals for need-based and targeted educational interventions to achieve both effective and sustainable effects in all communities.

Acknowledgments: The author acknowledges all members of the University of Iowa Health Care's Human Milk Equity Taskforce for their ongoing efforts to facilitate the provision of human milk for all infants throughout their hospitalizations and within their communities.

Conflicts of Interest: The authors declare no conflicts of interest.

List of Contributions

1. Elgzar, W.; Al-Thubaity, D.; Alshahrani, M.; Essa, R.; Ibrahim, H. The Relationship between maternal ideation and exclusive breastfeeding practice among Saudi nursing mothers: a cross-sectional study. *Nutrients* **2023**, *15*, 1719. https://doi.org/10.3390/nu15071719.
2. Olcina Simón, M.; Rotella, R.; Soriano, J.; Llopis-Gonzalez, A.; Peraita-Costa, I.; Morales-Suarez-Varela, M. Breastfeeding-related practices in rural ethiopia: Colostrum avoidance. *Nutrients* **2023**, *15*, 2177. https://doi.org/10.3390/nu15092177.
3. D'Adamo, E.; Peila, C.; Strozzi, M.; Barolo, R.; Maconi, A.; Nanni, A.; Botondi, V.; Coscia, A.; Bertino, E.; Gazzolo, F.; et al. Presepsin in human milk is delivery mode and gender dependent. *Nutrients* **2024**, *16*, 2554. https://doi.org/10.3390/nu16152554.
4. Vass, R.; Zhang, M.; Simon Sarkadi, L.; Üveges, M.; Tormási, J.; Benes, E.; Ertl, T.; Vari, S. Effect of Holder pasteurization, mode of delivery, and infant's gender on fatty acid composition of donor breast milk. *Nutrients* **2024**, *16*, 1689. https://doi.org/10.3390/nu16111689.
5. Verea-Nuñez, C.; Novoa-Maciñeiras, N.; Suarez-Casal, A.; Vazquez-Lago, J. Factors associated with exclusive breastfeeding during admission to a baby-friendly hospital initiative hospital: A cross-sectional study in Spain. *Nutrients* **2024**, *16*, 1679. https://doi.org/10.3390/nu16111679.
6. Al-Thubaity, D.; Alshahrani, M.; Elgzar, W.; Ibrahim, H. Determinants of high breastfeeding self-efficacy among nursing mothers in Najran, Saudi Arabia. *Nutrients* **2023**, *15*, 1919. https://doi.org/10.3390/nu15081919.
7. Bizon, A.; Giugliani, C.; Giugliani, E. Women's satisfaction with breastfeeding and risk of exclusive breastfeeding interruption. *Nutrients* **2023**, *15*, 5062. https://doi.org/10.3390/nu15245062.
8. Vila-Candel, R.; Soriano-Vidal, F.; Franco-Antonio, C.; Garcia-Algar, O.; Andreu-Fernandez, V.; Mena-Tudela, D. Factors influencing duration of breastfeeding: Insights from a prospective study of maternal health literacy and obstetric practices. *Nutrients* **2024**, *16*, 690. https://doi.org/10.3390/nu16050690.
9. Rodríguez-Gallego, I.; Corrales-Gutierrez, I.; Gomez-Baya, D.; Leon-Larios, F. Effectiveness of a postpartum breastfeeding support group intervention in promoting exclusive breastfeeding and perceived self-efficacy: A multicentre randomized clinical trial. *Nutrients* **2024**, *16*, 988. https://doi.org/10.3390/nu16070988.
10. Rodríguez-Gallego, I.; Vila-Candel, R.; Corrales-Gutierrez, I.; Gomez-Baya, D.; Leon-Larios, F. Evaluation of the impact of a midwife-led breastfeeding group intervention on prevention of postpartum depression: A multicentre randomised clinical trial. *Nutrients* **2024**, *16*, 227. https://doi.org/10.3390/nu16020227.
11. Melov, S.; Elhindi, J.; White, L.; McNab, J.; Lee, V.; Donnolley, K.; Alahakoon, T.; Padmanabhan, S.; Cheung, N.; Pasupathy, D. Previous high-intensity breastfeeding lowers the risk of an abnormal fasting glucose in a subsequent pregnancy oral glucose tolerance test. *Nutrients* **2024**, *16*, 28. https://doi.org/10.3390/nu16010028.

12. Libuda, L.; Filipiak-Pittroff, B.; Standl, M.; Schikowski, T.; von Berg, A.; Koletzko, S.; Bauer, C.; Heinrich, J.; Berdel, D.; Gappa, M. Full breastfeeding and allergic diseases—Long-term protection or rebound effects? *Nutrients* **2023**, *15*, 2780. https://doi.org/10.3390/nu15122780.

References

1. Victora, C.G.; Bahl, R.; Barros, A.J.; França, G.V.; Horton, S.; Krasevec, J.; Murch, S.; Sankar, M.J.; Walker, N.; Rollins, N.C. Breastfeeding in the 21st century: Epidemiology, mechanisms, and lifelong effect. *Lancet* **2016**, *387*, 475–490. [CrossRef] [PubMed]
2. Bernardo, H.; Cesar, V.; World Health Organization. *Long-Term Effects of Breastfeeding: A Systematic Review*; World Health Organization: Geneva, Switzerland, 2013. Available online: https://iris.who.int/handle/10665/79198 (accessed on 5 September 2024).
3. Chowdhury, R.; Sinha, B.; Sankar, M.J.; Taneja, S.; Bhandari, N.; Rollins, N.; Bahl, R.; Martines, J. Breastfeeding and maternal health outcomes: A systematic review and meta-analysis. *Acta Paediatr.* **2015**, *104*, 96–113. [CrossRef] [PubMed]
4. Tschiderer, L.; Seekircher, L.; Kunutsor, S.K.; Peters, S.A.E.; O'Keeffe, L.M.; Willeit, P. Breastfeeding is associated with a reduced maternal cardiovascular risk: Systematic review and meta-analysis involving data from 8 Studies and 1 192 700 parous women. *J. Am. Heart Assoc.* **2022**, *11*, e022746. [CrossRef] [PubMed]
5. World Health Organization (WHO). *Implementation Guidance: Protecting, Promoting and Supporting Breastfeeding in Facilities Providing Maternity and Newborn Services: The Revised Baby-Friendly Hospital Initiative*; World Health Organization: Geneva, Switzerland, 2018. Available online: https://www.who.int/publications/i/item/9789241513807 (accessed on 5 September 2024).

Disclaimer/Publisher's Note: The statements, opinions and data contained in all publications are solely those of the individual author(s) and contributor(s) and not of MDPI and/or the editor(s). MDPI and/or the editor(s) disclaim responsibility for any injury to people or property resulting from any ideas, methods, instructions or products referred to in the content.

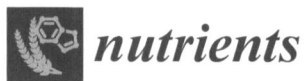

Article

The Relationship between Maternal Ideation and Exclusive Breastfeeding Practice among Saudi Nursing Mothers: A Cross-Sectional Study

Wafaa T. Elgzar [1], DaifAllah D. Al-Thubaity [1], Mohammed A. Alshahrani [2], Rasha M. Essa [3] and Heba A. Ibrahim [1,*]

1. Department of Maternity and Childhood Nursing, Nursing College, Najran University, Najran 66441, Saudi Arabia; wtelgzar@nu.edu.sa (W.T.E.)
2. Department of Clinical Laboratory Sciences, Applied Medical Sciences College, Najran University, Najran 66441, Saudi Arabia
3. Department of Obstetrics and Gynecologic Nursing, Nursing College, Damanhour University, Damanhour 22514, Egypt
* Correspondence: heaibrahim@nu.edu.sa

Abstract: All mortality risk factors are higher in non-breastfed infants compared to infants under five months of age who receive Exclusive Breastfeeding (EBF). Examining the predicting role of maternal ideation in EBF practices can help to direct and strengthen the cooperation between multidisciplinary healthcare providers to formulate multidisciplinary breastfeeding enhancement strategies. Methods: This correlational cross-sectional study investigates the relationship between maternal ideation and EBF practice among Saudi nursing mothers at Maternal and Children's Hospital (MCH) in Najran, Saudi Arabia. The study incorporated 403 Saudi nursing mothers aged 6–12 months with healthy infants. The data collected using a questionnaire comprises demographic characteristics and obstetric history, the EBF Practice scale, and a maternal ideation scale. The data was collected from the beginning of November 2022 to the end of January 2023 and analyzed using I.B.M. version 22. Results: Breastfeeding initiation within one hour occurred among 85.1% of women, while 39.2% fed their newborn only colostrum during the first three days. EBF until six months was practiced by 40.9% of the participants day and night and on-demand (38.7%). Furthermore, 60.8% of the study participants had satisfactory overall EBF practices. The cognitive part of maternal ideation shows that 68.2% of the participants had adequate knowledge and 63.5% had positive beliefs regarding EBF practice. The maternal psychological ideation dimensions show that 81.4% had high EBF self-efficacy. The maternal social ideation dimensions showed that high injunctive and descriptive norms were present among 40.9% and 37.5%, respectively. In addition, healthcare providers (39.2%) had the most significant social influence, followed by husbands (30.5%). Binary logistic regression shows that the mother's age, occupation, and education are the significant demographic predictors of satisfactory EBF practices ($p < 0.05$). All maternal ideation constructs were positive predictors of satisfactory EBF practices ($p < 0.05$). Conclusion: Maternal ideation constructs are positive predictors of satisfactory EBF practice and can be used to predict high-risk groups and plan for further intervention.

Keywords: exclusive breastfeeding; maternal ideation; knowledge; beliefs; self-efficacy; Saudia Arabia

Citation: Elgzar, W.T.; Al-Thubaity, D.D.; Alshahrani, M.A.; Essa, R.M.; Ibrahim, H.A. The Relationship between Maternal Ideation and Exclusive Breastfeeding Practice among Saudi Nursing Mothers: A Cross-Sectional Study. Nutrients 2023, 15, 1719. https://doi.org/10.3390/nu15071719

Academic Editor: Robert D. Roghair

Received: 12 March 2023
Revised: 28 March 2023
Accepted: 30 March 2023
Published: 31 March 2023

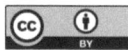

Copyright: © 2023 by the authors. Licensee MDPI, Basel, Switzerland. This article is an open access article distributed under the terms and conditions of the Creative Commons Attribution (CC BY) license (https://creativecommons.org/licenses/by/4.0/).

1. Introduction

The fourth-millennium development goal is concerned with decreasing child mortality. The World Health Organization (WHO) reported that 40% of under-five mortality occurred in under one month, and most occurred in the first week of age [1]. Sankar et al. conducted a systemic review to explore the relationship between satisfactory breastfeeding practice and infant and child mortality. They found that all mortality risk factors were higher in non-breastfed infants than in infants exclusively breastfed under five months of age.

Furthermore, the risk for infection-related mortality is twofold higher in the non-breastfed infant than in the exclusively breastfed [2]. Breastfeeding has unquestionable benefits for infants and mothers, whether rich or poor. The infant breastfeeding-related benefits are numerous and long-lasting, such as decreasing infectious disease risk, a decreased risk for type 2 diabetes mellitus and obesity, a decreased risk for respiratory asthma, and increased child intelligence and adulthood intelligence later on [3–5]. In other words, breastfeeding is a child's first inoculation against death, disease, and poverty and the most important and permanent investment in human physical, cognitive, and social capability [6]. Maternal benefits of breastfeeding include decreased breast and ovarian cancer risk, increased birth spacing, and decreased risk for type 2 diabetes and obesity.

Spotting on the breastfeeding benefits, which recommended only breastfeeding as the sole nutrient for the infant in the first six months of life with the allowance of prescribed medications, minerals, vitamins, and oral rehydration therapy. Complementary foods are introduced after six months, besides breastfeeding until two years of age [7]. The Saudi Ministry of Health issued policies to enhance the early initiation and continuation of breastfeeding exclusively until six months and complementarily until two years [8]. Saudi Arabia is a Muslim country; therefore, the Quran and Hadith are the main sources of legalization. In the Holy Quran, breastfeeding is a granted right for the infant until two years of age [9]. Although the Saudi Ministry of Health paid great attention to the early initiation and continuation of EBF, the rate is still lower than expected. In Saudi Arabia, the EBF rate varied by region, ranging from 0.8% to 43.9%; in a systemic review involving 17 studies [10] worldwide, the WHO stated that less than 50% of infants have EBF [7].

The Saudi Ministry of Health paid great attention to increasing public awareness of breastfeeding, but the rate is still low. This may highlight a question about the effectiveness of such educational interventions. The educational interventions have to be built on strong subject-related factors and address the target group's needs. Therefore, the most important step in a successful educational program is determining the target group's needs and the predictors of satisfactory breastfeeding practice. Factors associated with EBF practices are multiple and have a complicated nature. Some factors are not modifiable, such as demographic and obstetrical variables, and many others are modifiable. Modifiable factors are breastfeeding knowledge, beliefs, self-efficacy, the common norms and patterns of EBF in the community, social norms, and significant others who can influence the women's behaviors [11]. Modifiable factors are the milestones that can help educational programs produce behavior changes and stick to satisfactory EBF practices.

The maternal ideation model is one of the most important models that can be used to predict satisfactory EBF practice. Specifically, women with low maternal ideation, inadequate knowledge, negative beliefs, low self-efficacy, and low injunctive and descriptive norms are at a higher risk of unsatisfactory outcomes. The EBF ideation model tried to explain how new behaviors or practices can spread throughout the community through social interactions and communication among individuals and groups [12]. The ideation model of strategic communication and behavior change primarily focuses on behavioral and social changes toward positive health behaviors [13]. Interventions for improving breastfeeding based on the ideation model should focus on predicting the cognitive, psychological, and social dimensions of breastfeeding. Cognitive aspects of behavior change include women's knowledge and beliefs regarding breastfeeding. Psychological aspects include breastfeeding self-efficacy, or how the mother evaluates her ability to practice EBF effectively. Lastly, the social dimension of the ideation models includes injunctive norms, descriptive norms, and social influences. The injunctive norms evaluated the woman's trust in the benefits of breastfeeding for herself and her infant. Descriptive norms evaluated the women's perceptions of community norms regarding breastfeeding. The social influence evaluation evaluated the significant person or social network who may influence the women's breastfeeding practices. These people may be the husband, mother-in-law, friends, and health care provider. The ideation model is based on the assumption that a person with more enabling ideation factors can effectively manage behavior change to a more positive one [11].

The roles of ideation factors in predicting behavior change were examined for cancer care [13], contraceptive use [14], suicide [15], and malaria care [16], but rarely for breastfeeding in Nigeria [11]. Examining the predicting role of maternal ideation in EBF practices can help direct and strengthen the cooperation between multidisciplinary healthcare providers in formulating multidisciplinary breastfeeding enhancement strategies. Breastfeeding enhancement strategies can be implemented with the cooperation of breastfeeding specialists, pediatricians, psychologists, nurses, and social workers. The maternal ideation cognitive part (knowledge and beliefs) can be enhanced through educational programs provided by breastfeeding specialists, pediatricians, and nurses. Furthermore, the psychological maternal ideation dimension (breastfeeding self-efficacy) can be improved through educational and psychological interventions provided by psychologists. Lastly, the social part of the maternal ideation model (social influence, injunctive, and descriptive norms) can be enhanced through a social and educational intervention provided by social workers in cooperation with breastfeeding specialists, pediatricians, and nurses, all using different media. It can also help with EBF enhancement at national and subnational levels by accessing the whole community through all dimensions of the ideation model of strategic communication and behavioral change.

2. Materials and Methods

2.1. Study Design

This correlational cross-sectional study investigated the relationship between maternal ideation and EBF practice among Saudi nursing mothers in the Maternal and Children's Hospital (MCH).

The operational definitions are: EBF gives the infant breast milk only for the first six months of life, in addition to prescribed medications, minerals, oral rehydration therapy, and vitamins [17].

Unsatisfactory EBF practice is below-average (≤ 10) on the EBF practice scale, and satisfactory EBF practice is above-average (>10).

Maternal ideation is the complex and unique decision-making process that leads to behavioral changes, and it incorporates cognitive (knowledge and beliefs), psychological (self-efficacy), and social (injunctive norms, descriptive norms, and social influence) dimensions related to EBF [11].

2.2. Study Setting

The study was conducted in the outpatient department of the MCH Hospital in Najran, Saudi Arabia. The included clinics are immunization, pediatrics, and breastfeeding counseling. MCH is the only hospital in Najran City that provides maternal and child health care; therefore, it serves a large population. Najran city is the capital of the Najran region in southwestern Saudi Arabia. Najran City has many cultural and traditional beliefs about the maternity cycle and breastfeeding [18].

2.3. Study Participants

The study incorporated 403 Saudi nursing mothers with infants free from breastfeeding contraindications and aged 6–12 months; those aged 18 years and older can read, write, and accept participation in the study.

2.3.1. Sample Size and Sampling Procedures

The sample size was calculated using the Cohran formula [19]. The EBF prevalence in Saudi Arabia varies by region; it ranges from 0.8 to 43.9%, according to a systemic review by Al Junaid et al. [10]. Therefore, the EBF rate used in the sample size calculation is 43.9%. The formula used in the calculation is:

$$n = \frac{Z^2 Pq}{e^2}$$

where n is the required sample size, Z is the normal standard deviation at a 95% confidence level (1.96), and P is the estimated proportion of the target population, estimated to be 43.9%; according to Al Junaid et al., the sample size is 378 after adding 15% to compensate for the anticipated sample loss of n = 435.

2.3.2. Sampling Technique and Procedures

A systemic random sampling was utilized to recruit the participants. The suitable clinics for data collection were three pediatric clinics, an immunization clinic, and a breastfeeding counseling clinic. According to the clinic registry system, there are a total of 5 clinics with an average follow-up rate of 75 cases (15 for each clinic) per day in the morning and afternoon shifts. The data collection team was composed of three researchers; each researcher determined that he could collect a minimum of five cases daily; the total is 15 cases per day for the whole team, three days per week. The sampling interval was determined by dividing the follow-up rate by the expected total recruited cases daily, and it was 75/5 = 5. The starting point was picked randomly from a ball containing papers numbered 1–5, then an interval of 5 was applied. The participants were picked from the waiting area for the five clinics, which ran three days per week for 12 weeks from November 2022 to January 2023. If the selected participant refused participation or was illegible, the next case was included, and the sample interval was maintained. The study participants were distributed according to the following chart (Figure 1).

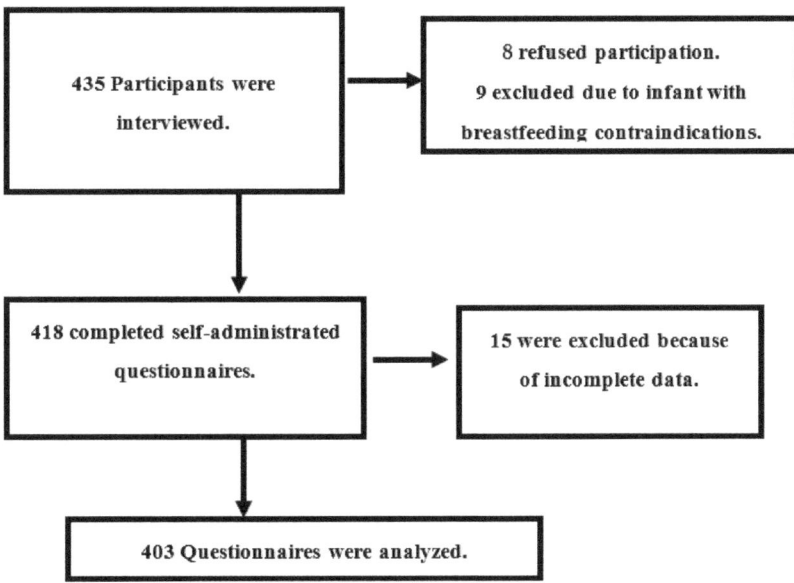

Figure 1. Participants' flow chart.

2.4. Study Measurement Tools

The study measurement tools are organized in a self-reported questionnaire that was developed after an intensive literature review. The questionnaire comprises three parts: demographic characteristics and obstetric history; EBF practice scale; and maternal ideation scale.

Part I consists of demographic characteristics and obstetric histories. It collects the mothers' age, occupation, education, and husband's education, as well as their monthly income. Obstetric history includes parity, mode of delivery, complications of the last delivery, duration of pregnancy for the last child, and the number of living children.

Part II is the self-reported EBF practice scale. It was developed by researchers and comprises ten statements that evaluated the initiation and different aspects of breastfeeding practices, guided by previous studies [17,20]. The scale items were dichotomous (yes or no) questions, where yes scored "one" and no scored "zero", The total scale score was 10, and the participant was considered to have unsatisfactory (0–5) or satisfactory (6–10) practice based on her score. Cronbach's alpha coefficient for the practice scale was 0.87, indicating high reliability.

Part III is the maternal ideation evaluation scale. Maternal ideation is composed of three main categories, which are cognitive (knowledge and beliefs), psychological (self-efficacy), and social (injunctive norms, descriptive norms, and social influence) [11].

The maternal breastfeeding knowledge was assessed using the Gender-Friendly Breastfeeding Knowledge Scale (GFBKS). It was validated by Gupta et al. and found to be highly reliable ($r = 0.787$). The scale incorporated 18 items rated on a 5-point Likert scale as false = 1, maybe false = 2, do not know = 3, may be true = 4, and true = 5. The total score for the 18 items ranged from 18 to 90. Based on her score, the mother was classified as having inadequate (18–54) or adequate knowledge (55–90) [21].

Mothers' beliefs regarding breastfeeding are adapted from the beliefs about breastfeeding questionnaire. The questionnaire consisted of 8 items rated on a 5-point Likert scale ranging from strongly disagreeing (1 point) to strongly agreeing (5 points). The total questionnaire score ranged from 8 to 40; the negative belief score ranged from 8 to 24; and the positive belief ranged from 25 to 40. The questionnaire indicated good internal consistency, which ranged from ($r = 0.73$–0.77) [22].

The psychological part of maternal ideation, mainly self-efficacy, was evaluated using the Breastfeeding Self-Efficacy Scale—Short Form (BSES-SF). Dennis created it in 2003 to evaluate postpartum women's breastfeeding confidence. The BSES-SF was rated on a 5-point Likert scale ranging from 1 (not at all confident) to 5 (always confident). The total score ranged from 14–70; low self-efficacy is considered from 14–42 and high self-efficacy from 43–70 [23]. According to Amini et al., the BSES-SF internal consistency was ($r = 0.910$) [24].

The injunctive norms evaluated the mother's trust in breastfeeding benefits for herself and her infant. The injunctive norms were evaluated using four items rated on a five-point Likert scale, resulting in a total injunctive norms score (4–20). The mother was considered to have low (4–12) or high (13–20) injunctive norms according to her total score for the four items [11].

Descriptive norms evaluated the mother's perception of the community norms regarding breastfeeding. It was evaluated through three items rated on a 5-point Likert scale ranging from strongly disagreeing (1 point) to strongly agreeing (5 points). The total descriptive norms score ranged from 3–15, and the woman was considered to have low (3–9) or high (10–15) descriptive norms according to her total score for the three items [11].

The social influence is evaluated using one multiple-choice question to evaluate who, besides the mother, can affect her decision regarding breastfeeding. The answers were no one, husband, mother-in-law, and health care provider [11].

2.5. Data Collection Procedures and Techniques

The data was collected from the beginning of November to the end of January 2023. At the beginning of the data collection interview, the researcher explained the study purpose, expected outcome, participants' role, data confidentiality, and the right to refuse participation without any penalties or consequences on the care provided. If the mother accepted participation, the questionnaire was given to her after she signed the informed consent. The data collector was present during the data collection process to clarify concerns and answer the participants' questions. After completing the questionnaire, the participant's medical records were used to confirm the basic data.

2.6. Data Quality Control

The three data collectors were researchers with good experience in data collection, sampling techniques, and research ethics. Before data analysis, the questionnaires were carefully checked for missing data; 15 cases were excluded.

2.7. Ethical Approval

At first, the research proposal was approved by the deanship of scientific research at Najran University; then, another approval was obtained from the Najran Health Affairs Ethics Committee, an ethical approval (I.R.B. Log Number 2023-02 E). Approval to start data collection was also obtained from the MCH head. In addition, during data collection, informed consent was obtained from each participant after explaining the study's purpose. Data confidentiality, anonymity, and the right to refuse participation without any penalties were emphasized to the participants.

2.8. Data Analysis

Data analysis was performed using the Statistical I.B.M. software, version 23 (I.B.M. Corp., Armonk, NY, USA). The data were checked for normal distribution and missing data. Sheets containing missing data were omitted from the analysis. The participants' basic data, obstetric history, and maternal ideation constructs were described using numbers, percentages, and mean $\pm$ SD. The total EBF knowledge, beliefs, self-efficacy, injunctive norms, and descriptive norms were obtained by summing items. The predictors of satisfactory EBF practice were examined using binary logistic regression. Among the independent variables, the participant's age, total B.F. knowledge, total B.F. beliefs, self-efficacy, injunctive norms, descriptive norms, gravidity, and the number of living children are continuous. Furthermore, occupation, mother's education, husband's education, monthly income, gravidity, mode of delivery of the last child, social influence, and duration of pregnancy are all categorical variables. The first category was the reference for all categorical variables. All factors were tested for multicollinearity before the regression model. The final model was tested with the Cox and Snell R-Squared goodness of fit test. Statistically significant findings were considered at $p < 0.05$.

3. Results

The participants' demographic characteristics are illustrated in Table 1. More than three-quarters (82.1%) of the study participants were aged 20–35, with a mean age of 28.95. Furthermore, 62.5%, 66.3%, and 67.7% are working, university-educated mothers and married to highly educated husbands, respectively. In addition, more than half (52.4%) of the study participants had enough monthly income, but only 10.2% could save.

Table 1. Participants' sociodemographic data ($n = 403$).

Sociodemographic Data	n (403)	%
Age (years)		
– <20 year	14	3.5
– 20–35	331	82.1
– ≥36	58	14.4
Mean $\pm$ SD	28.95 $\pm$ 7.64	
Occupational status		
– Housewife	151	37.5
– Working	252	62.5

Table 1. Cont.

Sociodemographic Data	n (403)	%
Woman's education		
− Read and write	20	5.0
− Secondary school	116	28.8
− University or postgraduate	267	66.3
Husband's education		
− Read and write	10	2.5
− Secondary school	120	29.8
− University or postgraduate	273	67.7
Monthly income		
− Not enough	151	37.5
− Enough	211	52.4
− Enough and can save	41	10.2

Obstetric history shows that 67.7% and 70.2% of the participants were multiparous and had a history of previous vaginal delivery, respectively. Furthermore, 83.1% and 90.6% of women suffered from complications during the last delivery and had full-term pregnancies, respectively. The mean number of living children for the study participants was 2.732 (Table 2).

Table 2. Participants' obstetric history and breastfeeding practice (n = 403).

Participants' Obstetric History and Breastfeeding Practices	n	%
Parity		
- Primiparous	130	32.3
- Multiparous	273	67.7
Mode of delivery		
- Vaginal delivery	283	70.2
- Cesarean section	120	29.8
Complications of last delivery		
- No	335	83.1
- Yes	68	16.9
Duration of pregnancy with the last child		
- Full-term	365	90.6
- Preterm	38	9.4
Number of living children (mean ± SD)	2.732 ± 2.024	

Self-reported EBF practices are illustrated in Table 3. Breastfeeding initiation within one hour occurred among 85.1% of women, while 39.2% fed their newborns only colostrum during the first three days of their lives. EBF until six months of life was practiced by 40.9% of the participants. Breastfeeding was practiced by 38.7% of women at all hours of the day and night. Nearly two-thirds of the participants ensured that their infant was properly latched on for the whole feeding (65%), determined that the baby got enough milk (64%), and fed their infant from the two breasts interchangeably (63.5%). In addition, 54.6% can comfortably breastfeed in the presence of family members. Lastly, 67.2% and 65.3% of the study participants maintained comfortable positions and performed eructation after each feeding, respectively. Furthermore, 60.8% of the study participants had satisfactory EBF practices, and 39.2% had unsatisfactory practices.

Table 3. Self-reported EBF practice (*n* = 403).

	Practice Items	Yes		No	
		N	%	N	%
1	I started to breastfeed my infant during the first hour of postpartum.	343	85.1	60	14.9
2	I fed my infant only colostrum during the first three days.	158	39.2	245	60.8
3	I feed my infant only breast milk until 6 months of age.	165	40.9	238	59.1
4	I feed my infant day and night and on demand.	156	38.7	247	61.3
5	During feeding, I ensured that my infant was properly latched on for the whole feeding.	262	65.0	141	35.0
6	During feeding, I determined that my baby got enough milk.	258	64.0	145	36.0
7	I feed my infant from both breasts interchangeably.	256	63.5	147	36.5
8	I comfortably breastfeed with my family members present.	220	54.6	183	45.4
9	I maintained comfortable positions for my infant and me during feeding.	271	67.2	132	32.8
10	I performed eructation for my infant after each feeding.	263	65.3	140	34.7
		Unsatisfactory		Satisfactory	
	Total EBF practice.	158	39.2	245	60.8

The cognitive part of maternal ideation shows that 68.2% of the participants had adequate knowledge and 63.5% had positive beliefs regarding breastfeeding practice. The maternal psychological ideation dimension shows that 81.4% had high breastfeeding self-efficacy. The maternal social ideation dimensions showed that high injunctive and descriptive norms were present among 40.9% and 37.5%, respectively. In addition, the most significant social influence is provided by health care providers (39.2%), followed by husbands (30.5%) (Table 4).

Table 4. Participants' breastfeeding maternal ideation (*n* = 403).

Ideational Dimension	Domain	n	%
Cognitive	Knowledge		
	Inadequate (18–54)	128	31.8
	Adequate (55–90)	275	68.2
	Beliefs		
	Negative (8–24)	147	36.5
	Positive (25–40)	256	63.5
Psychological	Self-efficacy		
	Low (14–42)	75	18.6
	High (43–70)	328	81.4
Social	Injunctive norms		
	Low	238	59.1
	High	165	40.9
	Descriptive norms		
	Low	252	62.5
	High	151	37.5

Table 4. Cont.

Ideational Dimension	Domain	n	%
	Social influence		
	No one	69	17.1
	Husband	123	30.5
	Mother-in-law	53	13.2
	Health care provider	158	39.2

Binary logistic regression shows that the mother's age, occupation, and education are all significant demographic predictors of EBF practices. An increase in the maternal age by one year increases the probability of satisfactory EBF practice by 1.2 times [AOR = 1.267 (1.109–1.449), $p = 0.001$]. Furthermore, being a housewife and university educated too much increased the probability for satisfactory EBF [AOR = 13.341 (2.249–39.249), $p = 0.004$] and [AOR = 3.218 (1.861–10.682), $p = 0.008$]. Obstetric history, parity, previous delivery mode, last pregnancy duration, and the number of living children were predictors of satisfactory EBF practices. Previous history of cesarean delivery [AOR = 0.239 (0.104–0.547), $p = 0.001$] and having preterm infants [AOR = 0.846 (0.780–0.898), $p = 0.000$] decreased the probability of satisfactory EBF practices, when taking vaginal delivery and a full-term infant as a reference. Moreover, being multiparous increased the probability of satisfactory EBF practices compared to primiparous mothers [AOR = 3.716 (1.214–16.290), $p = 0.027$]. Furthermore, an increase in the number of children by one increases the probability of satisfactory EBF practices by 4.3 times [AOR = 4.317 (1.806–8.236), $p = 0.000$]. (Table 5).

Table 5. Binary logistic regression analysis of the demographic and obstetric history predictors of satisfactory EBF practice (n = 403).

Predictors	EBF Practice	
	AOR (95% CI)	p
Occupational status		
- Working	Ref	
- Housewife	13.341 (2.249–39.249)	0.004 *
Education		0.028
- Read and write	Ref	
- Secondary school	1.037 (0.964–1.116)	0.324
- University or postgraduate	3.218 (1.861–10.682)	0.008 *
Husband's education		0.621
- Read and write	Ref	
- Secondary school	0.958 (0.954–1.046)	0.652
- University or postgraduate	0.942 (0.964–1.133)	0.715
Monthly income		0.814
- Enough and can save	Ref	
- Enough	0.928 (0.363–2.372)	0.775
- Not enough	1.114 (0.393–3.163)	0.839
Parity		
- Primiprous	Ref	
- Multiparous	3.716 (1.214–16.290)	0.027 *

Table 5. Cont.

Predictors	EBF Practice	
	AOR (95% CI)	p
Mode of delivery		
- Vaginal delivery	Ref	
- Cesarean section	0.239 (0.104–0.547)	0.001 *
Complications during last delivery		
- Yes	Ref	
- No	1.169 (0.484–2.823)	0.729
Duration of pregnancy		
- Full-term	Ref	
- Preterm	0.846 (0.780–0.898)	0.000 **
Age	1.267 (1.109–1.449)	0.001 *
Number of living children (mean ± SD)	4.317 (1.806–8.236)	0.000 **

AOR: Adjusted Odd Ratio. CI: Confidence Interval. * significant at $p < 0.05$. ** significant at $p < 0.001$.

Binary logistic regression shows that all maternal ideation constructs were positive predictors of satisfactory EBF practices. For the cognitive diminution of maternal ideation, an increase in maternal knowledge [AOR = 5.96 (1.968–17.787), $p = 0.002$] and beliefs [AOR = 1.76 (1.016–1.821), $p = 0.033$] increases the mother's probability to practice satisfactory EBF by 5.9 and 1.7 times, respectively. For the psychological dimension of maternal ideation, an increase in self-efficacy [AOR = 1.877 (1.201–1.939), $p = 0.000$] of one degree nearly doubled the probability of practicing EBF. For the social dimension, the husband's [AOR = 1.612 (0.732–3.877), $p = 0.038$] and health care provider's [AOR = 1.661 (1.066–4.016), $p = 0.047$] influence increased the mother's probability to have satisfactory EBF practice when compared to having none. Lastly, a one-degree increase of injunctive [AOR = 4.132 (1.656–8.874), $p = 0.000$] and descriptive norms [AOR = 5.547 (2.018–10.815), $p = 0.000$] increased the mother's probability of practicing satisfactory EBF by 4.13 and 5.54 times, respectively. Cox and Snell R-Square showed that the current model could predict 57.8% of the satisfactory EBF practices (Table 6).

Table 6. Binary logistic regression analysis for the predictive relation of the maternal ideation model on the satisfactory EBF practice ($n = 403$).

	Predictors	EBF Practice	
		AOR (95% CI)	p
Cognitive	- Knowledge	5.916 (1.968–17.787)	0.002 *
	- Beliefs	1.76 (1.016–1.821)	0.033 *
Psychological	Self-efficacy	1.877 (1.201–1.939)	0.000 **
Social	Social influence		0.016 *
	- No one	Ref	
	- Husband	1.612 (0.732–3.877)	0.038 *
	- Mother-in-law	0.581 (0.268–1.268)	0.171
	- Health care provider	1.661 (1.066–4.016)	0.047 *
	Injunctive norms	4.132 (1.656–8.874)	0.000 **
	Descriptive norms	5.547 (2.018–10.815)	0.000 **
	−2 Log likelihood (357.778)	Cox and Snell R-Square (0.578)	Nagelkerke R-Square (0.802)

AOR: Adjusted Odd Ratio. CI: Confidence Interval. * significant at $p < 0.05$. ** significant at $p < 0.001$.

4. Discussion

Breastfeeding in Saudi Arabia is influenced by a range of religious and cultural factors [9]. In addition, the benefits of breastfeeding are undeniable and supported by the Ministry of Health's educational efforts. Therefore, the challenge is to achieve and maintain satisfactory EBF practices, not only initiation. Satisfactory EBF practices were found among approximately two-thirds of the current study participants, with a relatively high early initiation rate among a large proportion of the study participants. However, there is a discrepancy between a very high breastfeeding initiation rate within the first hour (85.1%) and exclusive breastfeeding being continued only in 40.9% of cases, despite a generally positive maternal approach to breastfeeding supported by Muslim religious beliefs. The discrepancy between the early initiation rate and continuation of EBF can be explained by two main factors. First, in MCH, numerous policies support early initiation of EBF within one hour; therefore, early initiation of breastfeeding is an important task for healthcare providers in the delivery room and must be documented in the patient record. The second factor that may negatively affect EBF continuation is related to some traditions related to breastfeeding, such as giving some herbal teas for baby colic. Significant people in the woman's social network may advise her to give some herbal remedies or complementary bottle feeding during the first six months of life because they think that breast milk is insufficient [25]. Previous studies have reported the initiation rate to be high in different Saudi regions, but the continuation rate is still much lower than recommended [26–28]. Saudi women are guided by their religious beliefs to initiate breastfeeding but have challenges with its continuation. Most Saudi women discontinued breastfeeding against their wishes due to work and social barriers. It is worthy of note that in Saudi Arabia, the maternity leave period is limited to only 45–70 days (1.5–2.3 months) by law, which is too short for an employed mother to practice EBF for six months, which may force the mother to appoint babysitters and make their EBF continuation a challenge. The social challenge for lactating mothers who want to continue breastfeeding is how to handle social pressure and traditions related to EBF. Their close relatives mostly advise them to give herbs or bottle-feed the infant to promote better growth. Colostrum is fed to about two-fifths of the current study participants, and EBF is practiced day and night. Saudi women were found to have good knowledge about colostrum and reported a high preference to give only colostrum during the first three days of the newborn's life [29,30]. However, they may be pushed by baby illness, maternal exhaustion, a lack of social support, and some traditions to give the baby herbal drinks or formula milk and decrease the amount of colostrum feeding or avoid feeding it at all. The women also reported giving bottle feeding with breastfeeding from three months of age, and they reported insufficient breast milk or returned work as the main factors for introducing bottle feeding [28,29]. Therefore, the factors associated with EBF practices are multiple and complicated, containing cognitive, psychological, and social dimensions, which are the main components of the maternal ideation model.

In the current study, maternal ideations play an important role in EBF practices, where all maternal ideation constructs are positive predictors of satisfactory EBF practices. Specifically for the cognitive domain, an increase in maternal knowledge and beliefs regarding breastfeeding by one grade increases the women's probability to practice satisfactory EBF by 5.9 and 1.7 times, respectively. The maternal ideation role in breastfeeding was investigated by Anaba et al. in Nigeria. They reported on the important role of maternal ideation in predicting E.P.F. practice. They added that various cognitive, emotional, and social dimensions of maternal ideation significantly influenced the woman's breastfeeding decisions. Maternal knowledge regarding breastfeeding benefits, appropriate timing, and their beliefs regarding colostrum benefits (cognitive), women's breastfeeding self-efficacy (emotional), and perceived breastfeeding norms (social) were the most significant predictors of breastfeeding initiation in Nigeria [11].

Knowledge is well documented in previous national [31,32] and international studies [17,33,34] to be strongly linked to satisfactory EBF practices. The link between breastfeeding knowledge and satisfactory EBF practices seems logical because if the woman has to adopt any behavior, she should have sufficient knowledge to fit in and gain harmony with her previous mental schema. Therefore, many previous studies reported significant improvements in EBF practices after an educational program [17,35]. Most studies that evaluated breastfeeding knowledge also evaluated beliefs and may explore the link between breastfeeding knowledge and attitude [17,35]. This unique link presents the cognitive part of maternal ideation as an important component of breastfeeding practices. A previous study concluded that in an ambiguous situation that requires a decision, like EBF, there is a unique mediating role for knowledge in belief formulation, which consequently affects breastfeeding practice [36]. Saudi women's beliefs regarding breastfeeding are strongly affected by religious instructions from the Holy Quran and Hadith. In the Holy Quran, the infant is granted the right to breastfeed for two years; therefore, Muslim women have positive beliefs regarding breastfeeding, even if there are barriers to it [9].

Psychological readiness for breastfeeding is an important pillar in achieving satisfactory EBF practices, which reflects the importance of the psychological dimension of the maternal ideation model [11]. Breastfeeding self-efficacy reflects the woman's confidence in her ability to exclusively breastfeed her infant, and it acts as an important modifiable factor for satisfactory EBF practices. The current study showed that an increase of one grade in the woman's breastfeeding self-efficacy score could nearly double the probability of EBF practices. In this regard, Brockway et al. conducted a systemic review and meta-analysis of eleven studies exploring breastfeeding self-efficacy's role in EBF practices. They found that a one-point increase in the breastfeeding self-efficacy score can increase the probability of EBF by 10% compared with the control group [37]. In addition, breastfeeding self-efficacy was identified as a golden factor associated with the early initiation and continuation of EBF [38]. Psychological parts of the maternal ideation model (breastfeeding self-efficacy) represent the internal power that can help a woman use the available resources and support systems to enhance her EBF practices. Therefore, there is a connection between breastfeeding self-efficacy and the social part of the maternal ideation model.

The social part of the maternal ideation model incorporates social influence, injunctive norms, and descriptive norms. Social influencers represent the mother's support network, and they, other than herself, influence her decision to practice EBF. In the current study, husbands and health care providers' support increased the women's probability of having satisfactory EBF practices when compared to having none. A previous interventional study explored the role of husband support in breastfeeding practice. They found that increasing the husband's knowledge could improve the mother's knowledge and attitude toward EBF. On the other side, a motivated husband can provide physical and psychological support to his wife and help her overcome breastfeeding challenges [39]. Therefore, improving couples' knowledge and attitude can significantly improve satisfactory EBF practices. Another study elaborated that the husband's role in breastfeeding is not limited to his knowledge and attitude toward breastfeeding but also extended to women's empowerment to provide satisfactory EBF practices. As the husband represents the power source in Saudi families, his positive attitude and support of EBF practices can shape the mother's subjective criteria related to breastfeeding [40]. Healthcare providers are the first influencers who can prepare the woman during pregnancy regarding breastfeeding and help the woman during the postpartum period to initiate it early. In addition, they are counselors, educators, and motivators for the woman for EBF. Healthcare providers can also tailor and apply breastfeeding-friendly policies [28]. The role of health care providers is not only limited to women's education regarding breastfeeding; it also extends to the husband, family, and the whole community. Healthcare providers conducted numerous health education and counseling interventions to increase community awareness and social support for breastfeeding. McFadden et al. explored the role of healthcare providers' support, education, and monitoring in EBF initiation and continuation. They concluded that education, counseling, and continuous home visits by trained healthcare providers during the antenatal and postnatal period significantly increased the percentage of satisfactory EBF practices [41].

Lastly, a one-degree increase in injunctive and descriptive norms increased women's probability of satisfactory EBF practices by 4.13 and 5.54 times, respectively. The injunctive norms evaluated the woman's trust in breastfeeding benefits for herself and her infant. Descriptive norms evaluated the women's perceptions of community norms regarding breastfeeding. Being a Muslim generates a positive perception and tradition regarding breastfeeding anywhere and generates a descriptive norm that all Muslim women should breastfeed their infants. Kamoun and Spatz conducted a study to investigate the Islamic tradition's influence on breastfeeding practice among African American Muslims in West Philadelphia compared to non-Muslim African Americans. They concluded that Muslim women have a higher perception of breastfeeding benefits for mothers and infants. Most Muslim women have a positive attitude and higher breastfeeding self-efficacy [42]. The present study results are also in line with Anaba et al., who reported a significant association between E.P.F. practices and injunctive norms [11].

Breastfeeding is common among Saudi women but not exclusive. Saudi tradition enforces the introduction of complementary feeding and traditional herbs for the infant. Therefore, most women feed their infants, as reflected in their injunctive and descriptive norms [43].

In conclusion, Cox and Snell R-Square showed that 57.8% of satisfactory EBF practices could be predicted by the maternal ideation model for behavior change. Therefore, this model needs to be considered while designing and implementing breastfeeding educational interventions. The model tackles the most important cognitive (knowledge and beliefs), psychological (breastfeeding self-efficacy), and social (social influences, injunctive norms, and descriptive norms) dimensions that may significantly enhance EBF practices. Anaba et al. recommended that the utilization of the maternal ideation model in breastfeeding programs can promote more sustainability of positive breastfeeding practices [11].

Strengths and Limitations

This study discussed an important behavior change model that is rarely studied concerning breastfeeding. The sample size was estimated based on a 95% confidence interval, and a systemic random sampling procedure was used to engage the participants, which improved the results' generalizability. The AOR was estimated to perfectly assess the role of each predictor in satisfactory EBF practice and the role of each maternal ideation construct. Yet, this research has some limitations. The data gathered in this study is self-reported, which raises the potential for recall bias or the desire for social acceptance. In addition, replication of the current study is important to compare the differences between the different Saudi regions.

5. Conclusions

Around two-thirds of the study participants had satisfactory EBF practices with a relatively high early initiation rate. The mother's age, occupation, and education are significant demographic variables for satisfactory EBF practices. Moreover, parity, previous delivery mode, duration of the last pregnancy, and the number of living children were predictors of satisfactory EBF practices. Furthermore, knowledge and beliefs under cognitive maternal ideation, self-efficacy under psychological maternal ideation, injunctive and descriptive norms, and social influence under social maternal ideation were positive predictors of satisfactory EBF practices. The maternal ideation model could provide important insight to healthcare providers, policymakers, and health program designers about important modifiable and satisfactory EBF predictors.

Author Contributions: Conceptualization, W.T.E. and H.A.I.; methodology, W.T.E.; software, D.D.A.-T.; validation, M.A.A., R.M.E. and H.A.I.; formal analysis, H.A.I.; investigation, D.D.A.-T.; resources, M.A.A.; data curation, R.M.E.; writing—original draft preparation, W.T.E.; writing—review and editing, H.A.I.; visualization, R.M.E.; supervision, M.A.A.; project administration, D.D.A.-T.; funding acquisition, D.D.A.-T. All authors have read and agreed to the published version of the manuscript.

Funding: This research was funded by the Deputy for Research and Innovation-Ministry of Education, Kingdom of Saudi Arabia, grant number NU/IFC/2/MRC/-/4 And The APC was funded by D.D.A.-T.

Institutional Review Board Statement: Upon approval of the research proposal from the deanship of scientific research, the proposal and data collection tools were evaluated by the Ethical Committee of Najran Health Affairs before starting data collection; ethical approval (I.R.B. Log Number 2023-02 E). Clearance to perform the study was also obtained from the MCH administration.

Informed Consent Statement: Informed consent was obtained from all subjects involved in the study.

Data Availability Statement: The data will be made available by the corresponding author upon reasonable request.

Acknowledgments: The authors would like to acknowledge the support of the Deputy for Research and Innovation- Ministry of Education, Kingdom of Saudi Arabia, for funding this research through a grant (NU/IFC/2/MRC/-/4) under the Institutional Funding Committee at Najran University, Kingdom of Saudi Arabia.

Conflicts of Interest: The authors declare no conflict of interest.

Abbreviations

AOR	Adjusted Odd Ratio
EBF	Exclusive Breastfeeding
GFBKS	Gender-Friendly Breastfeeding Knowledge Scale
MCH	Maternal and Children's Hospital

References

1. World Health Organization. Better Care for Newborns Crucial for Millennium Development Goal on Child Deaths. Available online: https://www.who.int/news/item/10-12-2010-better-care-for-newborns-crucial-for-millennium-development-goal-on-child-deaths (accessed on 13 December 2022).
2. Sankar, M.J.; Sinha, B.; Chowdhury, R.; Bhandari, N.; Taneja, S.; Martines, J.; Bahl, R. Optimal breastfeeding practices and infant and child mortality: A systematic review and meta-analysis. *Acta Paediatr.* **2015**, *104*, 3–13. [CrossRef]
3. Patro-Gołąb, B.; Zalewski, B.M.; Polaczek, A.; Szajewska, H. Duration of Breastfeeding and Early Growth: A Systematic Review of Current Evidence. *Breastfeed. Med.* **2019**, *14*, 218–229. [CrossRef] [PubMed]
4. Victora, C.G.; Bahl, R.; Barros, A.J.; França, G.V.; Horton, S.; Krasevec, J.; Murch, S.; Sankar, M.J.; Walker, N.; Rollins, N.C.; et al. Breastfeeding in the 21st century: Epidemiology, mechanisms, and lifelong effect. *Lancet* **2016**, *387*, 475–490. [CrossRef] [PubMed]
5. Horta, B.L.; Hartwig, F.P.; Victora, C.G. Breastfeeding and intelligence in adulthood: Due to genetic confounding? *Lancet. Glob. Health* **2018**, *6*, e1276–e1277. [CrossRef] [PubMed]
6. Hansen, K. Breastfeeding: A smart investment in people and conomies. *Lancet* **2016**, *387*, 416. [CrossRef] [PubMed]
7. World Health Organization. Breastfeeding. Available online: https://www.who.int/health-topics/breastfeeding#tab=tab_1 (accessed on 13 December 2022).
8. Saudi Ministry of Health. Breastfeeding. Available online: https://www.moh.gov.sa/en/HealthAwareness/EducationalContent/wh/Pages/Breastfeeding.aspx (accessed on 13 December 2022).
9. Al-Jassir, M.; Moizuddin, S.K.; Al-Bashir, B. A review of some statistics on breastfeeding in Saudi Arabia. *Nutr. Health* **2003**, *17*, 123–130. [CrossRef]
10. Al Juaid, D.A.; Binns, C.W.; Giglia, R.C. Breastfeeding in Saudi Arabia: A review. *Int. Breastfeed. J.* **2014**, *9*, 1. [CrossRef] [PubMed]
11. Anaba, U.C.; Johansson, E.W.; Abegunde, D.; Adoyi, G.; Umar-Farouk, O.; Abdu-Aguye, S.; Hewett, P.C.; Hutchinson, P.L. The role of maternal ideations on breastfeeding practices in northwestern Nigeria: A cross-section study. *Int. Breastfeed. J.* **2022**, *17*, 63. [CrossRef]
12. Abegunde, D.; Hutchinson, P.; Anaba, U.; Oyedokun-Adebagbo, F.; Johansson, E.W.; Feyisetan, B.; Mtiro, E. Socioeconomic inequality in exclusive breastfeeding behavior and ideation factors for social behavioral change in three north-western Nigerian states: A cross-sectional study. *Int. J. Equity Health* **2021**, *20*, 172. [CrossRef]
13. Kummer, S.; Walter, F.M.; Chilcot, J.; Scott, S. Measures of psychosocial factors that may influence help-seeking behaviour in cancer: A systematic review of psychometric properties. *J. Health Psychol.* **2019**, *24*, 79–99. [CrossRef]
14. Babalola, S.; John, N.; Ajao, B.; Speizer, I.S. Ideation and intention to use contraceptives in Kenya and Nigeria. *Demogr. Res.* **2015**, *33*, 211–238. [CrossRef] [PubMed]
15. Vayngortin, T.; Clark, K.; Hollenbach, K. Sexual History Documentation and Screening in Adolescent Females with Suicidal Ideation in the Emergency Department. *Int. J. Environ. Res. Public Health* **2022**, *19*, 13018. [CrossRef]

16. Olapeju, B.; Adams, C.; Wilson, S.; Simpson, J.; Hunter, G.C.; Davis, T.; Mitchum, L.; Cox, H.; James, K.; Orkis, J.; et al. Malaria care-seeking and treatment ideation among gold miners in Guyana. *Malar. J.* **2022**, *21*, 29. [CrossRef] [PubMed]
17. Abdulahi, M.; Fretheim, A.; Argaw, A.; Magnus, J.H. Breastfeeding Education and Support to Improve Early Initiation and Exclusive Breastfeeding Practices and Infant Growth: A Cluster Randomized Controlled Trial from a Rural Ethiopian Setting. *Nutrients* **2021**, *13*, 1204. [CrossRef] [PubMed]
18. Ministry of Municipal and Rural Affairs and United Nations Human Settlements Programme. 2018. Available online: https://unhabitat.org/sites/default/files/2020/04/cpi_profile_for_najran_2019.pdf (accessed on 5 January 2023).
19. Cronbach, L.J.; Shavelson, R.J. My Current Thoughts on Coefficient Alpha and Successor Procedures. *Educ. Psychol. Meas.* **2004**, *64*, 391–418. [CrossRef]
20. Li, J.; Duan, Y.; Bi, Y.; Wang, J.; Lai, J.; Zhao, C.; Fang, J.; Yang, Z. Predictors of exclusive breastfeeding practice among migrant and non-migrant mothers in urban China: Results from a cross-sectional survey. *BMJ Open* **2020**, *10*, e038268. [CrossRef] [PubMed]
21. Gupta, A.; Aravindakshan, R.; Sathiyanarayanan, S.; Naidu, N.K.; Santhoshi, K.N.K.S.; Kakkar, R. Validation of Gender Friendly Breastfeeding Knowledge scale among young adults. *J. Prev. Med. Hyg.* **2022**, *62*, E892–E903. [CrossRef]
22. Davie, P.; Bick, D.; Chilcot, J. The Beliefs About Breastfeeding Questionnaire (BAB-Q): A psychometric validation study. *Br. J. Health Psychol.* **2021**, *26*, 482–504. [CrossRef]
23. Dennis, C.L. The breastfeeding self-efficacy scale: Psychometric assessment of the short form. *J. Obstet. Gynecol. Neonatal Nurs.* **2003**, *32*, 734–744. [CrossRef]
24. Amini, P.; Omani-Samani, R.; Sepidarkish, M.; Almasi-Hashiani, A.; Hosseini, M.; Maroufizadeh, S. The Breastfeeding Self-Efficacy Scale-Short Form (BSES-SF): A validation study in Iranian mothers. *BMC Res. Notes* **2019**, *12*, 622. [CrossRef]
25. Murad, A.; Renfrew, M.J.; Symon, A.; Whitford, H. Understanding factors affecting breastfeeding practices in one city in the Kingdom of Saudi Arabia: An interpretative phenomenological study. *Int. Breastfeed. J.* **2021**, *16*, 9. [CrossRef] [PubMed]
26. Alshammari, M.B.; Haridi, H.K. Prevalence and Determinants of Exclusive Breastfeeding Practice among Mothers of Children Aged 6–24 Months in Hail, Saudi Arabia. *Scientifica* **2021**, *2021*, 2761213. [CrossRef] [PubMed]
27. Alzaheb, R.A. Factors Influencing Exclusive Breastfeeding in Tabuk, Saudi Arabia. *Clin. Med. Insights Pediatr.* **2017**, *11*, 1179556517698136. [CrossRef]
28. Ahmed, A.E.; Salih, O.A. Determinants of the early initiation of breastfeeding in the Kingdom of Saudi Arabia. *Int. Breastfeed. J.* **2019**, *14*, 13. [CrossRef]
29. Al-Jassir, M.S.; El-Bashir, B.M.; Moizuddin, S.K.; Abu-Nayan, A.A. Infant feeding in Saudi Arabia: Mothers' attitudes and practices. *EMHJ-East. Mediterr. Health J.* **2006**, *12*, 6–13. [PubMed]
30. Harakeh, B.; Almatrafi, M.; Bukhari, R.; Alamri, T.; Barnawi, S.; Joshi, S.; Al Muhayawi, M.; Basunbul, G.; Alazraqi, M.; Al-Khalidy, A.; et al. Colostrum knowledge among Saudi mothers in Jeddah, Saudi Arabia. *J. Pak. Med. Assoc.* **2020**, *70*, 2221–2225. [CrossRef] [PubMed]
31. Alsulaimani, N.A. Exclusive breastfeeding among Saudi mothers: Exposing the substantial gap between knowledge and practice. *J. Fam. Med. Prim. Care* **2019**, *8*, 2803–2809. [CrossRef] [PubMed]
32. Hegazi, M.A.; Allebdi, M.; Almohammadi, M.; Alnafie, A.; Al-Hazmi, L.; Alyoubi, S. Factors associated with exclusive breastfeeding concerning knowledge, attitude and practice of breastfeeding mothers in Rabigh community, Western Saudi Arabia. *World J. Pediatr.* **2019**, *15*, 601–609. [CrossRef] [PubMed]
33. Zielińska, M.A.; Sobczak, A.; Hamułka, J. Breastfeeding knowledge and exclusive breastfeeding of infants in first six months of life. *Rocz. Państwowego Zakładu Hig.* **2017**, *68*, 51–59. [PubMed]
34. Chekol Abebe, E.; Ayalew Tiruneh, G.; Asmare Adela, G.; Mengie Ayele, T.; Tilahun Muche, Z.; Tilahun Mulu, A.; Asmamaw Dejenie, T. Levels and Determinants of Prenatal Breastfeeding Knowledge, Attitude, and Intention Among Pregnant Women: A Cross-Sectional Study in Northwest Ethiopia. *Front. Public Health* **2022**, *10*, 920355. [CrossRef]
35. Hernández Pérez, M.C.; Díaz-Gómez, N.M.; Romero Manzano, A.M.; Díaz Gómez, J.M.; Rodríguez Pérez, V.; Jiménez Sosa, A. Eficacia de una intervención para mejorar conocimientos y actitudes sobre lactancia materna en adolescentes [Effectiveness of an intervention to improve breastfeeding knowledge and attitudes among adolescents]. *Rev. Española Salud Pública* (In Spanish). **2018**, *92*, e201806033. [PubMed]
36. Fabrigar, L.R.; Petty, R.E.; Smith, S.M.; Crites, S.L. Understanding knowledge effects on attitude-behavior consistency: The role of relevance, complexity, and amount of knowledge. *J. Personal. Soc. Psychol.* **2006**, *90*, 556–577. [CrossRef] [PubMed]
37. Brockway, M.; Benzies, K.; Hayden, K.A. Interventions to Improve Breastfeeding Self-Efficacy and Resultant Breastfeeding Rates: A Systematic Review and Meta-Analysis. *J. Hum. Lact.* **2017**, *33*, 486–499. [CrossRef] [PubMed]
38. Shafaei, F.S.; Mirghafourvand, M.; Havizari, S. The effect of prenatal counseling on breastfeeding self-efficacy and frequency of breastfeeding problems in mothers with previous unsuccessful breastfeeding: A randomized controlled clinical trial. *BMC Women's Health* **2020**, *20*, 94. [CrossRef] [PubMed]
39. Ouyang, Y.Q.; Nasrin, L. Father's Knowledge, Attitude and Support to Mother's Exclusive Breastfeeding Practices in Bangladesh: A Multi-Group Structural Equations Model Analysis. *Healthcare* **2021**, *9*, 276. [CrossRef] [PubMed]
40. Agrawal, J.; Chakole, S.; Sachdev, C. The Role of Fathers in Promoting Exclusive Breastfeeding. *Cureus* **2022**, *14*, e30363. [CrossRef] [PubMed]

41. McFadden, A.; Gavine, A.; Renfrew, M.J.; Wade, A.; Buchanan, P.; Taylor, J.L.; Veitch, E.; Rennie, A.M.; Crowther, S.A.; Neiman, S.; et al. Support for healthy breastfeeding mothers with healthy term babies. *Cochrane Database Syst. Rev.* **2017**, *2*, CD001141. [CrossRef] [PubMed]
42. Kamoun, C.; Spatz, D. Influence of Islamic Traditions on Breastfeeding Beliefs and Practices Among African American Muslims in West Philadelphia: A Mixed-Methods Study. *J. Hum. Lact.* **2018**, *34*, 164–175. [CrossRef] [PubMed]
43. Albar, S.A. Mothers' feeding practices among infants (4–12 months) and associated factors: A cross-sectional study in Saudi Arabia. *J. Nutr. Sci.* **2022**, *11*, e83. [CrossRef] [PubMed]

Disclaimer/Publisher's Note: The statements, opinions and data contained in all publications are solely those of the individual author(s) and contributor(s) and not of MDPI and/or the editor(s). MDPI and/or the editor(s) disclaim responsibility for any injury to people or property resulting from any ideas, methods, instructions or products referred to in the content.

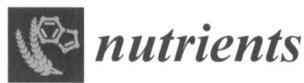

Article

Determinants of High Breastfeeding Self-Efficacy among Nursing Mothers in Najran, Saudi Arabia

DaifAllah D. Al-Thubaity [1], Mohammed A. Alshahrani [2], Wafaa T. Elgzar [1,3] and Heba A. Ibrahim [1,4,*]

[1] Department of Maternity and Childhood Nursing, Nursing College, Najran University, Najran 66441, Saudi Arabia
[2] Department of Clinical Laboratory Sciences, Applied Medical Sciences College, Najran University, Najran 66441, Saudi Arabia
[3] Department of Obstetrics and Gynecologic Nursing, Nursing College, Damanhour University, Damanhour 22514, Egypt
[4] Department of Obstetrics and Woman Health Nursing, Benha University, Benha 13511, Egypt
* Correspondence: heaibrahim@nu.edu.sa

Abstract: Many factors have been found to correlate with satisfactory Exclusive Breastfeeding (EBF) practices. The relationships between EBF practices and associated factors are complex and multidimensional; Breastfeeding Self-Efficacy (BSE) is the most important psychological factor that may help the mother to overcome any expected barriers. This study investigates the determinants of high breastfeeding self-efficacy among Saudi nursing mothers. Methods: This is a descriptive cross-sectional study investigating the determinant of BSE among 1577 nursing mothers in primary health centers in Najran City, Saudi Arabia. The study uses a cluster random sampling technique. Data collection was performed from June 2022 to January 2023 using a self-reported questionnaire that encompasses the Breastfeeding Self-Efficacy Scale—Short Form (BSES-SF), Gender Friendly Breastfeeding Knowledge Scale (GFBKS), Iowa Infant Feeding Attitude Scale (IIFAS), and a basic data questionnaire to assess women's demographic factors and obstetric history. Results: The mean score for all BSES-SF items was between 3.23–3.41, the highest mean score was in mothers who felt comfortable breastfeeding with family members present (3.41 ± 1.06), and the lowest mean was in mothers who could breastfeed their baby without using formula as a supplement (3.23 ± 0.94). The overall BSE score was high among 67% of the study participants. Binary logistic regression showed that being a housewife, being highly educated, having breastfeeding experience, and being multiparous are positive predictors for high BSE ($p \leq 0.001$). In addition, having adequate breastfeeding knowledge and positive breastfeeding attitudes were positively associated with higher BSE ($p = 0.000$). Conclusion: BSE can be predicted by modifiable predictors such as mothers' education, working status, parity, breastfeeding experience, adequate breastfeeding knowledge, and positive attitudes toward breastfeeding. If such predictors are considered during breastfeeding-related educational interventions, it could lead to more effective and sustainable effects in community awareness regarding breastfeeding.

Keywords: breastfeeding; self-efficacy; knowledge; attitude; Saudi Arabia

Citation: Al-Thubaity, D.D.; Alshahrani, M.A.; Elgzar, W.T.; Ibrahim, H.A. Determinants of High Breastfeeding Self-Efficacy among Nursing Mothers in Najran, Saudi Arabia. *Nutrients* 2023, 15, 1919. https://doi.org/10.3390/nu15081919

Academic Editor: Robert D. Roghair

Received: 31 March 2023
Revised: 12 April 2023
Accepted: 14 April 2023
Published: 15 April 2023

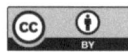

Copyright: © 2023 by the authors. Licensee MDPI, Basel, Switzerland. This article is an open access article distributed under the terms and conditions of the Creative Commons Attribution (CC BY) license (https://creativecommons.org/licenses/by/4.0/).

1. Introduction

Breastfeeding is the first and most important step toward healthy infants and communities. The World Health Organization recommends exclusive breastfeeding for the first 6 months of life, followed by the appropriate introduction of complementary foods with continued breastfeeding to two years and beyond [1]. Breastfeeding has evidence-based and well-known short- and long-term benefits for mothers and infants. Breast-milk composition is continually changed from one feed to another to meet the infant's body requirements. Human milk contains easily digested proteins such as glycoproteins, enzymes, and endogenous peptides, which help enhance immunity, cognitive development, and gut maturation, promote healthy infant development, and support healthy microbial colonization [2]. Furthermore, the fat in human milk is an essential source of energy and a facilitator of cell functions [3]. Long-term benefits of human milk include decreased risk for asthma [4], gastrointestinal infections, and adult diabetes [5]. For mothers, breastfeeding helps rapid weight loss [6], delayed fertility [7], and decreases the risk of diabetes, cardiovascular diseases, elevated blood cholesterol, and some types of cancers [8].

Despite the well-known benefits of breastfeeding, its rate is still much lower than expected. The World Health Organization stated that less than half of infants worldwide have EBF during the first six months of life [1]. The range of EBF in Saudi Arabia is much lower than reported by WHO and varies by region. EBF ranged from 0.8 to 43.9% according to a systemic review that surveyed 17 studies [9]. Many factors were found to be correlated with satisfactory EBF practices. In addition, the relationships between EBF practices and associated factors are complex and multidimensional; BSE is the most important psychological factor that may help the mother overcome any expected barriers and may correlate to other EBF-associated factors [10].

The term 'breastfeeding self-efficacy' (BSE) was first coined by Dennis in 1999 and is defined as maternal self-confidence in her ability to practice and master breastfeeding satisfactorily [11]. The research on breastfeeding has shown improvement in breastfeeding practices due to high BSE and has identified it as an essential factor in maternal ideation behavior regarding EBF [12,13]. If a woman has high BSE, she will make greater effort and demonstrate increased persistence to improve her breastfeeding practice, including searching for breastfeeding knowledge and seeking support from the health team and significant others. She will also work to overcome perceived barriers or challenges restricting her ability to breastfeed her infant satisfactorily [10]. Women with low BSE are three times more prone to terminate breastfeeding early [14].

Likewise, conclusions of previous systematic reviews reported a positive predictive relation between BSE and breastfeeding initiation and continuation. In addition, interventions to improve BSE improved breastfeeding initiation and continuation at one and two months postpartum [15,16]. Although numerous studies have investigated the association between BSE and breastfeeding practices, the relationship between the two variables still needs to be completely understood. Some international studies investigated the predictors of BSE during the immediate postpartum period or pregnancy [17–19]. However, few studies have investigated BSE among Saudi women during pregnancy [20,21]. No published studies have investigated BSE during the first six months of an infant's life, which is the most critical period in the breastfeeding span. Therefore, determining the BSE predictors during the first six months of life is crucial in anticipating breastfeeding initiation and continuity over time. Consequently, the current study investigates the determinants of high breastfeeding self-efficacy among Saudi nursing mothers.

2. Materials and Methods

2.1. Study Design and Setting

A descriptive cross-sectional study was conducted in four primary healthcare centers in Najran City, Saudi Arabia. Najran City is the largest city and capital of the Najran region. Najran region lies in southwestern the border with Yamen. The Najran population has numerous traditions and health beliefs related to breastfeeding, which may positively or negatively influence infant feeding practices. Najran City contains thirteen major primary health centers affiliated to the Ministry of Health [22].

2.2. Study Participants

The inclusion criteria were nursing mothers, with a child aged one day to less than six months, an absence of any breastfeeding contraindications such as HIV, or any condition that may hinder the continuity of EBF or affect milk production such as breast augmentation, lift, or reduction, or nipple surgery, aged 18 years or over, literate, and willing to participate in the study.

2.2.1. Sample Size Determinations and Sampling Procedures

The sample size was calculated based on the following formula:

$$n = \frac{(df)(t^2)P \times Q}{d^2} = \frac{(4)(1.96)^2 0.5 \times 0.5}{(0.05)^2} = 1536$$

where n = sample size, df = design effect of cluster sampling, t = the parameter related to the precision of obtaining the largest sample size (1.96 for an error risk of 5%) where the normal curve cuts off an area at the tails (the desired confidence level is 95%), p = expected prevalence of high BSE, $q = 1 - p$ the expected proportion of moderate or low BSE, d = maximum tolerable error (the desired level of precision). The sample size was 1689, after adding 10% to compensate the anticipated sample loss or non-response rate.

Najran City contains thirteen primary health centers; the researchers randomly selected 30% of the primary health centers (4 centers). The total sample size of 1689 was divided equally among the four primary health centers (422 participants from each center). In each center, all clinics dealing with children aged from 1 day to less than six months were included in the study. A proportional sample based on the follow-up rate was selected in each clinic, using the convenience sampling technique. The clinic nurse acted as a facilitator during the sampling process. Eight data collectors were distributed in the four centers (two in each center). Data collection took place from June 2022 to January 2023, three days per week from 9 a.m. until 2 p.m.

The study participants were allocated according to Figure 1.

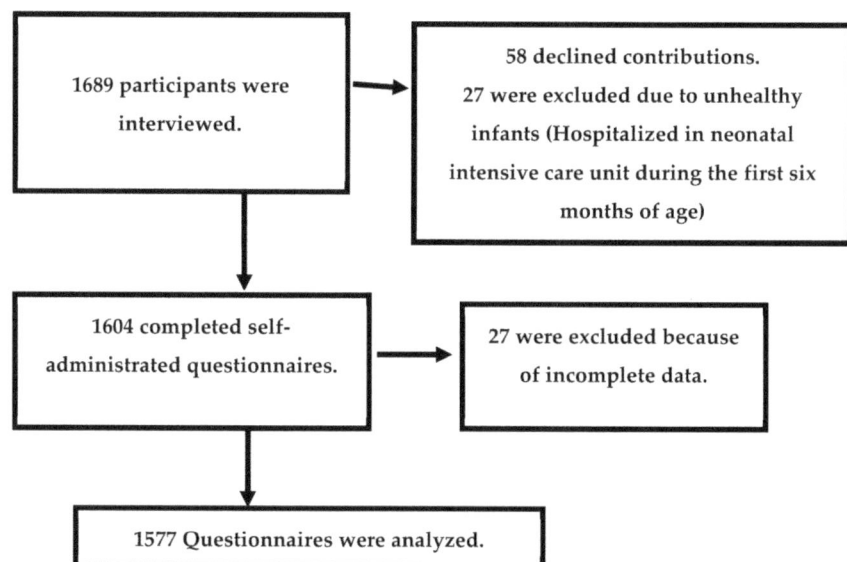

Figure 1. Participant flow chart.

2.2.2. Study Variables

The study's dependent variable was BSE, and the independent variables were women's demographic characteristics, obstetric history, previous breastfeeding experience, breastfeeding knowledge, and attitude.

2.3. Study Measurement Tools

BSE was evaluated using BSES-SF, developed by Dennis to assess breastfeeding confidence among puerperal women. The BSES-SF was rated on a 5-point Likert scale ranging from 1 (not at all confident) to 5 (always confident). The total scale score ranged from

14–70, classified as low self-efficacy from 14–42 and high self-efficacy from 43–70. Based on the study by Amini et al., the BSES-SF had good internal consistency (r = 0.910) [23]. The psychometric analysis of the BSES-SF Arabic version was tested in the United Arab Emirates and revealed a highly reliability measure (α = 0.95) [24].

The maternal breastfeeding knowledge was evaluated using the Gender Friendly Breastfeeding Knowledge Scale (GFBKS), created by Gupta et al. It comprised 18 statements rated on a 5-point Likert scale (scored as 1 = false, 2 = maybe false, 3 = don't know, 4 = maybe true, 5 = true). The GFBKS content validity was more than 0.80. The total scale score ranged from 18 to 90; the score for inadequate knowledge was 18–54, and adequate knowledge was from 55–90 [25]. The GFBKS Arabic version was validated by Tamim et al. and showed acceptable internal consistency (0.652) [26].

The Iowa Infant Feeding Attitude Scale (IIFAS) was utilized to evaluate women's attitudes to breastfeeding. IIFAS was created by De la Mora et al., and contains 17 items ranked on a 5-point Likert scale, from 1 (strongly disagree) to 5 (strongly agree). Overall IIFAS scores ranged from 17 to 85; each woman was considered to have a negative (17–51) or positive attitude (52–85) based on her score. IIFAS items' internal consistency ranged from 0.85 to 0.86 [27]. Charafeddine et al. assessed the psychometric properties of the IIFAS Arabic version with a sample of Lebanese women and found acceptable internal consistency (0.640) [28]. The scale was also validated in a study on Saudi pregnant women; the Cronbach alpha was 0.595 [29].

The researchers developed a basic data questionnaire to evaluate the women's demographic characteristics and obstetric history. Demographic data include age, occupation, residency, monthly income, and women's and their husbands' education. Obstetric history included gravidity, parity, number of living children, duration of pregnancy, complications during the most recent pregnancy and delivery, mode of delivery for the most recent child, and breastfeeding experience.

2.4. Data Collection Procedures and Technique

Data collection w from June 2022 to January 2023, three days weekly from 9 am until 2 pm. The data collection team comprised eight trained data collectors with previous experience in data collection. The data collectors were present in the waiting room in each clinic to identify the eligible participants based on the inclusion criteria. For each eligible participant, the data collector explained the study purpose and participant's role and obtained informed consent. A self-administered questionnaire was completed in the presence of the data collector. The data collector's role was to answer queries, clarify any concerns, and ensure data completeness in the questionnaire.

2.5. Data Quality Control

The data collectors have bachelor's degrees in nursing and previous data collection experience. Before data collection, the research team held two training sessions for the data collectors. The first session explained the research proposal, procedure, and ethics. At the end of the session, a copy of the data collection instrument was given to the data collectors to read before the next meeting. In the next session, one of the researchers provided a complete explanation of the questionnaire and clarified any queries. After data collection and during data entry, 27 questionnaires containing missing data were excluded from the analysis.

2.6. Ethical Approval

After research proposal approval from the deanship of scientific research, the proposal and data collection tools were assessed and approved by the Najran health affairs ethical committee; ethical approval 2023-02 E. Permission to start data collection was also obtained from the MCH administration. Informed consent was taken from each mother before starting data collection. Participant anonymity was applied, and data were utilized only for research purposes. The participants were informed about their rights to decline participation without any penalties or consequences for the care provided.

2.7. Data Analysis

Data analysis was performed using Statistical IBM, version 23 '(IBM Corp., Armonk, NY, USA)'. Data were described using numbers, percentages, means, and standard deviation. The total BSE, knowledge, and attitude scores were obtained by summing items. Chi-square (X^2) and Fisher exact tests (FET) were used to test group differences. Predictors of high BSE were examined through binary logistic regression. All the independent variables were categorical, and the first category was considered a reference. All factors were analyzed for multicollinearity in the regression model. The final model was checked with the Cox and Snell R-square goodness-of-fit test. Results were judged statistically significant at $p < 0.05$.

3. Results

The frequency distribution of nursing mothers by demographic characteristics and overall breastfeeding self-efficacy scores are illustrated in Table 1. More than three-quarters (78.8%) of the nursing mothers were between the ages of 20–35, and the majority (93.6%) were urban residents. More than half (55.9%) were housewives, and 51.4% reported insufficient family income. Regarding mothers' and their husbands' education, 55.0% and 66.6% had a university education, respectively. BSE was significantly high among housewives and university-educated mothers ($p = 0.000$).

Table 1. Frequency distribution of the nursing mothers by demographic characteristics and overall breastfeeding self-efficacy score.

Variables	Total Sample N = 1577		Breastfeeding Self-Efficacy				X^2/FET	p
			Low n = (520)		High n = (1057)			
	n	%	n	%	n	%		
Age (years)								
– <20	79	5.0	34	6.5	45	4.3	3.835	0.147
– 20–35	1242	78.8	404	77.7	838	79.3		
– ≥36	256	16.2	82	15.8	174	16.5		
Residence							0.081	0.775
– Rural	101	6.4	32	6.2	69	6.5		
– Urban	1476	93.6	488	93.8	988	93.5		
Occupational status							51.462	0.000 **
– Employee	696	44.1	296	56.9	400	37.8		
– Housewife	881	55.9	224	43.1	657	62.2		
Education							542.085	0.000 **
– University education	867	55.0	198	38.1	669	63.3		
– Secondary education	375	23.8	51	9.8	324	30.7		
– Read and write	335	21.2	271	52.1	64	6.1		
Husband education							3.267	0.195
– University education	1050	66.6	353	67.9	697	65.9		
– Secondary education	487	30.9	159	30.6	328	31.0		
– Read and write	40	2.5	8	1.5	32	3.0		

Table 1. Cont.

Variables	Total Sample N = 1577		Breastfeeding Self-Efficacy				X²/FET	p
			Low n = (520)		High n = (1057)			
	n	%	n	%	n	%		
Monthly income							5.445	0.066
- Sufficient and save	197	12.5	65	12.5	132	12.5		
- Sufficient	810	51.4	247	47.5	563	53.3		
- Insufficient	570	36.1	208	40.0	362	34.2		

X²: Chi-square FET Fisher exact tests ** significant at $p < 0.001$.

Approximately one-third (32.1%) of the nursing mothers breastfed exclusively, and 32.3% were primiparas. Around two-thirds (66.9%) delivered vaginally, and 19.7% reported complications during the most recent delivery. Concerning the participants' overall knowledge and attitudes toward BF, more than half (60.2%) had adequate breastfeeding knowledge and 56.9% had a positive breastfeeding attitude. Moreover, exclusive breastfeeding, parity, adequate knowledge, and positive attitude were associated with higher BSE ($p = 0.000$) (Table 2).

Table 2. Frequency distribution of nursing mothers by breastfeeding experience, obstetric history, overall breastfeeding knowledge, attitude, and self-efficacy scores.

Variables	Total Sample N = 1577		Breastfeeding Self-Efficacy				X²/FET	p
			Low n = (520)		High n = (1057)			
	n	%	n	%	n	%		
breastfeeding experience							15.085	0.000 **
- Exclusive	506	32.1	133	25.6	373	35.3		
- Nonexclusive	1071	67.9	387	74.4	684	64.7		
Parity							64.942	0.000 **
- Primiparous	510	32.3	228	43.8	282	26.7		
- Multiparous	1067	67.7	292	56.2	775	73.3		
Mode of delivery							0.804	0.370
- Vaginal delivery	1055	66.9	340	65.4	715	67.6		
- Cesarean section	522	33.1	180	34.6	342	32.4		
Complications during the last delivery							2.017	0.165
- No	1266	80.3	428	82.3	838	79.3		
- Yes	311	19.7	92	17.7	219	20.7		
Duration of pregnancy for the last child							2.469	0.116
- Full-term	1430	90.7	463	89.0	967	91.5		
- Preterm	147	9.3	57	11.0	90	8.5		
Overall knowledge							124.376	0.000 **
- Inadequate (18–54)	628	39.8	309	59.4	319	30.2		
- Adequate (55–90)	949	60.2	211	40.6	738	69.8		
Overall attitude							96.397	0.000 **
- Negative (17–51)	680	43.1	315	60.6	365	34.5		
- Positive (52–85)	897	56.9	205	39.4	692	65.5		

X²: Chi-square FET Fisher exact tests ** significant at $p < 0.001$.

The mean scores and standard deviation of BSES-SF items among nursing mothers are represented in Table 3. The overall mean BSES-SF score was 51.31 ± 10.79, with the mean score ranging from 3.23–3.41 for all BSES-SF items. As shown in the table, the highest mean score was for mothers who felt comfortable breastfeeding with family members present (3.41 ± 1.06), and the lowest mean was in mothers who could breastfeed their baby without using formula as a supplement (3.23 ± 0.94).

Table 3. Mean scores and standard deviation of BSES-SF items among nursing mothers.

	BSES-SF Items	Mean	SD
1.	Determine that my baby is getting enough milk	3.32	0.95
2.	Successfully cope with breastfeeding as I have with other challenging tasks	3.37	0.90
3.	Breastfeed my baby without using formula as a supplement	3.23	0.94
4.	Ensure that my baby is properly latched on for the whole feeding	3.33	0.99
5.	Manage the breastfeeding situation to my satisfaction	3.30	1.05
6.	Manage to breastfeed even if my baby is crying	3.25	0.97
7.	Keep wanting to breastfeed	3.38	1.07
8.	Comfortably breastfeed with my family members present	3.41	1.06
9.	Be satisfied with my breastfeeding experience	3.28	1.11
10.	Deal with the fact that breastfeeding can be time-consuming	3.40	1.05
11.	Finish feeding my baby on one breast before switching to the other breast	3.31	1.09
12.	Continue to breastfeed my baby for every feeding	3.24	1.09
13.	Manage to keep up with my baby's breastfeeding demands	3.26	1.07
14.	Tell when my baby is finished breastfeeding	3.24	1.11
	Overall mean of the BSES-SF score	51.31	10.79

Table 4 presents the binary logistic regression analysis of high BSE predictors. Occupational status was significantly associated with high BSE. Housewives had a 1.6 times higher probability of having high BSE (AOR 1.686; 95% CI 1.23–2.30, p = 0.001) when taking employed mothers as a reference. Educational level was also a significant predictor of high BSE. Higher odds ratios were found in mothers who had received university (OR 69.474; 95% CI 39.52–122.11, p = 0.000) and secondary education (OR 45.140; 95% CI 27.95–72.88, p = 0.000) compared with mothers who only could read and write. Furthermore, breastfeeding experience was significantly associated with high BSE. A mother who breastfed exclusively had a 5.9 times higher probability of having high BSE (OR 5.949; 95% CI 1.35–26.10, p = 0.000) compared with non-exclusively breastfeeding mothers. In addition, multiparous mothers had a 3.1 times higher probability of having high BSE (OR 3.170; 95% CI 1.96–5.120, p = 0.000) when compared with their primiparous counterparts. Finally, having adequate breastfeeding knowledge and positive attitudes were positively associated with higher BSE (OR 2.769; 95% CI 1.88–4.064, p = 0.000; and OR 4.803; 95% CI 2.60–8.85, p = 0.000, respectively).

Table 4. Binary logistic regression analysis of high BSE predictors.

Predictors	High Breastfeeding Self-Efficacy	
	AOR (95% CI)	p
Age (years)		0.167
− <20	Ref	
− 20–35	0.630 (0.18–2.12)	0.456

Table 4. *Cont.*

Predictors	High Breastfeeding Self-Efficacy	
	AOR (95% CI)	p
− ≥36	0.591 (0.34–1.02)	0.059
Residence		
− Rural	Ref	
− Urban	0.844 (0.48–1.48)	0.556
Occupational status		
− Employee	Ref	
− Housewife	1.686 (1.23–2.30)	0.001 *
Education		0.000 **
− Read and write	Ref	
− Secondary education	45.140 (27.95–72.88)	0.000 **
− University education	69.474 (39.52–122.11)	0.000 **
Husband education		0.223
− Read and write	Ref	
− Secondary education	1.180 (0.32–4.30)	0.803
− University education	0.857 (0.24–3.01)	0.810
Monthly income		0.055
− Insufficient	Ref	
− Sufficient	0.965 (0.69–1.33)	0.830
− Sufficient and save	1.909 (1.09–3.33)	0.033 *
breastfeeding experience		
- Nonexclusive	Ref	
- Exclusive	5.949 (1.35–26.10)	0.000 *
Parity		
- Primiparous	Ref	
- Multiparous	3.170 (1.96–5.120)	0.000 **
Mode of delivery		
- Vaginal delivery	Ref	
- Cesarean section	1.090 (0.77–1.532)	0.622
Complications during the last delivery		
- No	Ref	
- Yes	0.612 (0.34–1.10)	0.102
Duration of pregnancy for the last child		
- Full-term		
- Preterm	1.095 (0.28–4.160)	0.894
Overall knowledge		
- Inadequate (18–54)	Ref	
- Adequate (55–90)	2.769 (1.88–4.064)	0.000 **

Table 4. *Cont.*

Predictors	High Breastfeeding Self-Efficacy	
	AOR (95% CI)	p
Overall attitude		
- Negative (17–51)	Ref	
- Positive (52–85)	4.803 (2.60–8.85)	0.000 **
−2 Log likelihood (1263.883)	Cox and Snell R Square (0.374)	Nagelkerke R Square (0.519)

AOR: Adjusted odds ratio, CI: confidence interval, * significant at $p < 0.05$, ** significant at $p < 0.001$.

4. Discussion

The present study findings reveal that approximately two-thirds of the nursing mothers had a high BSE. The significant determinants of high BSE included high educational level, being a housewife, having adequate knowledge, and having positive attitudes regarding breastfeeding. Multiparous mothers and mothers who had previously exclusively breastfed their babies also had a high BSE. The current study findings can help health professionals and decision-makers to design and implement supportive interventions to improve maternal BSE. Increasing BSE will facilitate and accelerate the improvement of breastfeeding practices for the benefit of nursing mothers and their infants.

In the present study, the overall mean BSES-SF scores of 1577 Saudi nursing mothers were moderate, with a mean score of 51.31 ± 10.79 out of 70. The results indicate that Saudi nursing mothers are confident in breastfeeding their infants. Along the same lines, a cross-sectional study was conducted by Khresheh and Ahmad to evaluate the associated demographic variables of BSE among pregnant participants in Saudi Arabia. Their results indicated moderate to relatively high averages for a prenatal BSE scale of 70 out of 100. They also added that BSE is a significant variable affecting breastfeeding practice [21].

Similar mean scores were also reported among other participants in international studies using the same instrument: 50.80 ± 8.91 in Iran [23] and 49.7 in Cyprus [30]. In contrast, the BSE mean was much higher in Turkey (55.13 ± 8.39) than was documented in the current study [31], while a lower BSE mean (47.3 ± 10.50) was reported in China [32]. Among the aforementioned studies, the research by Mercan et al. [31] evaluated BSE in the first 42 days of the postpartum period. The research by Ip et al. [32] conducted a longitudinal cohort study and followed up to six months after delivery. The differences between the current study and the aforementioned studies may be attributed to the differences between the studies' designs and the data collection period.

This study revealed that a higher educational level significantly affected the BSE scale score. There is no doubt that educational level greatly affects breastfeeding knowledge and awareness. A high educational level may enhance BSE, empowering the mother in terms of health-seeking behavior and health education. Prior studies emphasized the important role of a high educational level in raising women's BSE and consequently enhancing successful breastfeeding practices [33,34]. In addition, cross-sectional surveys conducted in Taiwan suggested that educational level was positively associated with an increased likelihood of BSE, particularly among university-educated mothers [35].

According to Bandura's self-efficacy theory, if a person has good experience, their expectations will be higher [36]. In the current study, multiparous mothers with experience of exclusive breastfeeding had a higher probability of high BSE. According to Elgzar et al., previous experience of motherhood may initiate internal confidence in infant care and consequently shape maternal ideation behaviors regarding breastfeeding [37]. In several studies, higher BSE was related to previous positive breastfeeding experiences [37–39]. In addition, multi-parity was associated with successful breastfeeding among Saudi mothers in Al Hassa City [40]. The mediating role of BSE in successfully initiating and continuing breastfeeding practices has been documented in national and international studies [21,41–43].

Another important finding was the significant association between employment situation and the BSE score. Our findings revealed that housewives were 1.6 times more likely to have a high BSE compared with working mothers. This result was similar to other studies where working mothers outside their homes had low BSE and high barriers to optimal breastfeeding practices [44,45]. In addition, a recent qualitative study in Saudi Arabia showed that workplace policies and short periods of maternity leave (45–70 days) were connected with working mothers' early introduction of supplementary feeding or early weaning [46]. Therefore, it is necessary to establish supportive rules to ensure that breastfeeding breaks for working nursing mothers are available in the workplace. An Ethiopian study reported that increasing the period of breastfeeding leave from work and establishing childcare centers near workplaces significantly improved breastfeeding practices among employed mothers [47].

The present study found that adequate breastfeeding knowledge and positive attitudes predict higher BSE. At a national level, a recent Saudi study showed that mothers with gestational diabetes mellitus who had good breastfeeding knowledge were more likely to have higher BSE [33]. The significant role of knowledge in the current study indicates the importance of promoting strategies to improve nursing mothers' breastfeeding awareness and self-efficacy. Previous international studies have reported the benefits of educational interventions for enhancing mothers' BSE and breastfeeding rates [13,48]. Consistent with prior studies [18,49], positive attitudes toward breastfeeding among nursing mothers were also significantly linked with higher BSE in the present study. Attitude toward breastfeeding has also been recognized as a predictor of breastfeeding behavior among women in Western Saudi Arabia [50]. Thus, educating pregnant and postpartum mothers to improve their knowledge and develop positive attitudes toward breastfeeding may enhance BSE and improve breastfeeding practices among women in Saudi Arabia.

Strengths and Limitations

Our study has numerous strengths. A large sample size acquired using a random cluster sampling technique provides sufficient power to analyze the role of various predictors of BSE. Furthermore, this is the first study in Saudi Arabia to investigate the determinants of BSE in nursing mothers of babies under six months of age. Some limitations are also worthy to be mentioned. The current data were collected using a self-reported questionnaire, which may be susceptible to recall bias. In addition, it was not effectively possible to apply a random sampling technique to select the participants from each primary health center; therefore, we used a convenience sample.

5. Conclusions

The current study found that mothers' education, working status, parity, breastfeeding experience, adequate breastfeeding knowledge, and positive attitudes were predictors of BSE. If such predictors are considered during breastfeeding-related educational interventions, it could lead to more effective and sustainable effects in community awareness regarding breastfeeding. Despite the great efforts made by the Saudi Ministry of Health to raise community awareness regarding breastfeeding, multifaceted breastfeeding educational interventions, counseling, and support are needed to improve mothers' BSE and thereby enhance proper breastfeeding practices.

Author Contributions: Conceptualization, D.D.A.-T. and H.A.I.; methodology W.T.E.; software, D.D.A.-T.; validation, M.A.A. and H.A.I.; formal analysis, H.A.I.; investigation, D.D.A.-T.; resources, M.A.A.; data curation, D.D.A.-T.; writing—original draft preparation, W.T.E.; writing—review and editing, H.A.I.; visualization, M.A.A.; supervision, M.A.A.; project administration, D.D.A.-T.; funding acquisition, D.D.A.-T. All authors have read and agreed to the published version of the manuscript.

Funding: This research was funded by the Deputy for Research and Innovation- Ministry of Education, Kingdom of Saudi Arabia, grant number NU/IFC/2/MRC/-/-4 And The APC was funded by D.D.A.-T.

Institutional Review Board Statement: Upon approval of the research proposal from the deanship of scientific research, the proposal and data collection tools were evaluated by the Najran health affairs ethical committee before starting data collection; ethical approval IRB log number 2023-02 E. Clearance to perform the study was obtained from the MCH administration.

Informed Consent Statement: Informed consent was obtained from all subjects involved in the study.

Data Availability Statement: Data will be made available by the corresponding author upon reasonable request.

Acknowledgments: The authors would like to acknowledge the support of the Deputy for Research and Innovation- Ministry of Education, Kingdom of Saudi Arabia, for funding this research through a grant (NU/IFC/2/MRC/-/4) under the Institutional Funding Committee at Najran University, Kingdom of Saudi Arabia.

Conflicts of Interest: The authors declare no conflict of interest.

Abbreviations

AOR	Adjusted odds ratio
EBF	Exclusive breastfeeding
GFBKS	Gender-Friendly Breastfeeding Knowledge Scale
BSES-SF	Breastfeeding Self-Efficacy Scale—Short Form
BSE	Breastfeeding self-efficacy
IIFAS	Iowa Infant Feeding Attitude Scale

References

1. World Health Organization. WHO Breastfeeding [Internet]. Available online: https://www.who.int/health-topics/breastfeeding#tab=tab_1 (accessed on 25 January 2023).
2. Zhu, J.; Dingess, K.A. The Functional Power of the Human Milk Proteome. *Nutrients* **2019**, *11*, 1834. [CrossRef] [PubMed]
3. Wesolowska, A.; Brys, J.; Barbarska, O.; Strom, K.; Szymanska-Majchrzak, J.; Karzel, K.; Pawlikowska, E.; Zielinska, M.A.; Hamulka, J.; Oledzka, G. Lipid Profile, Lipase Bioactivity, and Lipophilic Antioxidant Content in High Pressure Processed Donor Human Milk. *Nutrients* **2019**, *11*, 1972. [CrossRef] [PubMed]
4. Oddy, W.H. Breastfeeding, Childhood Asthma, and Allergic Disease. *Ann. Nutr. Metab.* **2017**, *70* (Suppl. S2), 26–36. [CrossRef] [PubMed]
5. Nuzzi, G.; Trambusti, I.; DICicco, M.E.; Peroni, D.G. Breast milk: More than just nutrition! *Minerva Pediatr.* **2021**, *73*, 111–114. [CrossRef]
6. da Silva, M.d.C.; Oliveira Assis, A.M.; Pinheiro, S.M.; de Oliveira, L.P.; da Cruz, T.R. Breastfeeding and maternal weight changes during 24 months postpartum: A cohort study. *Matern. Child Nutr.* **2015**, *11*, 780–791. [CrossRef] [PubMed]
7. Calik-Ksepka, A.; Stradczuk, M.; Czarnecka, K.; Grymowicz, M.; Smolarczyk, R. Lactational Amenorrhea: Neuroendocrine Pathways Controlling Fertility and Bone Turnover. *Int. J. Mol. Sci.* **2022**, *23*, 1633. [CrossRef]
8. Binns, C.; Lee, M.; Low, W.Y. The Long-Term Public Health Benefits of Breastfeeding. *Asia-Pac. J. Public Health* **2016**, *28*, 7–14. [CrossRef]
9. Al Juaid, D.A.; Binns, C.W.; Giglia, R.C. Breastfeeding in Saudi Arabia: A review. *Int. Breastfeed J.* **2014**, *9*, 1. [CrossRef]
10. Rosenblad, A.K.; Funkquist, E.L. Self-efficacy in breastfeeding predicts how mothers perceive their preterm infant's state-regulation. *Int. Breastfeed J.* **2022**, *17*, 44. [CrossRef]
11. Dennis, C.L. Theoretical underpinnings of breastfeeding confidence: A self-efficacy framework. *J. Hum. Lact.* **1999**, *15*, 195–201. [CrossRef]
12. Anaba, U.C.; Johansson, E.W.; Abegunde, D.; Adoyi, G.; Umar-Farouk, O.; Abdu-Aguye, S.; Hewett, P.C.; Hutchinson, P.L. The role of maternal ideations on breastfeeding practices in northwestern Nigeria: A cross-section study. *Int. Breastfeed. J.* **2022**, *17*, 63. [CrossRef]
13. You, H.; Lei, A.; Xiang, J.; Wang, Y.; Luo, B.; Hu, J. Effects of breastfeeding education based on the self-efficacy theory on women with gestational diabetes mellitus: A CONSORT-compliant randomized controlled trial. *Medicine* **2020**, *99*, e19643. [CrossRef] [PubMed]
14. Vieira, E.S.; Caldeira, N.T.; Eugênio, D.S.; Lucca MM, D.; Silva, I.A. Breastfeeding self-efficacy and postpartum depression: A cohort study. *Rev. Lat.-Am. Enferm.* **2018**, *26*, e3035. [CrossRef] [PubMed]
15. Galipeau, R.; Baillot, A.; Trottier, A.; Lemire, L. Effectiveness of interventions on breastfeeding self-efficacy and perceived insufficient milk supply: A systematic review and meta-analysis. *Matern. Child Nutr.* **2018**, *14*, e12607. [CrossRef]
16. Maleki, A.; Faghihzadeh, E.; Youseflu, S. The Effect of Educational Intervention on Improvement of Breastfeeding Self-Efficacy: A Systematic Review and Meta-Analysis. *Obstet. Gynecol. Int.* **2021**, *2021*, 5522229. [CrossRef]

17. Melo, L.C.O.; Bonelli, M.C.P.; Lima, R.V.A.; Gomes-Sponholz, F.A.; Monteiro, J.C.D.S. Anxiety and its influence on maternal breastfeeding self-efficacy. *Rev. Lat.-Am. Enferm.* **2021**, *29*, e3485. [CrossRef]
18. Li, L.; Wu, Y.; Wang, Q.; Du, Y.; Friesen, D.; Guo, Y.; Dill, S.E.; Medina, A.; Rozelle, S.; Zhou, H. Determinants of breastfeeding self-efficacy among postpartum women in rural China: A cross-sectional study. *PLoS ONE* **2022**, *17*, e0266273. [CrossRef] [PubMed]
19. Piro, S.S.; Ahmed, H.M. Impacts of antenatal nursing interventions on mothers' breastfeeding self-efficacy: An experimental study. *BMC Pregnancy Childbirth* **2020**, *20*, 19. [CrossRef]
20. Mosher, C.; Sarkar, A.; Hashem, A.A.; Hamadah, R.E.; Alhoulan, A.; AlMakadma, Y.A.; Khan, T.A.; Al-Hamdani, A.K.; Senok, A. Self-reported breast feeding practices and the Baby Friendly Hospital Initiative in Riyadh, Saudi Arabia: Prospective cohort study. *BMJ Open* **2016**, *6*, e012890. [CrossRef] [PubMed]
21. Khresheh, R.M.; Ahmad, N.M. Breastfeeding self efficacy among pregnant women in Saudi Arabia. *Saudi Med. J.* **2018**, *39*, 1116–1122. [CrossRef]
22. Ministry of Municipal and Rural Affairs and United Nations Human Settlements Programme. 2018. Revised on: 5/1/2023. Available online: https://unhabitat.org/sites/default/files/2020/04/cpi_profile_for_najran_2019.pdf (accessed on 20 January 2023).
23. Amini, P.; Omani-Samani, R.; Sepidarkish, M.; Almasi-Hashiani, A.; Hosseini, M.; Maroufizadeh, S. The Breastfeeding Self-Efficacy Scale-Short Form (BSES-SF): A validation study in Iranian mothers. *BMC Res. Notes* **2019**, *12*, 622. [CrossRef] [PubMed]
24. Radwan, H.; Fakhry, R.; Boateng, G.O.; Metheny, N.; Bani Issa, W.; Faris, M.E.; Obaid, R.S.; Al Marzooqi, S.; Al Ghazal, H.; Dennis, C.L. Translation and Psychometric Evaluation of the Arabic Version of the Breastfeeding Self-Efficacy Scale-Short Form among Women in the United Arab Emirates. *J. Hum. Lact. Off. J. Int. Lact. Consult. Assoc.* **2023**, *39*, 40–50. [CrossRef] [PubMed]
25. Gupta, A.; Aravindakshan, R.; Sathiyanarayanan, S.; Naidu, N.K.; Santhoshi, K.N.K.S.; Kakkar, R. Validation of Gender Friendly Breastfeeding Knowledge scale among young adults. *J. Prev. Med. Hyg.* **2022**, *62*, E892–E903. [CrossRef] [PubMed]
26. Tamim, H.; Ghandour, L.A.; Shamsedine, L.; Charafeddine, L.; Nasser, F.; Khalil, Y.; Nabulsi, M. Adaptation and Validation of the Arabic Version of the Infant Breastfeeding Knowledge Questionnaire among Lebanese Women. *J. Hum. Lact.* **2016**, *32*, 682–688. [CrossRef]
27. De la Mora, A.; Russell, D.W.; Dungy, C.I.; Losch, M.; Dusdieker, L. The Iowa Infant Feeding Attitude Scale: Analysis of reli-ability and validity. *J. Appl. Soc. Psychol.* **1999**, *29*, 2362–2380. [CrossRef]
28. Charafeddine, L.; Tamim, H.; Soubra, M.; de la Mora, A.; Nabulsi, M. Research and Advocacy Breastfeeding Team. Validation of the Arabic Version of the Iowa Infant Feeding Attitude Scale among Lebanese Women. *J. Hum. Lact.* **2016**, *32*, 309–314. [CrossRef]
29. Almadani, M.; Vydelingum, V.; Lawrence, J. Saudi Mothers' Expected Intentions and Attitudes Toward Breast-Feeding. *Infant Child Adolesc. Nutr.* **2010**, *2*, 187–198. [CrossRef]
30. Economou, M.; Kolokotroni, O.; Paphiti-Demetriou, I.; Kouta, C.; Lambrinou, E.; Hadjigeorgiou, E.; Hadjiona, V.; Middleton, N. The association of breastfeeding self-efficacy with breastfeeding duration and exclusivity: Longitudinal assessment of the pre-dictive validity of the Greek version of the BSES-SF tool. *BMC Pregnancy Childbirth* **2021**, *21*, 421. [CrossRef]
31. Mercan, Y.; Tari Selcuk, K. Association between postpartum depression level, social support level and breastfeeding attitude and breastfeeding self-efficacy in early postpartum women. *PLoS ONE* **2021**, *16*, e0249538. [CrossRef]
32. Ip, W.Y.; Gao, L.L.; Choi, K.C.; Chau, J.P.; Xiao, Y. The Short Form of the Breastfeeding Self-Efficacy Scale as a Prognostic Factor of Exclusive Breastfeeding among Mandarin-Speaking Chinese Mothers. *J. Hum. Lact. Off. J. Int. Lact. Consult. Assoc.* **2016**, *32*, 711–720. [CrossRef]
33. Alyousefi, N.; Alemam, A.; Altwaijri, D.; Alarifi, S.; Alessa, H. Predictors of Prenatal Breastfeeding Self-Efficacy in Expectant Mothers with Gestational Diabetes Mellitus. *Int. J. Environ. Res. Public Health* **2022**, *19*, 4115. [CrossRef] [PubMed]
34. Colombo, L.; Crippa, B.L.; Consonni, D.; Bettinelli, M.E.; Agosti, V.; Mangino, G.; Bezze, E.N.; Mauri, P.A.; Zanotta, L.; Roggero, P.; et al. Breastfeeding Determinants in Healthy Term Newborns. *Nutrients* **2018**, *10*, 48. [CrossRef] [PubMed]
35. Waits, A.; Guo, C.Y.; Chien, L.Y. Evaluation of factors contributing to the decline in exclusive breastfeeding at 6 months postpartum: The 2011–2016 National Surveys in Taiwan. *Birth* **2018**, *45*, 184–192. [CrossRef]
36. Bandura, A.; Pastorelli, C.; Barbaranelli, C.; Caprara, G.V. Self-efficacy pathways to childhood depression. *J. Pers. Soc. Psychol.* **1999**, *76*, 258–269. [CrossRef] [PubMed]
37. Elgzar, W.T.; Al-Thubaity, D.D.; Alshahrani, M.A.; Essa, R.M.; Ibrahim, H.A. The Relationship between Maternal Ideation and Exclusive Breastfeeding Practice among Saudi Nursing Mothers: A Cross-Sectional Study. *Nutrients* **2023**, *15*, 1719. [CrossRef]
38. Gerhardsson, E.; Nyqvist, K.H.; Mattsson, E.; Volgsten, H.; Hildingsson, I.; Funkquist, E.L. The Swedish Version of the Breast-feeding Self-Efficacy Scale-Short Form: Reliability and Validity Assessment. *J. Hum. Lact. Off. J. Int. Lact. Consult. Assoc.* **2014**, *30*, 340–345. [CrossRef]
39. Tsaras, K.; Sorokina, T.; Papathanasiou, I.V.; Fradelos, E.C.; Papagiannis, D.; Koulierakis, G. Breastfeeding Self-efficacy and Related Socio-demographic, Perinatal and Psychological Factors: A Cross-sectional Study Among Postpartum Greek Women. *Mater. Socio-Med.* **2021**, *33*, 206–212. [CrossRef]
40. Amin, T.; Hablas, H.; Al Qader, A.A. Determinants of initiation and exclusivity of breastfeeding in Al Hassa, Saudi Arabia. *Breastfeed. Med. Off. J. Acad. Breastfeed. Med.* **2011**, *6*, 59–68. [CrossRef]

41. Rocha, I.S.; Lolli, L.F.; Fujimaki, M.; Gasparetto, A.; Rocha NB, D. Influence of maternal confidence on exclusive breastfeeding until six months of age: A systematic review. Influência da autoconfiança materna sobre o aleitamento materno exclusivo aos seis meses de idade: Uma revisão sistemática. *Cienc. Saude Coletiva* **2018**, *23*, 3609–3619. [CrossRef]
42. Monteiro, J.C.D.S.; Guimarães, C.M.S.; Melo, L.C.O.; Bonelli, M.C.P. Breastfeeding self-efficacy in adult women and its relationship with exclusive maternal breastfeeding. *Rev. Lat.-Am. Enferm.* **2020**, *28*, e3364. [CrossRef]
43. Moraes, G.G.W.; Christoffel, M.M.; Toso, B.R.G.O.; Viera, C.S. Association between duration of exclusive breastfeeding and nursing mothers' self-efficacy for breastfeeding. *Rev. Esc. Enferm. USP* **2021**, *55*, e03702. [CrossRef] [PubMed]
44. Titaley, C.R.; Dibley, M.J.; Ariawan, I.; Mu'asyaroh, A.; Alam, A.; Damayanti, R.; Do, T.T.; Ferguson, E.; Htet, K.; Li, M.; et al. Determinants of low breastfeeding self-efficacy amongst mothers of children aged less than six months: Results from the BADUTA study in East Java, Indonesia. *Int. Breastfeed. J.* **2021**, *16*, 12. [CrossRef]
45. Titaley, C.R.; Loh, P.C.; Prasetyo, S.; Ariawan, I.; Shankar, A.H. Socio-economic factors and use of maternal health services are associated with delayed initiation and non-exclusive breastfeeding in Indonesia: Secondary analysis of Indonesia Demographic and Health Surveys 2002/2003 and 2007. *Asia Pac. J. Clin. Nutr.* **2014**, *23*, 91–104. [CrossRef] [PubMed]
46. AlSedra, H.; AlQurashi, A.A. Exploring the Experience of Breastfeeding Among Working Mothers at Healthcare Facility in Saudi Arabia: A Qualitative Approach. *Cureus* **2022**, *14*, e25510. [CrossRef]
47. Awoke, N.; Tekalign, T.; Lemma, T. Predictors of optimal breastfeeding practices in Worabe town, Silte zone, South Ethiopia. *PLoS ONE* **2020**, *15*, e0232316. [CrossRef]
48. Dodt, R.C.; Joventino, E.S.; Aquino, P.S.; Almeida, P.C.; Ximenes, L.B. An experimental study of an educational intervention to promote maternal self-efficacy in breastfeeding. *Rev. Lat.-Am. Enferm.* **2015**, *23*, 725–732. [CrossRef]
49. Mirghafourvand, M.; Malakouti, J.; Mohammad-Alizadeh-Charandabi, S.; Faridvand, F. Predictors of Breastfeeding Self-efficacy in Iranian Women: A Cross-Sectional Study. *Int. J. Womens Health Reprod. Sci.* **2018**, *6*, 380–385. [CrossRef]
50. Hegazi, M.A.; Allebdi, M.; Almohammadi, M.; Alnafie, A.; Al-Hazmi, L.; Alyoubi, S. Factors associated with exclusive breastfeeding in relation to knowledge, attitude and practice of breastfeeding mothers in Rabigh community, Western Saudi Arabia. *World J. Pediatr. WJP* **2019**, *15*, 601–609. [CrossRef]

Disclaimer/Publisher's Note: The statements, opinions and data contained in all publications are solely those of the individual author(s) and contributor(s) and not of MDPI and/or the editor(s). MDPI and/or the editor(s) disclaim responsibility for any injury to people or property resulting from any ideas, methods, instructions or products referred to in the content.

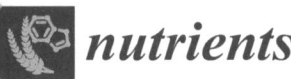

Article

Breastfeeding-Related Practices in Rural Ethiopia: Colostrum Avoidance

M. Ascensión Olcina Simón [1,2], Rosita Rotella [2], Jose M. Soriano [3,4], Agustin Llopis-Gonzalez [2,5], Isabel Peraita-Costa [2,5] and María Morales-Suarez-Varela [2,5,*]

1. MOS Solidaria, Avda. Blasco Ibáñez, 5-8º Puerta 16, 46400 Cullera, Spain; 7alenar@gmail.com
2. Unit of Preventive Medicine and Public Health, Department of Preventive Medicine and Public Health, Food Sciences, Toxicology and Forensic Medicine, University of Valencia, Avda. Vicent Andres Estelles s/n, 46100 Burjassot, Spain; rotella@alumni.uv.es (R.R.); agustin.llopis@uv.es (A.L.-G.); isabel.peraita@uv.es (I.P.-C.)
3. Observatory of Nutrition and Food Safety for Developing Countries, Food & Health Lab, Institute of Materials Science, University of Valencia, Carrer Catedrático Agustín Escardino 9, 46980 Paterna, Spain; jose.soriano@uv.es
4. Joint Research Unit on Endocrinology, Nutrition and Clinical Dietetics, University of Valencia-Health Research Institute La Fe, Avda. Fernando Abril Martorell, 106, 46026 Valencia, Spain
5. CIBER in Epidemiology and Public Health (CIBERESP), Institute of Health Carlos III, Avda. Monforte de Lemos 3-5, Pabellón 11, Planta 0, 28029 Madrid, Spain
* Correspondence: maria.m.morales@uv.es

Abstract: The practices of colostrum avoidance and prelacteal feeding, which are common in many developing countries, including Ethiopia, are firmly rooted in ancient traditions. The main objective of this work is to identify the prevalence of colostrum avoidance and study its associated factors among mothers of children aged less than 2 years old in the Oromia region of Ethiopia. A cross-sectional study on the practice of colostrum avoidance/prelacteal feeding was conducted in a rural community with 114 mothers of children under 2 years old. Our results reflected that colostrum avoidance and prelacteal feeding were practiced by 56.1% of mothers. The percentage of women who started breastfeeding in the first hour after birth, as recommended by the WHO, was 2.6%. Of the women who practiced colostrum avoidance, 67.2% gave birth at home, and 65.6% were attended by relatives. The likelihood of avoiding colostrum increases in mothers who have a lower educational level, who did not receive health care at the time of delivery, who think that colostrum is dirty and dangerous and who did not receive information about breastfeeding from healthcare professionals. The knowledge emanating from this work may be useful in designing new breastfeeding education programs and/or interventions in Ethiopia and other developing countries.

Keywords: colostrum; breastfeeding; prelacteal feeding; Ethiopia

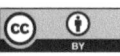

1. Introduction

Breastfeeding is an essential practice of optimal nutrition in the early life of a child and one of the most important factors for child survival and the prevention of childhood infections [1]. The World Health Organization (WHO) recommends that infants be exclusively breastfed for the first six months of life [2]. Exclusive breastfeeding is defined as giving no food or drink, not even water, except breastmilk [2]. The optimal breastfeeding practice includes initiation within the first hour after birth and continued breastfeeding for up to two years [3,4]. Colostrum is the first secretion produced by the mammary gland after childbirth, is available to the neonate in the first two to three days following birth [2] and is sometimes referred to as "golden milk" [5] due to its nutritional properties as a complete form of nutrition for newborns. It has been shown to be a protective factor against childhood malnutrition [6] and to deliver natural immunity against many bacteria and viruses by establishing microbiota in the newborn's gut [7,8]. Colostrum avoidance, which is defined as discarding colostrum within the first three days postpartum and entails the delayed initiation of breastfeeding, pumping and discarding colostrum, and/or wet nursing [9], deprives the neonate of nutrients and immunoglobulins, causing a reduction in the priming of the gastrointestinal tract and increasing the risk of infant morbidity and mortality [10]. Colostrum avoidance is a common practice in many developing countries of the world [11], including Ethiopia [9]. In Ethiopia, colostrum and breast milk are considered two distinctly separate substances known, respectively, as 'inger' and 'yetut wotet', and women will wait until they observe the characteristics of 'yetut wotet' to start breastfeeding [9]. During this period between birth and the establishment of breastfeeding, during which colostrum or 'inger' is discarded, a practice known as prelacteal feeding takes place. Prelacteal feeding, known in Amharic as 'makamesha', is the practice of feeding the child any solid or liquid foods other than breast milk during the first three days after birth [12]. Some of the solid foods given to the newborns include 'injera', 'shiro', 'genfo' and 'faffa'. The basis of any Ethiopian meal is a teff flour flatbread named 'injera or enjera'. 'Shiro' is a dish prepared with chickpea flour, water, oil, onions and a spice called 'berbere', which is very commonly used in Ethiopia. 'Genfo' is the Amharic name given to a breakfast porridge, and 'faffa' is a mix of fortified corn and soya bean flours used to supplement the diet of children suffering from malnutrition. It is estimated that 90% or more of children under ten years old are multidimensionally poor in Ethiopia [13]. Rural areas are particularly disadvantaged due primarily to their lack of access to safe drinking water, sanitation and/or electricity. Most of the inhabitants of these areas suffer from poor nutrition, repeated infection and inadequate psychosocial stimulation given to the lack of access to education making it particularly difficult to achieve an improvement of the situation [14]. The aim of this study was to identify the prevalence of the breastfeeding-related practice of colostrum avoidance and study its associated factors among mothers of children aged less than two years old in two rural villages of the Oromia region of Ethiopia.

2. Materials and Methods

2.1. Research Design

This cross-sectional community-based study carried out in two rural Ethiopian villages was approved by the Ethics Committee of Research in Humans of the Ethics Commission in Experimental Research of the University of Valencia (Register code: 1256147). It is in line with the ethical principles established by the Declaration of Helsinki [15], the U.S. National Bioethics Advisory Commission [16] and the European Commission [17]. It also follows the International Compilation of Human Research Standards applied to Ethiopia based on Proclamation 60/1999 (Section 21) and National Health Research Ethics Review Guidelines [18]. The design of the study is in line with its objective of determining the prevalence of colostrum avoidance and detecting associated factors. This work has been prepared in accordance with the STROBE guidelines for observational studies [19]. All the women participating in this study were recruited under the same inclusion and exclusion criteria. They were all interviewed in their homes following the same previously established protocol. The same interview questionnaire was used, which allows us to calculate the prevalence of the different variables studied. Subsequently, participants were stratified by WHO recommendations on the initiation of breastfeeding and the practice of prelacteal feeding. Those women who rejected colostrum in their lactation and practiced prelacteal feeding were considered the avoidance group, and those who did not reject colostrum during lactation and did not practice prelacteal feeding were considered the non-avoidance group. The outcome variable was colostrum avoidance during the early breastfeeding period.

2.2. Setting and Relevant Context

This study was carried out, in collaboration with The Missionary Community of Saint Paul the Apostle (MCSPA) [20], and the Spanish NGO MOS SOLIDARIA (MOSS) [21], in the villages of Andode and Muke Turi where MCSPA operates. Andode is found in the Anger Guten Valley in the Gida-Kiremu district of the Oromia region, 331 km from

Addis Ababa. Muke Turi is in the North Shoa region, 78 km northeast of Addis Ababa, and populated mainly by the Oromo ethnic people. The MCSPA has implemented a comprehensive program for development in the area comprising 3 health posts (Angar, Andode and Fite Bako) that care for an estimated 12,000 people and 3 nurseries (Guten, Gida and Andode) for around 450 children. It also runs the "Saint Joseph Mother and Child Center" in Muke Turi and a Nutritional Unit in Andode, where around 450 children 4 to 6 years old receive 2 nutritious meals per day, medical care and reading and writing lessons.

2.3. Participants

A sample size calculation was performed using the following values: 95% confidence level, 5% margin of error, 10% population proportion and 500 for population size. The value for the population proportion was chosen taking into consideration the prevalence of colostrum avoidance reported in previous studies in Ethiopia, and the population number is an estimation of the number of women of child-bearing age made using information collected by the MCSPA as no official demographic data for Andode and Muke Turi are available. The necessary sample was 109 women. The households that had potentially eligible study participants were identified by the MCSPA using the health extension workers' logbook. This helped to identify the initial convenience sample of woman that could meet the inclusion criteria of having a live child under 2 years of age and the exclusion criteria of not having given informed consent, providing unreliable responses and/or missing 30% of the responses. Once all potentially eligible women were identified from the population records kept by the MCSPA, a systematic random sampling technique (women that attended the MCSPA posts for any reason on days the project collaborators were present in each village) was used to choose which women would be invited to participate. The total number of potential participants (women of child-bearing age) was around 500; the actual number of women with a live child under 2 years of age is unknown as, as stated previously, no official demographic data are available for the studied populations. A total of 114 women were invited to participate in the study. All women invited to participate in the study accepted the offer, and, therefore, 114 mothers who had children aged less than 2 years old were included in the study. Participation was around 23%, which is about what was expected, taking into consideration previous experiences with this population.

2.4. Data Collection

Data were collected in situ in November 2020 by project collaborators from the University of Valencia with the aid of MCSPA, MOSS and local collaborators that served mainly as translators. Collection took place after the women were attended by the MCSPA and MOSS in a room ceded by the MCSPA within their installations in both villages for this specific purpose. A semi-structured questionnaire, which was not pre-tested, was used for data collection. It was created specifically for this study after reviewing the experiences of the local collaborators, the currently available literature on the topic and the possible association of breastfeeding practices with infant malnutrition. This questionnaire was administered during an individual face-to-face 30 min interview with the mothers. All possible participants were informed about the objectives of the study and the data confidentiality standards and had informed consent documents verbally translated by a native Ethiopian translator fluent in English and Amharic. For the women unable to write, an ink-stained fingerprint was used to indicate their agreement to the informed consent document in place of a signature. An identification number was given to every participant and collected data were anonymized in order to ensure confidentiality. Completed questionnaires were kept at all times by the collaborators from the University of Valencia in secure conditions (locked box) and are now stored under lock and key at the University of Valencia.

2.5. Measurement

The aim of the questionnaire was to collect data on if the mothers received antenatal care and/or infant nutritional guidance during pregnancy and to determine their infant feeding practices in the first three days postpartum. The data collection questionnaire used comprised three main sections. The first section included general personal and sociodemographic characteristics of the mothers such as their age, level of education, number of live children and delivery problems. The second section collected data specifically related to infant feeding practices, such as supplementary feeding, to understand when the child started to receive foods different from human milk and what kind of foods they received. The absence of a free-access hospital or conventional health care center in the area impeded the collection of any sort of official medical history. The third section of the questionnaire focused on the living conditions of the women such as building materials utilized for the construction of the home, sanitary conditions and the availability of drinking water. The overcrowding rate was calculated by dividing the square meters of the home by the number of people living in it. In this study, the outcome variable was the practice of colostrum avoidance among mothers of children aged less than two years old. The independent variables included the mother's characteristics, household characteristics and child's sex. Mothers were divided into two groups depending on their colostrum avoidance status. Women who avoided feeding colostrum to their infant formed the avoidance group, and the non-avoidance group was composed of the women who fed colostrum to their infant.

2.6. Data Analysis

After the quantitative data on the printed questionnaire form were completed and checked for consistency, the data were scrubbed, coded and entered into IBM SPSS Statistics (Version 26). Qualitative data were transcribed into English text. The data analysis, according to the project objective, was performed using a key question from the interview regarding colostrum avoidance at the initiation of breastfeeding. Frequencies and percentages were used to describe the prevalence of colostrum avoidance. Categorical variables were described with frequency and percentages, and the comparison among the groups, according to colostrum avoidance, was performed using Pearson's chi-square test with Yates's correction. Fisher's exact test was used when the expected count was less than 5. Continuous variables were described as means and standard deviation (SDs), after which normality was evaluated with the Kolmogorov–Smirnov test. An independent sample t-test was used to compare the groups. Crude odds ratios (ORs) were reported with 95% confidence interval (95% CI). Variables at p-value < 0.05 in the analysis were concluded as factors associated with colostrum avoidance.

3. Results

3.1. Characteristics of the Sample

The prevalence of colostrum avoidance was 56.1% (n = 64). The approximate age of the participants ranged from 18 to 45 years with a mean of 25.3 ± 5.0 years old. The mean in the avoidance group was 27.3 ± 6.6 years old, and the mean in the non-avoidance group was 27.4 ± 6.4 years old, with no significant differences (p = 0.870) between the groups. A general description of the participants is shown in Table 1.

Overall, 78.1% of the participants interviewed were illiterate and 7.0% had a secondary education. Among illiterate participants, 57.3% avoided colostrum, while the avoidance rate in literate participants was 52.0%. While the COR is higher for the illiterate participants than for those able to read and write, the sample is small and lacks the power to make any definitive conclusions regarding education. In addition, if the sample is collapsed into literate and illiterate groups, then the result does not differ based on education level. Significant differences were observed among the groups (p = 0.001) for parity. Most of the participants in the study were multiparous, and women who had more than one child more frequently avoided colostrum than participants who had one child, which was confirmed with a crude odds ratio (COR) > 1. The mean number of children was 3.5 ± 0.7 (3.9 ± 2.0

in the avoidance group and 4.0 ± 1.8 in the non-avoidance group). Overall, 84.2% of the participants were still breastfeeding their children, while 15.8% of the participants interviewed had stopped breastfeeding. No significant differences were observed among the groups. The only participants to follow WHO recommendations on the initiation of breastfeeding were in the avoidance group.

Table 1. Characteristics of mothers of children aged less than 24 months in a rural area of Ethiopia.

| Variable | Total ($n = 114$) | | Colostrum Avoidance | | | | p * | Crude Odds Ratio (95% CI) | p * |
| | | | Avoidance [1] ($n = 64$) | | Non-Avoidance [2] ($n = 50$) | | | | |
	n (%) **	95% CI	n (%) **	95% CI	n (%) **	95% CI			
Educational level									
Secondary school	8 (7.0%)	(3.30, 13.78)	1 (1.56%)	(0.1, 9.5)	7 (14.0%)	(6.3, 27.4)	0.121	1	-
Able to read and write	17 (14.9%)	(9.17, 23.08)	12 (18.8%)	(10.5, 30.8)	5 (10.0%)	(3.7, 22.6)		16.80 (1.62, 174.53)	0.022
Illiterate	89 (78.1%)	(69.15, 85.05)	51 (79.7%)	(67.4, 88.3)	38 (76.0%)	(62.8, 86.3)		9.39 (1.11, 79.61)	0.039
Parity									
Multiparous	85 (74.6%)	(65.36, 82.05)	45 (70.3%)	(57.4, 80.8)	40 (80.0%)	(65.9, 89.5)	0.001	1	
Primiparous	29 (24.5%)	(17.95, 34.61)	19 (29.7%)	(19.2, 42.6)	10 (20.0%)	(10.5, 34.1)		1.69 (0.70, 4.06)	0.336
Breastfeeding									
Still breastfeeding	96 (84.2%)	(75.92, 90.12)	50 (78.1%)	(65.7, 87.1)	46 (92.0%)	(79.9, 97.4)	0.292	1	-
Not breastfeeding	18 (15.8%)	(9.87, 24.07)	14 (21.9%)	(12.9, 34.3)	4 (8.0%)	(2.6, 20.1)	-	3.22 (0.99, 10.49)	0.079
Breastfeeding initiation time									
<1 h	3 (2.6%)	(0.68, 8.07)	3 (4.7%)	(1.2, 14.0)	0 (0.0%)	(0.00, 8.9)	-	-	-
>1 h	111 (97.4%)	(91.9, 99.3)	61 (95.3%)	(86.0, 98.8)	50 (100.0%)	(91.1, 100.0)	-	-	-

[1] Women who rejected colostrum in their lactation and practiced prelacteal feeding. [2] Women who did not reject colostrum during lactation and did not practice prelacteal feeding. * p value < 0.05 considered statistically significant. p value calculated using ANOVA or Chi-squared test. ** % by column.

3.2. Living Conditions

Table 2 presents the living conditions of the participants and their families who took part in the study. The quality of the flooring material was significantly different between the groups with most participants in the avoidance group stating that the flooring consisted of soil, while the value was lower but still constituted the majority for the non-avoidance group. Additionally, significant differences between the groups regarding the number of animals in the home were not found.

In both villages, more than 90% of the participants in the study were living in the traditional Ethiopian thatched-roof hut typical of the rural areas called 'tukul', in which any type of available wood, commonly eucalyptus planks, is used for wall construction and for the conical-shaped roof support and the floor of the house is plain earth. The mean number of people living in the house was 5.0 ± 1.9 (4.9 ± 0.9 in the avoidance group and 5.1 ± 1.8 in the non-avoidance group ($p = 0.527$)), while the square footage of the house was 15.5 ± 5.4 m^2 (16.6 ± 6.0 m^2 in the avoidance group and 14.0 ± 4.4 m^2 in the non-avoidance group ($p = 0.158$)). From the data collected, we estimated an average of 3.4 ± 1.4 m^2 (3.9 ± 1.6 m^2 in the avoidance group and 2.9 ± 0.8 m^2 in the non-avoidance group ($p = 0.001$)) of floor area per person, while the WHO literature suggests 9–10 m^2 of floor area per person. No differences were found in regard to toilet facility, the type of animal inside the house or main source of drinking water.

Table 2. Living conditions of the families who took part in the study.

Variable	Total (n = 114)		Colostrum Avoidance				p *	Crude Odds Ratio (95% CI)	p *
			Avoidance [1] (n = 64)		Non-Avoidance [2] (n = 50)				
	n (%) **	95% CI	n (%) **	95% CI	n (%) **	95% CI			
Flooring material of the house									
Soil	90 (81.8%)	(73.1, 88.3)	56 (88.9%)	(77.8, 95.0)	34 (72.3%)	(57.1, 83.9)	0.005	1	-
Cement	7 (6.4%)	(2.8, 13.1)	5 (7.9%)	(3.0, 18.3)	2 (4.3%)	(0.7, 15.7)		1.52 (0.28, 8.26)	0.231
Mud	13 (11.8%)	(6.7, 19.7)	2 (3.2%)	(0.6, 12.0)	11 (23.4%)	(12.8, 38.4)		0.11 (0.02, 0.53)	0.004
Toilet facility									
Pit latrine	85 (78.0%)	(68.8, 85.1)	48 (76.2%)	(63.5, 85.6)	37 (80.4%)	(65.6, 90.1)	0.297	1	-
No Facilities	24 (22.0%)	(14.9, 31.2)	15 (23.8%)	(14.4, 36.5)	9 (19.6%)	(9.9, 34.4)		1.28 (0.51, 3.26)	0.768
Animals inside the house									
Yes	33 (30%)	(21.8, 39.6)	19 (30.2%)	(19.6, 43.2)	14 (29.8%)	(17.8, 45.1)	0.002	1	-
No	77 (70%)	(60.4, 78.2)	44 (69.8%)	(56.8, 80.4)	33 (70.2%)	(54.9, 82.2)		1.02 (0.45, 2.32)	0.866
Number of people living in the house									
<4	58 (50.9%)	(41.4, 60.3)	33 (51.6%)	(38.8, 64.1)	25 (50.0%)	(35.7, 64.3)		1	-
4–8	48 (42.1%)	(33.0, 51.7)	27 (42.2%)	(30.2, 55.2)	21 (42.0%)	(28.5, 56.7)		0.97 (0.45, 2.11)	0.610
>8	8 (7.0%)	(3.3, 13.8)	4 (6.3%)	(2.0, 16.0)	4 (8.0%)	(2.6, 20.1)		0.76 (0.17, 3.33)	0.511
m² of the house									
<10	24 (21.1%)	(14.2, 29.9)	9 (14.1%)	(7.0, 25.5)	15 (30.0%)	(18.3, 44.8)		2.62 (1.03, 6.63)	0.041
>10	90 (78.9%)	(70.1, 85.8)	55 (85.9%)	(74.5, 93.0)	35 (70.0%)	(55.2, 81.7)		1	-
Overcrowding rate [3]									
<3	57 (50.0%)	(40.5, 59.5)	32 (50.0%)	(37.4, 62.6)	25 (50.0%)	(35.7, 64.3)		1.21 (0.58, 2.56)	0.401
>3	57 (50.0%)	(40.5, 59.5)	32 (50.0%)	(37.4, 62.6)	25 (50.0%)	(35.7, 64.3)		1	-
Kind of animals								0.534	
Chickens	19 (55.9%)	(38.1, 72.4)	11 (57.9%)	(33.9, 78.9)	8 (53.3%)	(27.4, 77,7)		1	-
Goats	2 (5.9%)	(1.0, 21.1)	1 (5.3%)	(0.3, 28.1)	1 (6.7%)	(0.3, 34.0)		0.73 (0.04, 13.45)	0.591
Cats	2 (5.9%)	(1.0, 21.1)	1 (5.3%)	(0.3, 28.1)	1 (6.7%)	(0.3, 34.0)		0.73 (0.04, 13.45)	0.591
Others	11 (32.4.0%)	(18.0, 50.6)	6 (31.6%)	(13.6, 56.5)	5 (33.3%)	(13.0, 61.3)		0.87 (0.20, 3.90)	0.838
Main source of drinking water									
Covered well	60 (54.5%)	(44.8, 64.0)	33 (54.1%)	(40.9, 66.7)	27 (55.1%)	(40.3, 69.1)	0.667	1	-
Open well	1 (0.9%)	(0.1, 5.7)	1 (1.6%)	(0.1, 10.0)	0 (0.0%)	(0.00, 9.1)		-	-
River	49 (44.5)	(35.2, 54.3)	27 (44.3%)	(31.8, 57.5)	22 (44.9%)	(30.9, 59.7)		1.00 (0.47, 2.14)	0.855

[1] Women who rejected colostrum in their lactation and practiced prelacteal feeding. [2] Women who did not reject colostrum during lactation and did not practice prelacteal feeding. [3] Overcrowding rate: m² of the house/number of people living in the house. * p value < 0.05 considered statistically significant. p value calculated using ANOVA or Chi-squared test. ** % by column.

3.3. Antenatal Care

The information collected on the health care received during pregnancy and delivery is shown in Table 3.

Table 3. Health care that the women interviewed received during pregnancy and information about delivery.

Variable	Total (n = 114)		Colostrum Avoidance				p *	Crude Odds Ratio (95% CI)	p *
			Avoidance [1] (n = 64)		Non-Avoidance [2] (n = 50)				
	n (%) **	95% CI	n (%) **	95% CI	n (%) **	95% CI			
Antenatal care									
Yes	70 (61.4%)	(51.8, 70.2)	36 (56.3%)	(43.3, 68.4)	34 (68.0%)	(53.2, 80.1)	0.635	1	-
No	44 (38.6%)	(29.8, 48.2)	28 (43.8%)	(31.6, 56,7)	16 (32.0%)	(19.9, 46.8)		1.65 (0.76, 3.58)	0.278
Delivery mode									
Caesarean section	7 (6.1%)	(2.71, 12.70)	4 (6.3%)	(2.0, 16.0)	3 (6.0%)	(1.6, 17.5)	0.003	1	-
Vaginal	107 (93.9%)	(87.31, 97.28)	60 (93.8%)	(84.0, 98.0)	47 (94,0%)	(82.5, 98.4)		0.96 (0.20, 4.29)	0.735
Delivery place									
Government hospital	18 (15.8%)	(9.87, 24.08)	9 (14.1%)	(7.0, 25.5)	9 (18.0%)	(9.0, 31.9)	0.060	1	-
Government health center	30 (26.3%)	(18.72, 35.54)	12 (18.8%)	(10.5, 30.8)	18 (36.0%)	(23.3, 50.9)		0.67 (0.21, 2.16)	0.988
Own home	66 (57.9%)	(48.28, 66.97)	43 (67.2%)	(54.2, 78.1)	23 (46.0%)	(32.1, 60.5)		1.87 (0.65, 5.36)	0.368

Table 3. Cont.

	Colostrum Avoidance								
Variable	Total (n = 114)		Avoidance [1] (n = 64)		Non-Avoidance [2] (n = 50)		p *	Crude Odds Ratio (95% CI)	p *
	n (%) **	95% CI	n (%) **	95% CI	n (%) **	95% CI			
Delivery attendance									
Health professional	48 (42.1%)	(33.03, 51.72)	21 (32.8%)	(21.9, 45.8)	27 (54.0%)	(39.4, 64.9)	0.001	1	-
Trained traditional birth attendant	6 (5.3%)	(2.16, 11.57)	0 (0.0%)	(0.00, 7.1)	6 (12.0%)	(5.0, 25.0)	-	-	-
Relatives	56 (49.1%)	(39.70, 58.60)	42 (65.6%)	(52.6, 76.8)	14 (28.0%)	(16.7, 42.7)		3.86 (1.68, 8.86)	0.002
Nobody	4 (3.5%)	(1.13, 9.27)	1 (1.6%)	(0.1, 9.5)	3 (6.0%)	(1.6, 17.5)		0.43 (0.04, 4.42)	0.839
Diet supplementation during pregnancy or breastfeeding									
Yes	7 (6.2%)	(2.74, 12.80)	3 (4.7%)	(1.2, 14.0)	4 (8.2%)	(2.6, 20.5)	0.577	1	-
No	106 (93.8%)	(87.20, 97.26)	61 (95.3%)	(86.0, 98.8)	45 (91.8%)	(79.5, 97.4)		1.81 (0.39, 8.48)	0.714

[1] Women who rejected colostrum in their lactation and practiced prelacteal feeding. [2] Women who did not reject colostrum during lactation and did not practice prelacteal feeding. * p value < 0.05 considered statistically significant. p value calculated using ANOVA or Chi-squared test. ** % by column.

More than half of all the participants received antenatal care during pregnancy. The percentage of participants who did not receive antenatal was higher in the avoidance group than in the non-avoidance group without a significant difference. Significant differences were observed for the mode of delivery and the delivery attendants. The participants who practice colostrum avoidance were more likely to have caesarean births and be attended by relatives. Around 7/10 of the participants who practice colostrum avoidance gave birth at home, while the percentage of home deliveries decreased, but not significantly, in the non-avoidance group. No differences were observed in diet supplementation.

3.4. Infant Feeding Practices and Beliefs

The main findings of the study regarding the participants' knowledge and attitudes about infant feeding practices are shown in Tables 4 and 5.

Table 4. Breastfeeding practices and beliefs.

	Colostrum Avoidance								
Variable	Total (n = 114)		Avoidance [1] (n = 64)		Non-Avoidance [2] (n = 50)		p *	Crude Odds Ratio (95% CI)	p *
	n (%) **	95% CI	n (%) **	95% CI	n (%) **	95% CI			
What does the woman think about colostrum?									
It is important	12 (10.5%)	(5.8, 18.0)	3 (4.7%)	(1.2, 14.0)	9 (18.0%)	(9.0, 31.9)	0.001	1	-
It stimulates milk production	5 (4.4%)	(1.6, 10.4)	0 (0.0%)	(0.0, 7.1)	5 (10.0%)	(3.7, 22.6)		-	-
It is not sufficient	7 (6.1%)	(2.7, 12.7)	4 (6.3%)	(2.0, 16.0)	3 (6.0%)	(1.6, 17.5)		4.00 (0.55, 29.18)	0.364
It is dirty and dangerous	74 (64.9%)	(55.4, 73.5)	51 (79.7%)	(67.4, 88.3)	23 (46.0%)	(32.1, 60.5)		6.65 (1.65, 26.88)	0.009
No idea	16 (14.0%)	(8.5, 22.1)	6 (9.4%)	(3.9, 19.9)	10 (20.0%)	(10.5, 34.1)		1.80 (0.34, 9.40)	0.770
Does the woman think colostrum should be discarded?									
Disagree	23 (20.0%)	(13.6, 29.1)	6 (9.4%)	(3.9, 19.9)	17 (34.7%)	(22.1, 49.7)	0.001	1	-
Agree	83 (73.0%)	(64.7, 81.1)	55 (85.9%)	(74.5, 93.0)	28 (57.1%)	(42.3, 70.9)		5.57 (1.98, 15.68)	0.001
No idea	7 (6.0%)	(2.7, 12.8)	3 (4.7%)	(1.2, 14.0)	4 (8.2%)	(2.7, 20.5)		2.13 (0.36, 12.39)	0.706

[1] Women who rejected colostrum in their lactation and practiced prelacteal feeding. [2] Women who did not reject colostrum during lactation and did not practice prelacteal feeding. * p value < 0.05 considered statistically significant. p value calculated using ANOVA or Chi-squared test. ** % by column.

Table 5. Infant feeding knowledge and practices.

Variable	Total ($n = 114$)		Colostrum Avoidance				p *	Crude Odds Ratio (95% CI)	p *
			Avoidance [1] ($n = 64$)		Non-Avoidance [2] ($n = 50$)				
	n (%) **	95% CI	n (%) **	95% CI	n (%) **	95% CI			
Did the woman receive information about infant feeding?									
About breastfeeding only	38 (33.3%)	(25.0, 42.9)	16 (25.0%)	(15.4, 37.7)	22 (44.0%)	(30.3, 58.7)		1	-
About suppl. feeding	3 (2.6%)	(0.7, 8.1)	1 (1.6%)	(0.1, 9.5)	2 (4.0%)	(0.7 14.9)	0.102	0.69 (0.06, 8.25)	0.755
No information	72 (63.2%)	(53.6, 71.9)	46 (71.9%)	(59.0, 82.1)	26 (52.0%)	(37.6 66.1)		2.43 (1.09, 5.43)	0.047
Information on other feeding practices	1 (0.9%)	(0.1, 5.5)	1 (1.6%)	(0.1, 9.5)	0 (0.0%)	(0.00, 9.0)		-	-
What was the main food that the child received during the first six months after birth?									
Breast milk	100 (87.8%)	(93.8, 99.9)	56 (98.2%)	(89.4, 99.9)	44 (100.0%)	(90.0, 100.0)	0.677	1	-
Other food	1 (0.99%)	(0.1, 6.2)	1 (1.8%)	(0.1, 10.6)	0 (0.0%)	(0.0, 10.0)		-	-
When did/will the woman start supplementary feeding?									
2 months	1 (0.9%)	(0.0, 5.5)	0 (0.0%)	(0.0,7.1)	1 (2.0%)	(0.1, 12.0)		0.42 (0.04, 4.82) ***	0.014
5 months	2 (1.8%)	(0.3, 6.8)	1 (1.6%)	(0.1, 9.5)	1 (2.0%)	(0.1, 12.0)			
6 months	96 (84.2%)	(75.9, 90.1)	52 (81.3%)	(69.2, 89.5)	44 (88.0%)	(75.0, 95.0)	0.302	1	-
7 months	12 (10.5%)	(5.8, 18.0)	9 (14.1%)	(7.0, 25.5)	3 (6.0%)	(1.6, 17.5)		2.33 (0.69, 7.82) ****	0.704
8 months	1 (0.9%)	(0.0, 5.5)	0 (0.0%)	(0.0,7.1)	1 (2.0%)	(1.6, 17.5)			
9 months	2 (1.8%)	(0.3, 6.8)	2 (3.1%)	(0.5, 11.8)	0 (0.0%)	(0.00, 8.9)			
What was the first food the child received/will receive?									
Enjera	30 (29.4%)	(21.0, 39.4)	17 (27.0%)	(17.0, 39.9)	13 (33.3%)	(19.6, 50.3)		1	-
Shiro	15 (14.7%)	(8.7, 23.4)	9 (14.3%)	(7.1, 25.9)	6 (15.4%)	(6.4, 31.2)		1.15 (0.33, 4.05)	0.915
Faffa	6 (5.9%)	(2.4, 12.9)	6 (9.5%)	(3.9, 20.3)	0 (0.0%)	(0.0, 11.2)		-	-
Whatever the mother eats	9 (8.8%)	(4.4, 16.5)	7 (11.1%)	(5.0, 22.1)	2 (5.1%)	(0.9, 18.6)	0.299	2.68 (0.47, 15.09)	0.452
Porridge	24 (23.5%)	(15.9, 33.2)	13 (20.6%)	(11.9, 33.0)	11 (28.2%)	(15.5, 45.1)		0.90 (0.31, 2.66)	0.927
Genfo	11 (10.8%)	(5.8, 18.9)	8 (12.7%)	(6.0, 24.0)	3 (7.7%)	(2.0, 22.0)		2.04 (0.45, 9.24)	0.567
Other foods	7 (6.9%)	(3.0, 14.1)	3 (4.8%)	(1.2, 14.2)	4 (10.3%)	(3.3, 25.2)		0.57 (0.11, 3.02)	0.811

[1] Women who rejected colostrum in their lactation and practiced prelacteal feeding. [2] Women who did not reject colostrum during lactation and did not practice prelacteal feeding. * p value < 0.05 considered statistically significant. p value calculated using ANOVA or Chi-squared test. ** % by column. *** Crude odds ratio (95% CI) for < 6 months. **** Crude odds ratio (95% CI) for >6 months.

Significant differences were observed among the groups in regard to breastfeeding beliefs but not for infant feeding practices. The percentage of participants who did not discard colostrum that said that colostrum stimulates milk production or that it is important for the infant was less than 30%, while less than 5% of those that did discard colostrum agreed with this statement. Among those that discarded colostrum, around 80% thought that colostrum was dirty and could be dangerous for the newborn. These beliefs are significantly associated with avoiding colostrum (COR = 6.65). The participants in this study declared that, during the first days after giving birth, they would wet their breast with hot water and manually massage it in order to extract the colostrum, which they would then discard. However, none of them could explain the reason for this practice; it was simply understood as traditional. The large percentage of participants who did not receive information about infant feeding during pregnancy learned how to feed their infants from popular traditions handed down from mother to daughter, and this characteristic makes these women have a significantly (COR = 2.43) higher probability of avoiding colostrum. This probability was similarly high in the participants who directly agreed with colostrum avoidance (COR = 5.27) or stated to not have an opinion (COR = 2.13). In general, a third of participants stated that they fed their infants with only human milk during the first three days after birth; within them, a quarter of the avoidance group had received information about breastfeeding, while in the non-avoidance group, the percentage was almost double. Of the 114 participants who answered and had children aged more than 6 months, almost all said that human milk was the main food that the infants received during the first 6 months of life. The results show that the majority of the participants started supplementary feeding at six months. The most commonly added foods to a child's diet were 'injera', 'shiro' and 'genfo'.

4. Discussion

This study revealed that the prevalence of colostrum avoidance was higher than that described by one study conducted in an urban area of Ethiopia, which reported an avoidance of 6.3% [22], and that described by studies performed in other different areas of Ethiopia, including Raya Kobo (13.5%) [23], Amibara (36.9%) [24], Goba Woreda (35.0%) [25], and rural northern Ethiopia (63%) [12]. Due to inaccessible health care, many of the mothers in our study did not receive adequate prenatal care and gave birth at home. In Andode, there is no hospital, only a health post without a pharmacy. The nearest hospital and pharmacy are 70 km away. While there is a small hospital in Muke Turi, it does not have the capability to treat any serious medical situation, and those requiring more specialized care must travel to Addis Ababa 80 km away. Additionally, health care is costly, and the majority of the women do not have insurance and are unable to cover the associated cost. In an emergency or a life or death case, the MCSPA will cover the health care cost, but antenatal care must be paid for by the women.

A lack of prenatal care contributes to inadequate breastfeeding education and reliance on maternally transmitted, traditional infant feeding beliefs and practices. Maternal education and antenatal care have been shown to be connected to the early initiation of breastfeeding (EIBF) and exclusive breastfeeding (EBF) rates [24,26–41]. Therefore, appropriate antenatal care that includes a maternal education component on adequate breastfeeding practices may help improve rates of EIBF and EBF. Given the structure of health care in Ethiopia and the difficulty of accessing it for some of its citizens, the use of health extension workers is recommended [42]. The rate of EBF in Ethiopia is significantly under the global recommendations [42]. There are recent scientific publications from Ethiopia regarding breastfeeding practices and their associated factors available that could be used as a basis for the design of interventions geared towards improving EIBF and EBF rates [41,43]. The advantages of EIBF for both mother and infant [44], such as lower neonatal mortality [45,46], have been clearly proven. It is difficult to establish a national rate of EIBF in Ethiopia as previous studies have shown results ranging from 40% to over 80% [24,26–36]. However, the results of this study in a rural area are in line with those of previous studies, which have shown lower EIBF rates in women from rural areas compared to women from urban centers [24,29,30,35,47].

Colostrum avoidance is a common practice in Ethiopia [12,22,23,48]; however, studies [49,50] have shown varying degrees of avoidance with different regions of the country presenting rates as high as 77% or as low as 11%. Colostrum avoidance (56.14%) in this study was higher than the estimated national Ethiopian average (39.8%) [51] and that found in more developed areas of the country [22,52]. This difference in incidence is significantly associated (COR = 9.39) with a low level of education in the same areas, where 78.1% were illiterate. The participating women stated that they would actively discard colostrum by wetting their breast with hot water and pumping in the days immediately after giving birth. When asked to explain the reasoning behind this practice, they stated they followed this practice because they believed colostrum to be dirty and dangerous for the newborn or to be insufficient for the newborn because it is too similar to water.

A systematic review and meta-analysis calculated the pooled prevalence of prelacteal feeding in Ethiopia at 25.29% with severe heterogeneity [53]. This traditional practice delays the initiation of breastfeeding and can affect the future success of breastfeeding [12,48,54,55]. This practice is more common in rural areas than in urban areas due to the lack of education regarding infant feeding and the lack of health care centers, which leads to high rates of homebirths [12,41,53,56]. The newborn intestinal tract is more permeable and vulnerable to pathogens, which may be carried in prelacteal foods [56]. This can lead to a microbial load too high to handle for the immature immune system of the infant, a situation made worse due to colostrum avoidance. Colostrum, the perfect food for a newborn to receive after birth, is essential to compensate for the immunological immaturity of the newborn intestinal tract, is low in fat [57,58] and improves the gut microbiome of the newborn [59,60].

This study has certain limitations that must be taken into consideration. The cross-sectional design has some inherent limitations regarding the nature of the association between the different factors and colostrum avoidance. While factors associated with colostrum avoidance can be determined, the nature of the relationship of these factors and the practice of colostrum avoidance cannot be established. This is the first scientific study carried out in these particular areas regarding breastfeeding practices. The questionnaire administered during the face-to-face interviews was not pre-tested and had to be adapted in situ due to limitations regarding date availability. One of the main limitations related to data availability was the fact that most of the women did not become aware of their pregnancy until the third/fourth month, and no official medical histories were available for review. The information obtained from mothers might be subject to recall bias. The sample size is also a limitation. This limitation arises mainly due to the limited time that the research team was permitted to stay in either village, the travel time between locations and the length of the interviews, which needed simultaneous translation.

5. Conclusions

This study allows us to identify that mothers are not well educated about correct infant feeding practices and that colostrum avoidance is still widely practiced in this rural region at a higher rate than found in previous studies carried out in other parts of Ethiopia. A low level of education and limited health care are the main factors for colostrum avoidance. Education and quality health care are central for development at every level. Education is an essential tool for improving living conditions, reducing poverty and building a food-secure world. Adequate infant feeding information and care from health professionals during and after pregnancy is still a luxury in these rural areas that most women will not be able to access. An intervention aimed at improving access to nutritional education and health care could help reduce the prevalence of colostrum avoidance in a sustainable way that could lead to improved overall infant and community health and development.

Author Contributions: Conceptualization, methodology, formal analysis and investigation, M.A.O.S., R.R., A.L.-G., I.P.-C., J.M.S. and M.M.-S.-V.; data curation and writing—original draft preparation, M.A.O.S., A.L.-G., I.P.-C. and M.M.-S.-V.; writing—review and editing, J.M.S. All authors have read and agreed to the published version of the manuscript.

Funding: This research received no external funding.

Institutional Review Board Statement: The study was conducted in accordance with the Declaration of Helsinki and approved by the Ethics Committee of the University of Valencia (Spain) (protocol and register code: 1256147; date of approval: 16 June 2020).

Informed Consent Statement: Informed consent was obtained from all subjects involved in the study. Written informed consent has been obtained from the patient to publish this paper.

Data Availability Statement: The data are not publicly available due to ethical and privacy restrictions.

Acknowledgments: The authors wish to thank The Missionary Community of Saint Paul the Apostle (MCSPA) for hosting and helping during data collection as well as all the participating women.

Conflicts of Interest: The authors declare no conflict of interest.

References

1. Hossain, S.; Mihrshahi, S. Exclusive breastfeeding and childhood morbidity: A narrative review. *Int. J. Environ. Res. Public Health.* **2022**, *19*, 14804. [CrossRef] [PubMed]
2. World Health Organization. *Definition of Skilled Health Personnel Providing Care during Childbirth: The 2018 Joint Statement by WHO, UNFPA, UNICEF, ICM, ICN, FIGO and IPA (No. WHO/RHR/18.14)*; World Health Organization: Geneva, Switzerland, 2018.
3. Abdulahi, M.; Fretheim, A.; Argaw, A.; Magnus, J.H. Breastfeeding education and support to improve early initiation and exclusive breastfeeding practices and infant growth: A cluster randomized controlled trial from a rural Ethiopian setting. *Nutrients* **2021**, *13*, 1204. [CrossRef] [PubMed]
4. Rodriguez-Gallego, I.; Leon-Larios, F.; Corrales-Gutierrez, I.; Gonzalez-Sanz, J.D. Impact and effectiveness of group strategies for supporting breastfeeding after birth: A systematic review. *Int. J. Environ. Res. Public Health.* **2021**, *18*, 2550. [CrossRef] [PubMed]

5. Liben, M. *Colostrum: The Golden Milk for Infants' Health*; Juniper Publishers: Simi Valley, CA, USA, 2017.
6. Das, J.K.; Salam, R.A.; Saeed, M.; Kazmi, F.A.; Bhutta, Z.A. Effectiveness of interventions for managing acute malnutrition in children under five years of age in low-income and middle-income countries: A systematic review and meta-analysis. *Nutrients* **2020**, *12*, 116. [CrossRef] [PubMed]
7. Lyons, K.E.; Ryan, C.A.; Dempsey, E.M.; Ross, R.P.; Stanton, C. Breast milk, a source of beneficial microbes and associated benefits for infant health. *Nutrients* **2020**, *12*, 1039. [CrossRef]
8. Beghetti, I.; Biagi, E.; Martini, S.; Brigidi, P.; Corvaglia, L.; Aceti, A. Human milk's hidden gift: Implications of the milk microbiome for preterm infants' health. *Nutrients* **2019**, *11*, 2944. [CrossRef]
9. Biset, G.; Dagnaw, K.; Abebaw, N. A systematic review and meta-analysis of colostrum avoidance practice among breastfeeding mothers in Ethiopia, December 2021. *J. Neonatal Nurs.* **2022**, *29*, 33–42. [CrossRef]
10. Ayalew, T.; Asmare, E. Colostrum avoidance practice among primipara mothers in urban Northwest Ethiopia. A cross-sectional study. *BMC Pregnancy Childbirth.* **2021**, *21*, 123. [CrossRef]
11. Alemu, S.M.; Alemu, Y.M.; Habtewold, T.D. Association of age and colostrum discarding with breast-feeding practice in Ethiopia: Systematic review and meta-analyses. *Public Health Nutr.* **2019**, *22*, 2063–2082. [CrossRef]
12. Rogers, N.L.; Abdi, J.; Moore, D.; Nd'iangui, S.; Smith, L.J.; Carlson, A.J.; Carlson, D. Colostrum avoidance, prelacteal feeding and late breast-feeding initiation in rural northern Ethiopia. *Public Health Nutr.* **2011**, *14*, 2029–2036. [CrossRef]
13. Ghosh, S.; Suri, D.; Hiko, D.; Fentahun, N.; Griffiths, J.K. *Factors Associated with Stunting in Ethiopian Children under Five*; Save the Children: Addis Ababa, Ethiopia, 2014.
14. Olcina Simón, M.A.; Soriano, J.M.; Morales-Suarez-Varela, M. Assessment of malnutrition among children presenting in a Nutrition Center in Gimbichu, Ethiopia. *Children* **2023**, *10*, 627. [CrossRef]
15. World Medical Association. WMA Declaration of Helsinki—Ethical Principles for Medical Research Involving Human Subjects. Available online: https://www.wma.net/policies-post/wma-declaration-of-helsinkiethical-principles-for-medical-research-involving-human-subjects (accessed on 12 April 2023).
16. U.S. National Bioethics Advisory Commission. Ethical and Policy Issues Research: Clinical Trials in Developing Countries. Available online: http://bioethics.georgetown.edu/nbac/clinical/Vol1.pdf (accessed on 12 April 2023).
17. European Commission. EU Directive 2001/20/EC. *Off. J. Eur. Communities* **2001**, *121*, 34–44.
18. Office for Human Research Protections (OHRP); Office of the Assistant Secretary for Health (OASH); U.S. Department of Health and Human Services (HHS). International Compilation of Human Research Standards. Available online: https://www.hhs.gov/sites/default/files/ohrp-international-compilation-2021-africa.pdf (accessed on 12 April 2023).
19. Vandenbroucke, J.P.; Von Elm, E.; Altman, D.G.; Gøtzsche, P.C.; Mulrow, C.D.; Pocock, S.J.; Poole, C.; Schlesselman, J.J.; Egger, M. Strobe Initiative. Strengthening the reporting of observational studies in epidemiology (STROBE): Explanation and elaboration. *Ann. Intern. Med.* **2007**, *147*, 163–194. [CrossRef]
20. The Missionary Community of Saint Paul the Apostle. Available online: https://mcspa.org (accessed on 12 April 2023).
21. Olcina Simón, M.A.; Morales-Suarez-Varela, M.; San Onofre, N.; Soriano, J.M. Approach to Development Cooperation 3.0: From the statutes to the praxis in a NGDO. *Int. J. Eng. Res. Technol.* **2023**, *12*, 81–88.
22. Weldesamuel, G.T.; Atalay, H.T.; Zemichael, T.M.; Gebre, H.G.; Abraha, D.G.; Amare, A.K.; Gidey, E.B.; Alemayoh, T.T. Colostrum avoidance and associated factors among mothers having children less than 2 years of age in Aksum town, Tigray, Ethiopia: A cross-sectional study 2017. *BMC Res. Notes* **2018**, *11*, 7. [CrossRef]
23. Legesse, M.; Demena, M.; Mesfin, F.; Haile, D. Factors associated with colostrum avoidance among mothers of children aged less than 24 months in Raya Kobo district, north-eastern Ethiopia: Community-based cross-sectional study. *J. Trop. Pediatr.* **2015**, *61*, 357–363. [CrossRef]
24. Liben, M.L.; Yesuf, E.M. Determinants of early initiation of breastfeeding in Amibara district, northeastern Ethiopia: A community based cross-sectional study. *Int. Breastfeed. J.* **2016**, *11*, 7. [CrossRef]
25. Setegn, T.; Gerbaba, M.; Belachew, T. Determinants of timely initiation of breastfeeding among mothers in Goba Woreda, south east Ethiopia: A cross sectional study. *BMC Public Health* **2011**, *11*, 217. [CrossRef]
26. Habtewold, T.D.; Mohammed, S.H.; Endalamaw, A.; Mulugeta, H.; Dessie, G.; Berhe, D.F.; Birhanu, M.M.; Islam, M.A.; Teferra, A.A.; Asefa, N.G.; et al. Higher educational and economic status are key factors for the timely initiation of breastfeeding in Ethiopia: A review and meta-analysis. *Acta Paediatr.* **2020**, *109*, 2208–2218. [CrossRef]
27. John, J.R.; Mistry, S.K.; Kebede, G.; Manohar, N.; Arora, A. Determinants of early initiation of breastfeeding in Ethiopia: A population-based study using the 2016 demographic and health survey data. *BMC Pregnancy Childbirth* **2019**, *19*, 69. [CrossRef]
28. Tariku, A.; Biks, G.A.; Wassie, M.M.; Worku, A.G.; Yenit, M.K. Only half of the mothers practiced early initiation of breastfeeding in northwest Ethiopia, 2015. *BMC Res. Notes* **2017**, *10*, 501. [CrossRef] [PubMed]
29. Lakew, Y.; Tabar, L.; Haile, D. Socio-medical determinants of timely breastfeeding initiation in Ethiopia: Evidence from the 2011 nationwide demographic and health survey. *Int. Breastfeed. J.* **2015**, *10*, 24. [CrossRef] [PubMed]
30. Alebel, A.; Dejenu, G.; Mullu, G.; Abebe, N.; Gualu, T.; Eshetie, S. Timely initiation of breastfeeding and its association with birth place in Ethiopia: A systematic review and meta-analysis. *Int. Breastfeed. J.* **2017**, *12*, 44. [CrossRef] [PubMed]
31. Belachew, A. Timely initiation of breastfeeding and associated factors among mothers of infants age 0-6 months old in Bahir Dar city, northwest, Ethiopia, 2017: A community based cross-sectional study. *Int. Breastfeed. J.* **2019**, *14*, 5. [CrossRef]

32. Ayalew, T.; Tewabe, T.; Ayalew, Y. Timely initiation of breastfeeding among first time mothers in Bahir Dar city, north west, Ethiopia, 2016. *Pediatr. Res.* **2019**, *85*, 612–616. [CrossRef]
33. Bimerew, A.; Teshome, M.; Kassa, G.M. Prevalence of timely breastfeeding initiation and associated factors in Dembecha district, north west Ethiopia: A cross-sectional study. *Int. Breastfeed. J.* **2016**, *11*, 28. [CrossRef]
34. Tewabe, T. Timely initiation of breastfeeding and associated factors among mothers in Motta town, East Gojjam zone, Amhara regional state, Ethiopia, 2015: A cross-sectional study. *BMC Pregnancy Childbirth* **2016**, *16*, 314. [CrossRef]
35. Mekonen, L.; Seifu, W.; Shiferaw, Z. Timely initiation of breastfeeding and associated factors among mothers of infants under 12 months in South Gondar zone, Amhara regional state, Ethiopia; 2013. *Int. Breastfeed. J.* **2018**, *13*, 17. [CrossRef]
36. Hunegnaw, M.T.; Gezie, L.D.; Teferra, A.S. Exclusive breastfeeding and associated factors among mothers in Ggozamin district, northwest Ethiopia: A community based cross-sectional study. *Int. Breastfeed. J.* **2017**, *12*, 30. [CrossRef]
37. Adugna, B.; Tadele, H.; Reta, F.; Berhan, Y. Determinants of exclusive breastfeeding in infants less than six months of age in Hawassa, an urban setting, Ethiopia. *Int. Breastfeed. J.* **2017**, *12*, 45. [CrossRef]
38. Azeze, G.A.; Gelaw, K.A.; Gebeyehu, N.A.; Gesese, M.M.; Mokonnon, T.M. Exclusive breastfeeding practice and associated factors among mothers in Boditi town, Wolaita zone, Southern Ethiopia, 2018: A community-based cross-sectional study. *Int. J. Pediatr.* **2019**, *2019*, 1483024. [CrossRef]
39. Asemahagn, M.A. Determinants of exclusive breastfeeding practices among mothers in Azezo district, Northwest Ethiopia. *Int. Breastfeed. J.* **2016**, *11*, 22. [CrossRef]
40. Tariku, A.; Alemu, K.; Gizaw, Z.; Muchie, K.F.; Derso, T.; Abebe, S.M.; Yitayal, M.; Fekadu, A.; Ayele, T.A.; Alemayehu, G.A.; et al. Mothers' education and ANC visit improved exclusive breastfeeding in Dabat Health and Demographic Surveillance System Site, northwest Ethiopia. *PLoS ONE* **2017**, *12*, e0179056. [CrossRef]
41. Seyoum, K.; Tekalegn, Y.; Teferu, Z.; Quisido, B.J.E. Determinants of prelacteal feeding practices in Ethiopia: Unmatched case-control study based on the 2016 Ethiopian Demographic and Health Survey Data. *Midwifery* **2021**, *99*, 103009. [CrossRef]
42. Alebel, A.; Tesma, C.; Temesgen, B.; Ferede, A.; Kibret, G.D. Exclusive breastfeeding practice in Ethiopia and its association with antenatal care and institutional delivery: A systematic review and meta-analysis. *Int. Breastfeed. J.* **2018**, *13*, 31. [CrossRef]
43. Habtewold, T.D.; Sharew, N.T.; Alemu, S.M. Evidence on the effect of gender of newborn, antenatal care and postnatal care on breastfeeding practices in Ethiopia: A meta-analysis and meta-regression analysis of observational studies. *BMJ Open.* **2019**, *9*, e023956. [CrossRef]
44. Rollins, N.C.; Bhandari, N.; Hajeebhoy, N.; Horton, S.; Lutter, C.K.; Martines, J.C.; Piwoz, E.G.; Richter, L.M.; Victora, C.G.; Lancet Breastfeeding Series Group. Why invest, and what it will take to improve breastfeeding practices? *Lancet* **2016**, *387*, 491–504. [CrossRef]
45. NEOVITA Study Group. Timing of initiation, patterns of breastfeeding, and infant survival: Prospective analysis of pooled data from three randomised trials. *Lancet Glob. Health* **2016**, *4*, e266–e275. [CrossRef]
46. Smith, E.R.; Hurt, L.; Chowdhury, R.; Sinha, B.; Fawzi, W.; Edmond, K.M.; Neovita Study Group. Delayed breastfeeding initiation and infant survival: A systematic review and meta-analysis. *PLoS ONE* **2017**, *12*, e0180722. [CrossRef]
47. Woldeamanuel, B.T. Trends and factors associated to early initiation of breastfeeding, exclusive breastfeeding and duration of breastfeeding in Ethiopia: Evidence from the Ethiopia Demographic and Health Survey 2016. *Int. Breastfeed. J.* **2020**, *15*, 3. [CrossRef]
48. Gedamu, H.; Tsegaw, A.; Debebe, E. The prevalence of traditional malpractice during pregnancy, child birth, and postnatal period among women of childbearing age in Meshenti town, 2016. *Int. J. Reprod. Med.* **2018**, 5945060. [CrossRef] [PubMed]
49. Mose, A.; Dheresa, M.; Mengistie, B.; Wassihun, B.; Abebe, H. Colostrum avoidance practice and associated factors among mothers of children aged less than six months in Bure district, Amhara region, north west, Ethiopia: A community-based cross-sectional study. *PLoS ONE* **2021**, *16*, e0245233. [CrossRef] [PubMed]
50. Gebretsadik, G.G.; Tkuwab, H.; Berhe, K.; Mulugeta, A.; Mohammed, H.; Gebremariam, A. Early initiation of breastfeeding, colostrum avoidance, and their associated factors among mothers with under one year old children in rural pastoralist communities of Afar, northeast Ethiopia: A cross sectional study. *BMC Pregnancy Childbirth* **2020**, *20*, 448. [CrossRef] [PubMed]
51. Ethiopian Health and Nutrition Research Institute (EHNRI). *Nutritional Baseline Survey Report for the National Nutrition Program of Ethiopia*. Addis Ababa, Ethiopia; Ethiopian Health and Nutrition Research Institute (EHNRI): Addis Ababa, Ethiopia, 2010.
52. Tamiru, D.; Belachew, T.; Loha, E.; Mohammed, S. Sub-optimal breastfeeding of infants during the first six months and associated factors in rural communities of Jimma Arjo Woreda, Southwest Ethiopia. *BMC Public Health* **2012**, *12*, 363. [CrossRef] [PubMed]
53. Temesgen, H.; Negesse, A.; Woyraw, W.; Getaneh, T.; Yigizaw, M. Prelacteal feeding and associated factors in Ethiopia: Systematic review and meta-analysis. *Int. Breastfeed. J.* **2018**, *13*, 49. [CrossRef]
54. Wolde, T.F.; Ayele, A.D.; Takele, W.W. Prelacteal feeding and associated factors among mothers having children less than 24 months of age, in Mettu district, Southwest Ethiopia: A community based cross-sectional study. *BMC Res. Notes* **2019**, *12*, 9. [CrossRef]
55. Amele, E.A.; Demissie, B.W.; Desta, K.W.; Woldemariam, E.B. Prelacteal feeding practice and its associated factors among mothers of children age less than 24 months old in Southern Ethiopia. *Ital. J. Pediatr.* **2019**, *45*, 15. [CrossRef]
56. Tewabe, T. Prelacteal feeding practices among mothers in Motta town, Northwest Ethiopia: A cross-sectional study. *Ethiop. J. Health Sci.* **2018**, *28*, 393–402. [CrossRef]

57. Zhao, P.; Zhang, S.; Liu, L.; Pang, X.; Yang, Y.; Lu, J.; Lv, J. Differences in the triacylglycerol and fatty acid compositions of human colostrum and mature milk. *J. Agric. Food Chem.* **2018**, *66*, 4571–4579. [CrossRef]
58. Li, R.; Zhou, Y.; Xu, Y. Comparative analysis of oligosaccharides in breast milk and feces of breast-fed infants by using LC-QE-HF-MS: A communication. *Nutrients* **2023**, *15*, 888. [CrossRef]
59. Stinson, L.F.; George, A.D. Human milk lipids and small metabolites: Maternal and microbial origins. *Metabolites* **2023**, *13*, 422. [CrossRef]
60. Taylor, R.; Keane, D.; Borrego, P.; Arcaro, K. Effect of maternal diet on maternal milk and breastfed infant gut microbiomes: A Scoping review. *Nutrients* **2023**, *15*, 1420. [CrossRef]

Disclaimer/Publisher's Note: The statements, opinions and data contained in all publications are solely those of the individual author(s) and contributor(s) and not of MDPI and/or the editor(s). MDPI and/or the editor(s) disclaim responsibility for any injury to people or property resulting from any ideas, methods, instructions or products referred to in the content.

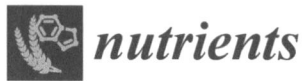 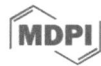

Article

Full Breastfeeding and Allergic Diseases—Long-Term Protection or Rebound Effects?

Lars Libuda [1,2,*,†], Birgit Filipiak-Pittroff [2,3,†], Marie Standl [4,5], Tamara Schikowski [6], Andrea von Berg [3], Sibylle Koletzko [7,8], Carl-Peter Bauer [9], Joachim Heinrich [5,10,11], Dietrich Berdel [3] and Monika Gappa [2]

1. Institute of Nutrition, Consumption and Health, Faculty of Natural Sciences, Paderborn University, Warburger Straße 100, 33098 Paderborn, Germany
2. Children's Hospital, Evangelisches Krankenhaus Düsseldorf, 40217 Düsseldorf, Germany
3. Formerly Department of Pediatrics, Research Institute, Marien-Hospital Wesel, 46483 Wesel, Germany
4. Institute of Epidemiology, Helmholtz Zentrum München, German Research Center for Environmental Health, 85764 Neuherberg, Germany
5. Comprehensive Pneumology Center Munich (CPC-M), German Center for Lung Research (DZL), 81377 Munich, Germany
6. IUF-Leibniz Research Institute for Environmental Medicine, 40225 Düsseldorf, Germany
7. Department of Pediatrics, Dr. von Hauner Children's Hospital, University Hospital, LMU Munich, 80337 Munich, Germany
8. Department of Pediatrics, Gastroenterology and Nutrition, School of Medicine Collegium Medicum, University of Warmia and Mazury, 10-719 Olsztyn, Poland
9. Department of Pediatrics, Technical University of Munich, 80804 Munich, Germany
10. Institute and Clinic for Occupational, Social and Environmental Medicine, University Hospital, LMU Munich, 80336 Munich, Germany
11. Allergy and Lung Health Unit, Melbourne School of Population and Global Health, The University of Melbourne, Melbourne 3010, Australia
* Correspondence: lars.libuda@uni-paderborn.de; Tel.: +49-5251-603835
† These authors contributed equally to the study.

Abstract: A previous follow-up of the GINIplus study showed that breastfeeding could protect against early eczema. However, effects diminished in adolescence, possibly indicating a "rebound effect" in breastfed children after initial protection. We evaluated the role of early eczema until three years of age on allergies until young adulthood and assessed whether early eczema modifies the association between breastfeeding and allergies. Data from GINIplus until 20-years of age (N = 4058) were considered. Information on atopic eczema, asthma, and rhinitis was based on reported physician's diagnoses. Adjusted Odds Ratios (aOR) were modelled by using generalized estimating equations. Early eczema was associated with eczema (aORs = 3.2–14.4), asthma (aORs = 2.2–2.7), and rhinitis (aORs = 1.2–2.7) until young adulthood. For eczema, this association decreased with age (p-for-interaction = 0.002–0.006). Longitudinal models did not show associations between breastfeeding and the respective allergies from 5 to 20 years of age. Moreover, early eczema generally did not modify the association between milk feeding and allergies except for rhinitis in participants without family history of atopy. Early eczema strongly predicts allergies until young adulthood. While preventive effects of full breastfeeding on eczema in infants with family history of atopy does not persist until young adulthood, the hypothesis of a rebound effect after initial protection cannot be confirmed.

Keywords: GINIplus; breastfeeding; atopic diseases; allergy prevention; early nutrition; long-term effects; rebound

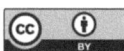

1. Introduction

Dietary guidelines in Germany recommend exclusive breastfeeding in the first six months of life and an introduction in complementary foods not before the fifth month of life [1]. German guidelines for allergy prevention recently also suggested exclusive breastfeeding for the first four to six month after birth, but this recommendation was not based on evidence of a preventive effect of breastfeeding on allergies, but general health-promoting effects of breastfeeding for mother and child [2]. The evidence regarding allergy prevention was classified as inconsistent considering that the majority of recent studies did not point to protective effects [3–7].

However, the guidelines mention an analysis of the GINIplus study which indicates that the benefits of breastfeeding for allergy prevention might be restricted to children with a family history of atopy in first-degree relative, i.e., those children considered at risk to develop an allergic disease [8]. The cumulative incidence of early eczema up to three years of age was lower in high-risk children who were fully breastfed for at least four months compared to their counterparts who received conventional cow's milk formula (CMF) in this period, either as part of partial breastfeeding or as the only source of food. Protective effects of breastfeeding compared with CMF on atopic eczema during the first years of life were already reported in previous analyses of the GINIplus study [9,10]. However, after age three until 15 years of age, the observed differences in cumulative incidences of eczema in the GINIplus study attenuated [8]. This finding is in line with results from a meta-analysis considering data from 24 cohort studies, 17 cross-sectional studies, and one case-control study [11]. The authors reported protective effects of breastfeeding on eczema until the age of two years of life, but disappearing effects thereafter. Moreover, results from studies covering the age between three and 20 years seem to indicate a slightly increased risk for eczema, although the pooled estimate was not significant. Accordingly, the decrease in group differences in GINIplus upon inclusion of data until 15 years of age might indicate a rebound effect after initial protection, i.e., that eczema manifests more frequently after the age of three years in fully breastfed children without early eczema compared to their counterparts fed with CMF. Following this hypothesis, early eczema would modify the long-term preventive effect of full breastfeeding. Accordingly, breastfed children without early eczema might represent a vulnerable group for allergic disease manifestation with increasing age and would, thus, be a target group for additional preventive measures and regular clinical assessments.

An analysis of the GINI intervention cohort after 20-years follow-up recently demonstrated heterogeneous long-term effects of different infant CMF on allergies [12], but long-term effects of full breastfeeding remain to be evaluated. Moreover, early eczema in the first three years was only considered in pathway analysis for different types of hydrolyzed formulae [12]. Thus, the meaning of early eczema protection for long-term effects of full breastfeeding is still unclear. Extending the analysis to data from the non-intervention cohort in the GINIplus study, we aimed to examine the following questions:

i. Is early eczema a determinant of the course of allergic diseases until early adulthood which should be considered in long-term analysis of breastfeeding effects?
ii. Does early eczema modify potential long-term associations of milk feeding with the development of atopic diseases?

2. Materials and Methods

2.1. Study Design of the GINIplus Study

The current data analysis considered data from the GINIplus study from birth until the age of 20 years. Details of the study design of the GINIplus study have previously been described [8,13–15]. In short, 5991 healthy term newborns were initially recruited from 16 maternity wards in two regions of Germany (rural Wesel and urban Munich) between September 1995 and June 1998 and either participated in the GINI intervention study (I cohort) or the GINI non-intervention study (NI cohort). Mothers with a chronic, immunological relevant disease other than allergies (e.g., HIV, autoimmune disease, diabetes) were excluded [15]. The baseline characteristics from the families (e.g., allergies in parents and siblings and parental education) were assessed by questionnaires at birth or before. Written informed consent was obtained from the participating families. The study protocol was approved by the local ethics committees.

In the prospective, double-blind intervention trial only infants with a high family risk of atopy defined as having a family history (FH+) with at least one parent or biologic sibling with a history of allergic disease were included. If parents agreed to participate in the intervention study (I cohort, $N = 2252$), the newborns were randomly allocated at birth to one of four blinded study formulae, i.e., three different hydrolyzed formulae (partially hydrolyzed whey (pHF-W); extensively hydrolyzed whey (eHF-W); extensively hydrolyzed casein (eHF-C)) and one formula based on intact cow's milk protein (CMF). Mothers in the I cohort received written recommendations for feeding of the infants. Mothers were, e.g., encouraged to exclusively breastfeed for at least four months and not to introduce solid foods during this period. The respective formula was used during the first four months of life as a milk substitute only if exclusive breastfeeding was not possible [16]. Infants with a negative family history of allergy in a first degree relative (FH−, $N = 2507$) or those with positive risk whose parents did not want to participate in the intervention trial (FH+, $N = 1232$) were allocated to the NI-cohort. Their parents did not receive any feeding recommendations.

2.2. Definition of Outcome and Exposure Variables

Both cohorts have regularly been followed from birth onwards and recently participated in the 20-years follow-up. Self-administered questionnaires were sent to the parents around their child's 1st, 2nd, 3rd, 4th, 6th, 10th, and 15th birthdays and to the study participants themselves around their 20th birthdays to collect information on the child's health, allergic symptoms, physician diagnoses of allergic diseases, and further information such as nutrition and several lifestyle factors. The definition of the main outcomes in the GINI study was continuously based on the same set of questions, which have been used since the first year of life. Until age 15 years, the following question was asked to the parents separately for each year of life: "Did a doctor diagnose your child with one of the following diseases [eczema, asthma, allergic rhinitis, hay fever] in 1st [2nd, . . . , 15th] year of life?" For the 20-year-questionnaire covering the period from 16–20 years of age, this question was directly addressed to the participants themselves. We further considered a question on disease treatment ("Have you (your child) been treated for [asthma, hay fever, allergic rhinitis, atopic eczema] in the past 12 months?").

The primary outcomes of the present analyses are period prevalence of eczema, asthma, and allergic rhinitis/hay fever as well as the cumulative incidence of these up to 20 years of age. Any "yes" response to physician's diagnosis in the period and/or treatment in the last 12 months was used to determine period prevalence. Any positive reply during the lifetime of the child was used to determine cumulative incidence. Early eczema was defined considering physician's diagnosis of eczema in the 1st, 2nd, and 3rd year of life as answered by the parents in the respective questionnaires.

In the I-cohort, information on milk feeding was derived from weekly diaries. Full breastfeeding was defined if "breast milk only" was reported as milk feeding for each of the first 16 weeks. Accordingly, one documented bottle of the randomized study formula sufficed for the definition "mixed fed with breast milk and study formula". In the NI-cohort the mode of milk feeding was retrospectively assessed at the age of 1 year using the question "What kind of milk did your child drink during 1st, 2nd, . . . 6th month of life?" The child was classified as "fully breastfed" if parents selected "breast milk only" for all of months 1 to 4, infants receiving formula during this period were labelled as "not fully breastfed".

2.3. Statistics

Statistical analyses were performed using the statistical software SAS for Windows, Release 9.4 (SAS Institute, Cary, NC, USA). To determine associations between the status of early eczema and the prevalence of specified allergies in pre-defined periods, logistic regression analyses were performed and odds ratios (OR) for period prevalence are reported. Cumulative incidence was estimated by the life table method [17] and analyzed by generalized estimating equations (GEE) [18] using a complementary log-log link and independent correlation structure in PROC GENMOD. The results are presented as relative risks (RR) for the specified contrasts (Full breastfeeding in comparison to randomized formula feeding for the I-cohort and to non-full breastfeeding for the NI-cohort).

To examine the course of allergies, i.e., period prevalences from the 5th to 20th years, considering the status of early eczema and the mode of milk feeding, longitudinal analyses (GEE models with logit link, PROC GENMOD) were performed. The backward selection method (threshold $p < 0.05$) was used to find the best fit for the data and started with all two-factor interaction terms between the terms: time-period, status of early eczema, and mode of milk feeding. Accordingly, the interaction term between early eczema and breastfeeding which would indicate a potential rebound effect was tested for every outcome in every cohort. Only significant interaction terms were retained in the final model. The main factors of interest, i.e., milk feeding and early eczema as well as time period and the set of confounders were fixed in the models (and excluded from elimination process). Results from the final models are given as OR for the interesting terms.

The analyses were conducted for each cohort separately and the models were adjusted for a fixed set of known risk factors or confounders. To avoid multicollinearity the chosen set was reduced to family history of the corresponding outcome (eczema, asthma, and allergic rhinitis, respectively) and heredity of family allergy in the cohorts with family risk of atopy (I-cohort and NI FH+) as well as sex, study region, parental education and older siblings in all cohorts. Parental education was used as a proxy for socio-economic status and study region as a proxy for environmental determinants. Results of the adjusted models are given as adjusted OR or RR (aOR, aRR). p values less than 0.05 were considered statistically significant and estimates of OR and RR were given with 95% confidence intervals (95%CI).

3. Results

3.1. Study Population and Characteristics

For the present analysis, all participants with complete information on early eczema were considered (Table S1). Of the 2252 recruited infants in the I-cohort the status of eczema during the first three years was available for 1661. The NI-cohort comprises 2397 infants, 40 of whom were excluded from the analysis on effects of milk feeding due to missing information. Further details regarding number of subjects at the different stages of follow-ups are presented in Table S1.

Early eczema was more prevalent in children "at risk": While the prevalence was similar in children with positive family history (FH+) in the I- and NI-cohorts (I-cohort: 453 children (27.3%), NI-cohort: 207 (25.7%)), children in the NI-cohort without family history less often develop early eczema (FH−, 240 children (15.1%), chi-square test $p < 0.0001$ for group differences) (Table 1 and Table S1). Nearly half of the analysis population was fully breastfed for four months, with slightly lower rates in the I-cohort (I-cohort: 44.1%, NI FH+: 51.0%, NI FH−: 47.9%, chi-square test $p = 0.004$ for group differences). Additionally, children in the I-cohort had siblings less often (chi-square $p < 0.0001$ for group differences) while parental education was higher (chi-square $p < 0.0001$ for group differences), the latter especially upon comparison with the NI cohort with negative family history. Additionally, number of siblings and parental education differed in three cohorts (chi-square tests $p < 0.0001$).

Table 1. Characteristics of the analysis population, stratified by study cohorts * and eczema during the first three years.

		Intervention Cohort			Non-Intervention Cohort FH+			Non-Intervention Cohort FH−		
		Early Eczema − N = 1208 n (%)	Early Eczema + N = 453 n (%)	Chi² test p-value	Early Eczema − N = 597 n (%)	Early Eczema + N = 207 n (%)	Chi² test p-value	Early Eczema − N = 1353 n (%)	Early Eczema + N = 240 n (%)	Chi² test p-value
Family history of allergy	no	846 (70.0)	291 (64.2)	0.024	503 (84.3)	159 (76.8)	0.016	1353 (100)	240 (100)	-
	single	362 (30.0)	162 (35.8)		94 (15.7)	48 (23.2)				
	double	0	0		0	0				
Family risk for	eczema	419 (34.7)	249 (55.0)	<0.001	155 (26.0)	96 (46.4)	<0.001	-	-	
	asthma	329 (27.2)	141 (31.1)	0.117	108 (18.1)	40 (19.3)	0.693	-	-	
	AR	1033 (85.5)	370 (81.7)	0.055	453 (75.9)	154 (74.4)	0.669	-	-	
Sex	male	615 (50.9)	244 (53.9)	0.284	294 (49.2)	114 (55.1)	0.149	687 (50.8)	119 (49.6)	0.733
Study region	Munich	635 (52.6)	239 (52.8)	0.944	364 (61.0)	122 (58.9)	0.606	469 (34.7)	104 (43.3)	0.010
Siblings #	0	719 (59.5)	252 (55.6)	0.246	262 (43.9)	78 (37.7)	0.256	675 (49.9)	141 (58.8)	0.037
	1	373 (30.9)	145 (32.0)		241 (40.4)	96 (46.4)		520 (38.4)	78 (32.5)	
	>1	113 (9.4)	53 (11.7)		94 (15.7)	33 (15.9)		158 (11.7)	21 (8.8)	
Parental education #	low (<10 years)	76 (6.3)	28 (6.2)	0.707	59 (9.9)	19 (9.2)	0.923	176 (13.0)	34 (14.2)	0.641
	middle (10–12 years)	328 (27.2)	132 (29.1)		166 (27.8)	60 (29.0)		462 (34.1)	74 (30.8)	
	high (>12 years)	804 (66.6)	292 (64.5)		372 (62.3)	128 (61.8)		714 (52.8)	129 (53.8)	
Full breastfeeding for 4 months #		533 (44.1)	200 (44.2)	0.992	302 (51.5)	102 (49.5)	0.618	633 (47.5)	116 (50.0)	0.479

[1] FH+: children with family risk of atopy; FH−: children without family risk of atopy; early eczema+: children with eczema up to the 3rd year of life; early eczema−: children without eczema up to the 3rd year of life; * chi² test revealed significant differences between the three cohorts for all parameters (all p < 0.01) except for sex (p = 0.797). # 3 missing values regarding siblings, 5 missing values regarding parental education; 12 and 28 missing values regarding full breastfeeding in the Non-intervention FH+ and Non-intervention FH−.

3.2. Development of Atopic Diseases up to Young Adulthood Depending on Early Eczema during the First Three Years of Life

The illustration of the period prevalence of atopic diseases stratified by the state of early eczema (Figure 1) gives a first description of the potential meaning of early eczema for the development of atopic diseases in later life. Early eczema was apparently accompanied by a higher eczema period prevalence up to young adulthood. Moreover, for asthma and AR, the prevalence was constantly higher in participants with early eczema compared with those without early eczema. This finding was not only observed in subjects with a high risk of atopic diseases, i.e., the I cohort (Figure 1a) and the NI cohort with positive family history (Figure 1b), but also in the NI cohort with a negative family history (Figure 1c).

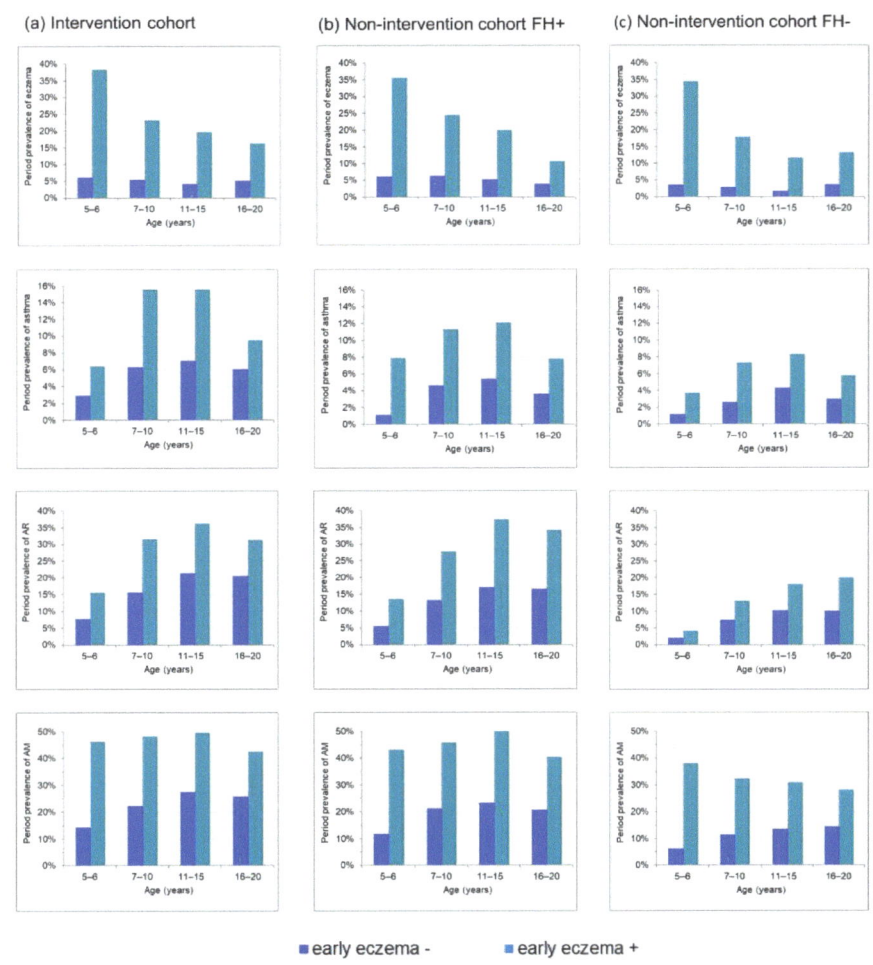

Figure 1. Prevalence of allergic diseases from childhood to young adulthood stratified by eczema during the first 3 years for (**a**) the intervention cohort, (**b**) the non-intervention cohort with family risk of atopy and (**c**) the non-intervention cohort without family risk of atopy.

Statistical analyses using logistic regression models confirmed this conclusion since early eczema was not only a significant predictor of eczema prevalence up to young adulthood, but also of asthma and AR (Table 2). While the highest aORs were generally found for eczema compared with the other atopic phenotypes, the association of early eczema for this phenotype attenuated with increasing age as illustrated by decreasing aORs (Table 2). This is also reflected by decreasing prevalence differences in Figure 1 due to strictly monotonous falling eczema period prevalence with increasing age in those participants with early eczema, but constant levels in those without early eczema (Figure 1). For asthma and AR, a more parallel course was observed in participants with or without early eczema (Figure 1) and also aORs remained relatively constant (Table 2). Longitudinal GEE models with eczema as outcome confirmed that aORs for early eczema decrease with age in the I-cohort and the NI-cohort without family history, while the effect for asthma and also for AR did not change over time in all cohorts (Table 3).

Table 2. Association between eczema during the first three years and prevalence of allergies in life periods up to age 20 years in the intervention-cohort and for the non-intervention-cohort with family risk of atopy family risk of atopy (FH+) and without family risk of atopy (FH−). OR [a] and adjusted OR (aOR [b,c]) with 95%CI from logistic models for those with eczema during the first three years in comparison to those without.

		Prevalence eczema							
		5 to 6th Year		7 to 10th Year		11 to 15th Year		16 to 20th Year	
Intervention	OR	9.5	(6.9–13.2)	5.3	(3.6–7.8)	5.5	(3.6–6.6)	3.6	(2.3–5.8)
	aOR [b]	8.7	(6.2–12.2)	5.0	(3.4–7.6)	5.0	(3.2–7.9)	3.4	(2.1–5.5)
Non-intervention FH+	OR	8.5	(5.2–13.7)	4.8	(2.8–8.2)	4.6	(2.6–8.1)	2.9	(1.3–6.5)
	aOR [b]	8.1	(4.9–13.4)	4.4	(2.5–7.6)	4.1	(2.2–7.4)	2.4	(1.0–5.6)
Non-intervention FH−	OR	14.6	(9.4–22.6)	7.4	(4.3–12.8)	8.3	(4.1–16.9)	4.0	(2.2–7.5)
	aOR [c]	14.7	(9.5–22.8)	7.4	(4.2–12.9)	8.2	(4.0–16.9)	4.7	(2.4–9.1)
		Prevalence asthma							
		5 to 6th year		7 to 10th year		11 to 15th year		16 to 20th year	
Intervention	OR	2.3	(1.3–4.0)	2.7	(1.8–4.1)	2.5	(1.6–3.7)	1.6	(1.0–2.7)
	aOR [b]	2.1	(1.2–3.8)	2.6	(1.7–4.0)	2.4	(1.6–3.6)	1.6	(0.95–2.7)
Non-intervention FH+	OR	7.4	(2.8–19.8)	2.6	(1.4–5.1)	2.4	(1.3–4.5)	2.2	(0.93–5.4)
	aOR [b]	6.8	(2.5–18.6)	2.5	(1.3–5.0)	2.2	(1.2–4.3)	1.9	(0.78–4.8)
Non-intervention FH−	OR	3.0	(1.2–7.6)	3.0	(1.5–6.1)	2.0	(1.1–3.9)	2.0	(0.87–4.5)
	aOR [c]	2.9	(1.1–7.3)	3.2	(1.5–6.5)	2.1	(1.1–4.1)	2.1	(0.89–4.7)
		Prevalence allergic rhinitis/hay fewer							
		5 to 6th year		7 to 10th year		11 to 15th year		16 to 20th year	
Intervention	OR	2.2	(1.5–3.2)	2.5	(1.9–3.4)	2.1	(1.6–2.8)	1.8	(1.3–2.4)
	aOR [b]	2.2	(1.5–3.1)	2.6	(1.9–3.5)	2.1	(1.6–2.8)	1.7	(1.2–2.4)
Non-intervention FH+	OR	2.7	(1.5–4.8)	2.5	(1.6–4.0)	2.9	(1.9–4.4)	2.6	(1.6–4.3)
	aOR [b]	2.8	(1.5–5.0)	2.4	(1.6–3.9)	2.9	(1.9–4.4)	2.6	(1.6–4.3)
Non-intervention FH−	OR	2.0	(0.89–4.5)	1.9	(1.1–3.2)	1.9	(1.2–3.1)	2.2	(1.4–3.6)
	aOR [c]	2.0	(0.87–4.5)	1.9	(1.1–3.2)	2.0	(1.2–3.1)	2.1	(1.3–3.4)
		Prevalence allergic diseases (Eczema, asthma or rhinitis/hay fewer)							
		5 to 6th year		7 to 10th year		11 to 15th year		16 to 20th year	
Intervention	OR	5.1	(3.9–6.7)	3.3	(2.5–4.3)	2.6	(2.0–3.4)	2.1	(1.6–2.9)
	aOR [b]	5.0	(3.8–6.6)	3.4	(2.5–4.5)	2.6	(2.0–3.5)	2.1	(1.5–2.8)
Non-intervention FH+	OR	5.7	(3.8–8.5)	3.1	(2.1–4.6)	3.3	(2.2–4.9)	2.6	(1.6–4.1)
	aOR [b]	5.6	(3.6–8.6)	3.1	(2.1–4.7)	3.2	(2.1–4.9)	2.5	(1.6–4.1)
Non-intervention FH−	OR	9.2	(6.3–13.4)	3.7	(2.5–5.4)	2.8	(1.9–4.1)	2.3	(1.5–3.5)
	aOR [c]	9.1	(6.2–13.4)	3.7	(2.5–5.5)	2.8	(1.9–4.2)	2.3	(1.5–3.5)

[a] OR of <1 indicates a decreased risk of disease, that is lower risk in the early eczema group than in the compared feeding group, whereas OR >1 indicates higher risk in early eczema group than in the compared non-early eczema group; [b] adjusted for family history of corresponding disease, heredity of family allergy, sex, study region, siblings, parental education; [c] no family history per definition, therefore adjusted for sex, study region, siblings, parental education.

3.3. Short- and Long-Term Risk of Allergies in Fully-Breastfeed Children

The 20-year data confirm that the risk reducing effect of breastfeeding on eczema compared with CMF in the I-cohort diminished after early protection and became non-significant when cumulative incidence up to 20 years of life was considered (Table S2). In contrast, high-risk children in the I-cohort fed with eHF-C constantly had an even lower risk of eczema compared with breastfed children not only until 3 years of age, but up to young adulthood. This association remained significant upon adjustment for several confounders. In both groups of the NI-cohort, i.e., children with or without family history, full breastfeeding was not associated with lower cumulative incidences of any atopic outcome compared with non-fully-breastfeeding. Moreover, longitudinal models using period prevalence from five to 20 years as outcome did not reveal general breastfeeding effects on any outcome (Table 3). The adjusted ORs for eczema ranged from 0.92 to 1.1, for asthma from 0.78 to 1.2 and for AR from 0.77 to 1.7 (all n.s.).

3.4. Examination of a Potential Rebound Effect in Fully-Breastfed Children without Early Eczema

If there was a rebound effect of full breastfeeding, a higher period prevalence in later life would be expected in fully breastfed children without early eczema compared to their counterparts who were fed at least partly with CMF. In general, descriptive illustrations of crude period prevalence in Figure 2 do not indicate such higher period prevalence in fully breastfed children without early eczema (red bars) compared with CMF fed children without early eczema (black bars). Eczema prevalence was slightly higher in the period between 5 and 10 years in the I-cohort (Figure 2a, red bar and black bar) and up to 6 years of age in the NI-cohort in children with family history (Figure 2b) only.

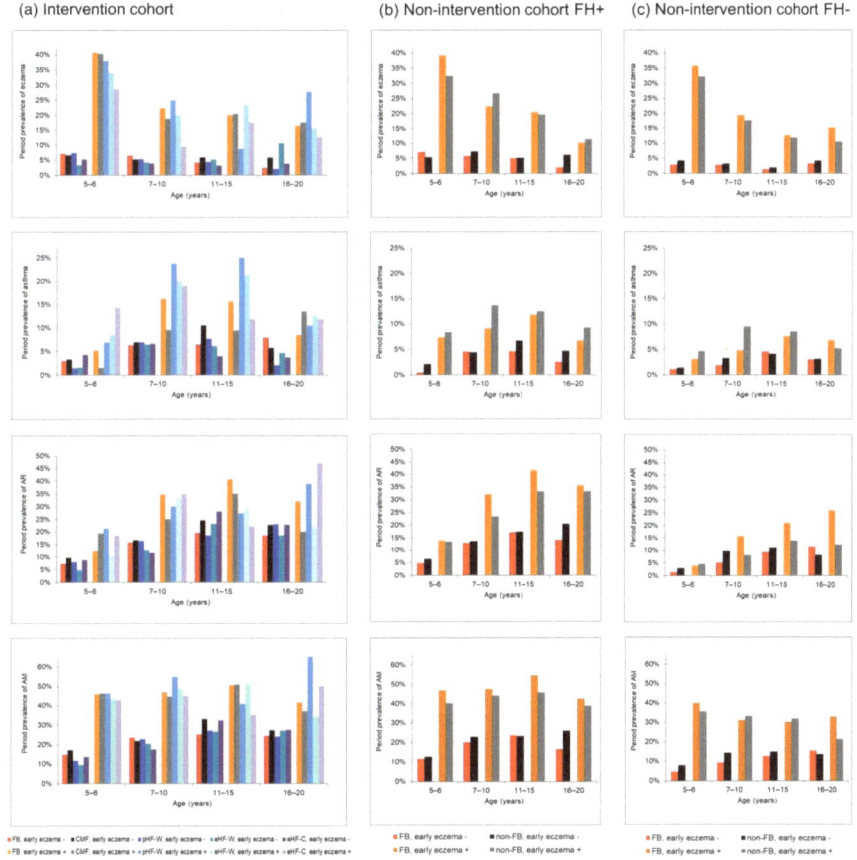

Figure 2. Prevalence of allergic diseases from childhood to young adulthood by eczema during the first three years and feeding groups (**a**) in the intervention-cohort stratified for the full breastfeeding group (FB) and for the four groups supplemented only with their randomized formula, (**b**) in the non-intervention-cohort with family risk (FH+) and (**c**) without risk (FH−) both cohorts stratified by full breastfeeding.

Statistical analyses using longitudinal models included an interaction term between infant milk feeding and early eczema in order to examine the hypothesis of early eczema as a potential modifier (Table 3). These models confirm the impression from the descriptive evaluation of crude prevalence in Figure 2: The analyses did not reveal a significant modifying effect of early eczema on milk feeding effects on the development of eczema, asthma and AR in children with family history of allergies. Differences in breastfeeding effects depending on early eczema were only observed for AR in children without family risk of allergic diseases (NI cohort FH−, p for interaction = 0.04): in those without early eczema breastfeeding tended to be associated with lower long-term AR risk compared with CMF (OR= 0.77, 95%CI (0.53–1.1)), while breastfeeding in those with early eczema was associated with a (non-significantly) higher rhinitis risk compared with CMF (OR = 1.7, 95%CI (0.84–3.4), Table 3). Sensitivity analyses including introduction in solid foods as additional covariate did not substantially change these results (results not shown).

Table 3. Association of full breastfeeding with allergic diseases from 5 to 20 years under consideration of status of eczema during first three years. Results from adjusted longitudinal GEE models [#] for the intervention cohort and non-intervention cohort with family risk of atopy (FH+) and without family risk of atopy (FH−).

		Intervention Cohort (N = 1661)	Non-Intervention FH+ (N = 792)	Non-Intervention FH− (N = 1565)
Eczema				
Interaction feeding with early eczema *	p-value	0.987	0.738	0.174
Final Model		M1	M2	M1
FB vs. CMF/non FB	aOR (95%CI)	1.1 (0.72–1.6)	0.92 (0.62–1.3)	0.94 (0.65–1.3)
eHF-C vs. CMF	aOR (95%CI)	0.64 (0.34–1.2)	−[1]	−[1]
Interaction early eczema with time-periods	p-value	0.002	−	0.006
Early eczema effect at 5–6th years	aOR (95%CI)	8.8 (6.3–12.3)		14.4 (9.2–22.7)
Early eczema effect at 7–10th years	aOR (95%CI)	4.7 (3.2–7.0)		7.7 (4.4–13.4)
Early eczema effect at 11–15th years	aOR (95%CI)	4.9 (3.1–7.7)		8.6 (4.2–17.4)
Early eczema effect at 16–20th years	aOR (95%CI)	3.2 (2.0–5.1)		3.9 (2.1–7.4)
Early eczema effect	aOR (95%CI)	-	5.0 (3.4–7.4)	-
Time-period 7–10th vs. 5–6th years	aOR (95%CI)		0.76 (0.57–1.02)	
11–15th vs. 5–6th years	aOR (95%CI)		0.58 (0.42–0.80)	
16–20th vs. 5–6th years	aOR (95%CI)		0.34 (0.21–0.52)	
Asthma				
Interaction feeding with early eczema *	p-value	0.405	0.698	0.923
Final model		M2	M2	M2
FB vs. CMF/non FB	aOR (95%CI)	1.2 (0.72–2.1)	0.78 (0.45–1.3)	0.95 (0.59–1.5)
eHF-C vs. CMF	aOR (95%CI)	1.1 (0.52–2.1)	−[1]	−[1]
Early eczema effect	aOR (95%CI	2.2 (1.6–3.1)	2.7 (1.6–4.9)	2.4 (1.4–4.1)
Time-period 7–10th vs. 5–6th years	aOR (95%CI)	2.5 (1.9–3.3)	2.4 (1.6–3.6)	2.0 (1.3–3.1)
11–15th vs. 5–6th years	aOR (95%CI)	2.7 (2.0–3.6)	2.8 (1.7–4.5)	3.1 (2.0–4.9)
16–20th vs. 5–6th years	aOR (95%CI)	1.9 (1.4–2.7)	1.7 (1.0–3.0)	2.2 (1.3–3.9)
AR				
Interaction feeding with early eczema *	p-value	0.471	0.186	0.040
Final model		M2	M2	M3
FB vs. CMF/non FB	aOR (95%CI)	0.96 (0.68–1.3)	0.98 (0.71–1.4)	-
eHF-C vs. CMF	aOR (95%CI)	1.1 (0.69–1.7)	−[1]	−[1]
FB vs. non FB at early eczema -	aOR (95%CI)			0.77 (0.53–1.1)
FB vs. non FB at early eczema +	aOR (95%CI)			1.7 (0.84–3.4)
Early eczema effect	aOR (95%CI	2.1 (1.7–2.7)	2.7 (1.9–3.8)	
Early eczema effect at FB	aOR (95%CI)			2.7 (1.7–4.5)
Early eczema effect at non FB	aOR (95%CI)			1.2 (0.71–2.2)
Interaction feeding with time-periods	p-value	-	-	0.004
FB vs. non FB at 5–6th years	aOR (95%CI)			0.68 (0.33–1.5)
FB vs. non FB at 7–10th years	aOR (95%CI)			0.90 (0.55–1.5)
FB vs. non FB at 11–15th years	aOR (95%CI)			1.3 (0.81–2.0)
FB vs. non FB at 16–20th years	aOR (95%CI)			2.2 (1.3–3.6)
Time-period 7–10th vs. 5–6th years	aOR (95%CI)	2.3 (1.9–2.8)	2.5 (1.9–3.4)	
11–15th vs. 5–6th years	aOR (95%CI)	3.3 (2.7–4.0)	3.6 (2.7–4.9)	
16–20th vs. 5–6th years	aOR (95%CI)	2.9 (2.4–3.6)	3.4 (2.4–4.8)	

Table 3. Cont.

		Intervention Cohort (N = 1661)	Non-Intervention FH+ (N = 792)	Non-Intervention FH− (N = 1565)
AM				
Interaction * feeding with early eczema	p-value	0.558	0.169	0.177
Final Model		M1	M1	M4
FB vs. CMF/non FB	aOR (95%CI)	0.96 (0.72–1.3)	1.0 (0.76–1.4)	−
eHF-C vs. CMF	aOR (95%CI)	0.90 (0.61–1.3)	−[1]	−[1]
Interaction feeding with time-periods	p-value	−	−	0.040
FB vs. non FB at 5–6th years	aOR (95%CI)			0.81 (0.55−1.2)
FB vs. non FB at 7–10th years	aOR (95%CI)			0.70 (0.50–0.99)
FB vs. non FB at 11–15th years	aOR (95%CI)			0.90 (0.64–1.3)
FB vs. non FB at 16–20th years	aOR (95%CI)			1.3 (0.92–1.9)
Interaction early eczema with time-periods	p-value	0.001	0.027	0.001
Early eczema effect at 5–6th years	aOR (95%CI)	5.2 (3.9–6.9)	5.5 (3.6–8.4)	9.1 (6.2–13.4)
Early eczema effect at 7–10th years	aOR (95%CI)	3.2 (2.4–4.2)	3.0 (2.0–4.5)	3.6 (2.4–5.4)
Early eczema effect at 11–15th years	aOR (95%CI)	2.5 (1.9–3.3)	3.2 (2.2–4.8)	2.8 (1.9–4.2)
Early eczema effect at 16–20th years	aOR (95%CI)	2.1 (1.5–2.8)	2.6 (1.6–4.2)	2.2 (1.4–3.4)

[1] not to be determined in the non-intervention cohort; # All models were adjusted for family history of corresponding disease, heredity of family allergy, sex, study region, siblings, parental education in the intervention and non-intervention FH+ cohort and for sex, study region, siblings, parental education in the non-intervention FH− cohort; * test of interaction-term whether early eczema modify the feeding association, started with all two-factor interaction terms and used backward selection modelling. p-values for the interaction between feeding and early eczema were derived from the last step, where the interesting term was deleted or from final model. Final models: Only significant interaction terms were retained as a result from backward selection modelling. The main interesting factors milk feeding and early eczema as well as time-period and the set of confounders were fixed in the models (and excluded from elimination process). M1: model includes variables for time-periods, status of early eczema, feeding groups and the interaction of status of early eczema with time-periods; M2: model includes variables for time-periods, status of early eczema, feeding groups; M3: model includes variables for time-periods, status of early eczema, FB feeding, interaction of status of early eczema with feeding and interaction of feeding with time-periods; M4: Model includes variables for time-periods, status of early eczema, feeding groups and the interaction of feeding with time-periods and interaction of status of early eczema with time-periods.

4. Discussion

Using data from the GINIplus study up to 20 years of age, we examined whether early eczema is a determinant of the course of allergic disease until early adulthood. Additionally, we examined the hypothesis of a potential rebound effect in breastfed children after initial protection against allergies in young childhood. Our analysis showed that early eczema is linked with a higher risk of all types of allergic diseases over the course of childhood up to 20 years of age. Odds ratios were generally highest for eczema, but decrease with increasing age. Additionally, our analysis provides evidence that preventive effects of full breastfeeding on eczema are restricted to subgroups and early childhood, attenuate over time and do not persist until young adulthood. However, since early eczema was not observed to modify the association between milk feeding and allergy risk, we did not find evidence of a rebound effect after initial protection in young childhood.

Our present analysis shows that early eczema is not only associated with eczema in later life, but also with rhinitis and asthma. This finding could be related to a "multimorbid" allergic cluster, which was identified as one of seven different clusters of allergic disease development from birth until adolescence in a combined analysis of the German GINIplus and LISAplus studies [19]. Our data also showed that eczema prevalence decreases over time in those subjects with early eczema, indicating a natural remission, i.e., an "early−resolving dermatitis" cluster [19]. Interestingly, Kilanowski et al. identified sex, parental history of allergies, and pet exposure as early life determinants for the different clusters, while breastfeeding did not differ between allergic cases and controls in their analysis [19].

Our finding that full breastfeeding does not decrease the risk of allergic diseases across subgroups and at different ages is completely in line with conclusions stated in the current S3-guidelines Allergy Prevention in Germany [2]. Focusing on data from a particularly vulnerable group, i.e., children with a family risk for allergic diseases, the GINIplus study indicates that full breastfeeding might only have transient preventive effects on allergy in early life. Indeed, the initial reduction in cumulative incidence of eczema lost its significance when considering data up to young adulthood, while lower risks of rhinitis or asthma were neither observed in the short- nor in the long-term in this subgroup. The Global Initiative for

Asthma (GINA) recently also concluded that breastfeeding decreases wheezing episodes in early life, but may not prevent the development of persistent asthma [20]. Interestingly, the hypothesis of attenuating effects on eczema and/or asthma does not seem to be transferable to infant nutrition in general. Using data from the I-cohort, we recently examined effects of different types of formulae [12]. We observed that the cumulative incidence of eczema until young adulthood was reduced in children fed with eHF-C or pHF-W compared to the CMF group. Additionally, asthma prevalence between 16 and 20 years was significantly lower in both groups compared to CMF.

Two very recent studies using data from large-scale population-based studies, i.e., National Health and Nutrition Examination Survey (NHANES, 833 cases and 5167 controls) [21] and UK Biobank (7157 cases with childhood-onset asthma and 158,253 controls) [22], could not yet be considered in the above-mentioned guidelines. Both showed potential protective effects: Breastfed children from the UK Biobank less frequently developed asthma until 12 years of age compared to their counterparts who were not breastfed [22]. The second study showed that in three to six year-old children participating in NHANES who were exclusively breastfed for at least four to six months asthma risk was reduced by 31% compared with children never breastfed [21]. Interestingly, Chen et al. also reported that protective effects seem to diminish in older children [21].

We hypothesized that diminishing protective effects could represent a rebound effect in fully breastfed children. This could be explained through less exposure to potential allergens in cow's milk formula which in turn might influence the development of tolerance and therefore affect development of allergic diseases in the long-term. Another explanation for the reduced protective effect could be that the early exposure to immune components found in breast milk such as antibodies, growth factors, cytokines, antimicrobial compounds, and specific immune cells [23] might only protect against allergies until young childhood. Over the years, other factors including environmental factors such as air pollution are likely to have an increasing effect on the immune system, overriding nutritional effects during infancy. However, longitudinal analyses over the course of childhood in our study did not generally support the hypothesis of a rebound effect. To the best of our knowledge, a rebound effect in fully breastfed children regarding allergies has not yet been examined in other studies. Most studies are limited in that they focused on relatively early periods of life potentially hampering identification of a rebound effect. Up to now, the 16-years follow-up of the cluster-randomized controlled study PROBIT conducted in Belarus provides the longest-term insights into this topic [24]. Focusing on effects of breastfeeding promotion on health development, PROBIT also assessed several allergy outcomes at the age of 16 years with mixed results: Flohr et al. reported a 50% risk reduction regarding flexural eczema on skin examination at 16 years of age, but no significant associations with self-reported eczema or asthma symptoms in the past year [24]. Rebound effects of breastfeeding were not reported.

While the findings in PROBIT based on self-reports are comparable with our GINIplus data, the reduction in the prevalence of flexural eczema based on clinical examination even seems to indicate long-term protective effects of full breastfeeding [24]. Accordingly, studies using self-reports on eczema such as GINIplus might underestimate long-term effects of breastfeeding. However, partly conflicting results between GINIplus and PROBIT may also be explained by differences in study design and populations. PROBIT was conducted in a setting with a low risk of allergic diseases: Prevalence of family risk of allergic diseases (5.2% in the intervention group and 3.7% in the control group) as well as the prevalence of eczema in study participants themselves (<1% in both study groups upon skin examination as well as self-reported symptoms) [24] were substantially lower compared with the population in our GINIplus study. It might be speculated that breastfeeding is more relevant in the long-term in populations where genetic risk and/or exposure to other risk factors is less pronounced. Even if protective effects of breastfeeding on eczema are restricted to early childhood in populations such as GINIplus, these effects could still be relevant for long-term health beyond allergies. A previous analysis of the GINI study revealed a higher risk for mental health problems at the age of 10 years in children with infant-onset eczema even if eczema was limited to infancy compared with children never diagnosed as having eczema [25]. Accordingly, full breastfeeding could have indirect long-term effects on mental health by protecting against infant onset eczema.

While our study in general did not reveal long-term effects of breastfeeding on allergies, an interesting finding is that we also observed potential long-term benefits in a subgroup with low allergy risk: In children without family risk of allergies and without early eczema, a subgroup that has not been in the focus so far, full breastfeeding was associated with a lower period prevalence of rhinitis between five and 20 years of age. Considering that this finding missed significance, more studies are needed to confirm a potential long-term preventive effect of breastfeeding particularly in children with a negative family history of atopy.

A strength of our analysis is that we considered data not only until adolescence, but up to young adulthood. Compared with previous results from GINIplus considering data until adolescence only [8], slightly decreasing effect sizes as well as the lack of significance regarding cumulative incidence of eczema in the current analysis indicate that the relevance of breastfeeding might attenuate further in young adulthood. A further strength of GINIplus is that the repeated allergy assessment is based on the same set of questions throughout the ages. Accordingly, these data provide the opportunity to conduct longitudinal data analysis which not only increases the statistical power, but also enables the evaluation of rebound effects of breastfeeding over time.

Several limitations of the study need to be considered. First of all, although GINIplus included an interventional study cohort, this part of the study was not a priori designed to assess the effects of breastfeeding. In the interventional study, mothers were encouraged to exclusively breast-feed for at least 4 months and preferably 6 months. The decision to include the specific study formula in their children's diet was exclusively made by the parents. In the NI cohort, parents did not receive dietary recommendations. Accordingly, the present data analysis represents an observational study design, which hampers conclusions on causality due to the general risk of reverse causation and residual confounding. Regarding the relationship between breastfeeding and atopic diseases, Lowe et al. hypothesized that the protective effects of breastfeeding could be masked due to prolonged breastfeeding in children with early signs of atopic diseases [26]. Accordingly, our study may underestimate the true preventive effects of breastfeeding. Regarding the risk of residual confounding, we observed that early eczema was associated with both, exposition (i.e., full breastfeeding) and outcome (i.e., allergic diseases). Accordingly, future studies investigating allergy prevention effects of breastfeeding should consider early eczema as potential mediator or confounder. Last but not least, the GINIplus sample is not representative for children in Germany, which might restrict the external validity of our results. However, e.g., full-breastfeeding prevalence was comparable to the representative SuSe I study conducted in 1997: in SuSe I, a prevalence of 48.5 % of breastfeeding only (exclusive and predominant breastfeeding, i.e., breastfeeding plus liquids) was found in West Germany at the age of 4 months [27]. We therefore believe that our results give a good impression on the relevance of breastfeeding for allergy prevention in the general population.

5. Conclusions

Preventive effects of breastfeeding seem to attenuate with increasing age at least in children with family risk of allergies. However, there is no rebound effect in fully breastfed children without early eczema with regard to allergies in later life. Accordingly, data from GINIplus confirm that breastfeeding should be recommended in terms of allergy prevention—at least for beneficial effects in early life. Potential long-term protection against rhinitis in children with low family risk of allergies needs to be confirmed in future studies.

Supplementary Materials: The following supporting information can be downloaded at: https://www.mdpi.com/article/10.3390/nu15122780/s1, Table S1: Number of participants during follow-up stratified by eczema during first 3 years and mode of milk feeding in the first 4 months in the intervention cohort and by early eczema and status of full-breastfeeding (FB) in the first 4 months in the non-intervention cohort with family risk of atopy (FH+) and without family risk of atopy (FH−); Table S2: Cumulative incidence of allergic diseases from birth to 20 years of age for fully breastfed infants in comparison with formula fed infants in the intervention-cohort and in comparison with non-fully breastfed infants with family risk of atopy (FH+) and without family risk of atopy (FH−) in the non-intervention-cohort.

Author Contributions: Conceptualization, L.L., B.F.-P. and M.G.; Formal analysis, B.F.-P.; Funding acquisition, A.v.B. and M.G.; Investigation, M.G.; Methodology, B.F.-P., M.S., T.S. and M.G.; Software, B.F.-P.; Supervision, M.G.; Visualization, B.F.-P.; Writing—original draft, L.L., B.F.-P. and M.G.; Writing—review and editing, M.S., T.S., J.H., A.v.B., D.B., C.-P.B. and S.K. All authors have read and agreed to the published version of the manuscript.

Funding: The GINI study was mainly supported for the first 3 years by the Federal Ministry for Education, Science, Research and Technology. The 4-year, 6-year, 10-year, 15-year, and 20-year follow-up examinations of the GINI study were covered from the respective budgets of the 5 study centers (Helmholtz Zentrum Munich (former GSF), Research Institute at Marien-Hospital Wesel, LMU Munich, TU Munich and from 6 years onwards also from IUF—Leibniz Research Institute for Environmental Medicine at the University of Düsseldorf) and a grant from the Federal Ministry for Environment (IUF Düsseldorf, FKZ 20462296). Further, the 15-year follow-up examination of the GINI study was supported by the Commission of the European Communities, the 7th Framework Program: MeDALL project. The 15-year and 20-year follow-up examinations were additionally supported by the companies Mead Johnson and Nestlé. The present data analysis was additionally supported by Nestlé. The funders had no role in the design of the study; in the collection, analyses, or interpretation of data; in the writing of the manuscript; or in the decision to publish the results". We acknowledge support for the publication cost by the Open Access Publication Fund of Paderborn University.

Institutional Review Board Statement: The study was conducted in accordance with the Declaration of Helsinki, and approved by the local ethics committees (20-year follow-up: Bavarian General Medical Council No. 10090 and Medical Council of North Rhine-Westphalia No. 2015491).

Informed Consent Statement: Written informed consent was obtained from all participating families.

Data Availability Statement: Data available on reasonable request due to restrictions of privacy, provided it is consistent with the consent given by the study participants. In some cases, ethical approval can be obtained for the release. Lastly, a data transfer agreement must be accepted and the request must be approved by the studies' steering committees. Requests should be addressed to MS (marie.standl@helmholtz-muenchen.de).

Acknowledgments: The authors thank all the families for their participation in the GINIplus study. Furthermore, we thank all members of the GINIplus Study Group for their excellent work. The GINIplus Study group consists of the following: Institute of Epidemiology I, Helmholtz Zentrum München, German Research Center for Environmental Health, Neuherberg (Heinrich, J., Brüske, I., Schulz, H., Flexeder, C., Zeller, C., Standl, M., Schnappinger, M., Ferland, M., Thiering, E., Tiesler, C.); formerly Department of Pediatrics, Marien-Hospital, Wesel (Berdel, D., von Berg, A.); Evangelisches Krankenhaus Düsseldorf (Gappa, M., Libuda, L.); Ludwig-Maximilians-University of Munich, Dr von Hauner Children's Hospital (Koletzko, S.); Child and Adolescent Medicine, University Hospital rechts der Isar of the Technical University Munich (Bauer, C.P., Hoffmann, U.); IUF- Environmental Health Research Institute, Düsseldorf (Schikowski, T., Link, E., Klümper, C., Krämer, U., Sugiri, D.).

Conflicts of Interest: L.L. is member of the German National Breastfeeding Committee. A.v.B. has received speakers' fees from Nestlé Nutrition Institute. The Research Institute at the Marien-Hospital has received a grant from Nestlé Vevey, Switzerland. S.K. received research support from BioGaia, Mead Johnson and Nestec Nutrition, and received honoraria or consultant fees from Abbvie, BerlinChemie, Celgene, Danone, Janssen, Mead Johnson, Nestlé, Pharmacosmos, Pfizer, Takeda, Vifor. M.G. received research funding from Boehringer and Nestlé Vevey, Switzerland; and received honoraria for lectures and consultant fees from ALK, Astra Zeneca, Boehringer, Chiesi, GSK, HAL, Novartis, Omron, Pari and Sanofi/Regeneron.

References

1. Koletzko, B.; Bauer, C.-P.; Cierpka, M.; Cremer, M.; Flothkötter, M.; Graf, C.; Heindl, I.; Hellmers, C.; Kersting, M.; Krawinkel, M.; et al. Ernährung und Bewegung von Säuglingen und stillenden Frauen. *Mon. Kinderheilkd* **2016**, *164*, 771–798. [CrossRef]
2. Kopp, M.V.; Muche-Borowski, C.; Abou-Dakn, M.; Ahrens, B.; Beyer, K.; Blümchen, K.; Bubel, P.; Chaker, A.; Cremer, M.; Ensenauer, R.; et al. S3 guideline Allergy Prevention. *Allergol. Sel.* **2022**, *6*, 61–97. [CrossRef] [PubMed]
3. Van Meel, E.R.; de Jong, M.; Elbert, N.J.; den Dekker, H.T.; Reiss, I.K.; de Jongste, J.C.; Jaddoe, V.W.V.; Duijts, L. Duration and exclusiveness of breastfeeding and school-age lung function and asthma. *Ann. Allergy Asthma Immunol.* **2017**, *119*, 21–26.e2. [CrossRef] [PubMed]
4. Groenwold, R.H.H.; Tilling, K.; Moons, K.G.M.; Hoes, A.W.; van der Ent, C.K.; Kramer, M.S.; Martin, R.M.; Sterne, J.A.C. Breast-feeding and health consequences in early childhood: Is there an impact of time-dependent confounding? *Ann. Nutr. Metab.* **2014**, *65*, 139–148. [CrossRef]
5. Ajetunmobi, O.M.; Whyte, B.; Chalmers, J.; Tappin, D.M.; Wolfson, L.; Fleming, M.; MacDonald, A.; Wood, R.; Stockton, D.L. Breastfeeding is associated with reduced childhood hospitalization: Evidence from a Scottish Birth Cohort (1997–2009). *J. Pediatr.* **2015**, *166*, 620–625.e4. [CrossRef]
6. Jelding-Dannemand, E.; Malby Schoos, A.-M.; Bisgaard, H. Breast-feeding does not protect against allergic sensitization in early childhood and allergy-associated disease at age 7 years. *J. Allergy Clin. Immunol.* **2015**, *136*, 1302–1308.e13. [CrossRef]
7. Leung, J.Y.Y.; Kwok, M.K.; Leung, G.M.; Schooling, C.M. Breastfeeding and childhood hospitalizations for asthma and other wheezing disorders. *Ann. Epidemiol.* **2016**, *26*, 21–27.e3. [CrossRef]
8. Filipiak-Pittroff, B.; Koletzko, S.; Krämer, U.; Standl, M.; Bauer, C.-P.; Berdel, D.; von Berg, A. Full breastfeeding and allergies from infancy until adolescence in the GINIplus cohort. *Pediatr. Allergy Immunol.* **2018**, *29*, 96–101. [CrossRef]
9. Laubereau, B.; Brockow, I.; Zirngibl, A.; Koletzko, S.; Gruebl, A.; von Berg, A.; Filipiak-Pittroff, B.; Berdel, D.; Bauer, C.P.; Reinhardt, D.; et al. Effect of breast-feeding on the development of atopic dermatitis during the first 3 years of life--results from the GINI-birth cohort study. *J. Pediatr.* **2004**, *144*, 602–607. [CrossRef]
10. Schoetzau, A.; Filipiak-Pittroff, B.; Franke, K.; Koletzko, S.; von Berg, A.; Gruebl, A.; Bauer, C.P.; Berdel, D.; Reinhardt, D.; Wichmann, H.-E. Effect of exclusive breast-feeding and early solid food avoidance on the incidence of atopic dermatitis in high-risk infants at 1 year of age. *Pediatr. Allergy Immunol.* **2002**, *13*, 234–242. [CrossRef]
11. Lodge, C.J.; Tan, D.J.; Lau, M.X.Z.; Dai, X.; Tham, R.; Lowe, A.J.; Bowatte, G.; Allen, K.J.; Dharmage, S.C. Breastfeeding and asthma and allergies: A systematic review and meta-analysis. *Acta Paediatr.* **2015**, *104*, 38–53. [CrossRef]
12. Gappa, M.; Filipiak-Pittroff, B.; Libuda, L.; von Berg, A.; Koletzko, S.; Bauer, C.-P.; Heinrich, J.; Schikowski, T.; Berdel, D.; Standl, M. Long-term effects of hydrolyzed formulae on atopic diseases in the GINI study. *Allergy* **2021**, *76*, 1903–1907. [CrossRef] [PubMed]
13. Berg, A.v.; Krämer, U.; Link, E.; Bollrath, C.; Heinrich, J.; Brockow, I.; Koletzko, S.; Grübl, A.; Filipiak-Pittroff, B.; Wichmann, H.-E.; et al. Impact of early feeding on childhood eczema: Development after nutritional intervention compared with the natural course—The GINIplus study up to the age of 6 years. *Clin. Exp. Allergy* **2010**, *40*, 627–636. [CrossRef]
14. Von Berg, A.; Filipiak-Pittroff, B.; Schulz, H.; Hoffmann, U.; Link, E.; Sußmann, M.; Schnappinger, M.; Brüske, I.; Standl, M.; Krämer, U.; et al. Allergic manifestation 15 years after early intervention with hydrolyzed formulas--the GINI Study. *Allergy* **2016**, *71*, 210–219. [CrossRef] [PubMed]
15. Heinrich, J.; Brüske, I.; Cramer, C.; Hoffmann, U.; Schnappinger, M.; Schaaf, B.; von Berg, A.; Berdel, D.; Krämer, U.; Lehmann, I.; et al. GINIplus and LISAplus—Design and selected results of two German birth cohorts about natural course of atopic diseases and their determinants. *Allergol. Sel.* **2017**, *1*, 85–95. [CrossRef] [PubMed]
16. Von Berg, A.; Koletzko, S.; Grübl, A.; Filipiak-Pittroff, B.; Wichmann, H.-E.; Bauer, C.P.; Reinhardt, D.; Berdel, D. The effect of hydrolyzed cow's milk formula for allergy prevention in the first year of life: The German Infant Nutritional Intervention Study, a randomized double-blind trial. *J. Allergy Clin. Immunol.* **2003**, *111*, 533–540. [CrossRef]
17. Kleinbaum, D.G. *Epidemiologic Research: Principles and Quantitative Methods*; John Wiley & Sons: Hoboken, NJ, USA, 1982; ISBN 047128985X.
18. Diggle, P. *Analysis of Longitudinal Data*, 2nd ed.; Oxford University Press: Oxford, UK, 2002; ISBN 0191664324.
19. Kilanowski, A.; Thiering, E.; Wang, G.; Kumar, A.; Kress, S.; Flexeder, C.; Bauer, C.-P.; Berdel, D.; von Berg, A.; Bergström, A.; et al. Allergic disease trajectories up to adolescence: Characteristics, early-life, and genetic determinants. *Allergy* **2022**, *78*, 836–850. [CrossRef]
20. Global Initiative for Asthma. Global Strategy for Asthma Management and Prevention 2022. Available online: https://ginasthma.org/wp-content/uploads/2022/07/GINA-Main-Report-2022-FINAL-22-07-01-WMS.pdf (accessed on 14 December 2022).
21. Chen, C.-N.; Lin, Y.-C.; Ho, S.-R.; Fu, C.-M.; Chou, A.-K.; Yang, Y.-H. Association of Exclusive Breastfeeding with Asthma Risk among Preschool Children: An Analysis of National Health and Nutrition Examination Survey Data, 1999 to 2014. *Nutrients* **2022**, *14*, 4250. [CrossRef]
22. Hou, W.; Guan, F.; Xia, L.; Xu, Y.; Huang, S.; Zeng, P. Investigating the influence of breastfeeding on asthma in children under 12 years old in the UK Biobank. *Front. Immunol.* **2022**, *13*, 967101. [CrossRef]
23. Paramasivam, K.; Michie, C.; Opara, E.; Jewell, A.P. Human breast milk immunology: A review. *Int. J. Fertil. Womens. Med.* **2006**, *51*, 208–217.

24. Flohr, C.; Henderson, A.J.; Kramer, M.S.; Patel, R.; Thompson, J.; Rifas-Shiman, S.L.; Yang, S.; Vilchuck, K.; Bogdanovich, N.; Hameza, M.; et al. Effect of an Intervention to Promote Breastfeeding on Asthma, Lung Function, and Atopic Eczema at Age 16 Years: Follow-up of the PROBIT Randomized Trial. *JAMA Pediatr.* **2018**, *172*, e174064. [CrossRef] [PubMed]
25. Schmitt, J.; Apfelbacher, C.; Chen, C.-M.; Romanos, M.; Sausenthaler, S.; Koletzko, S.; Bauer, C.-P.; Hoffmann, U.; Krämer, U.; Berdel, D.; et al. Infant-onset eczema in relation to mental health problems at age 10 years: Results from a prospective birth cohort study (German Infant Nutrition Intervention plus). *J. Allergy Clin. Immunol.* **2010**, *125*, 404–410. [CrossRef] [PubMed]
26. Lowe, A.J.; Carlin, J.B.; Bennett, C.M.; Abramson, M.J.; Hosking, C.S.; Hill, D.J.; Dharmage, S.C. Atopic disease and breast-feeding--cause or consequence? *J. Allergy Clin. Immunol.* **2006**, *117*, 682–687. [CrossRef] [PubMed]
27. Dulon, M.; Kersting, M.; Schach, S. Duration of breastfeeding and associated factors in Western and Eastern Germany. *Acta Paediatr.* **2001**, *90*, 931–935. [CrossRef] [PubMed]

Disclaimer/Publisher's Note: The statements, opinions and data contained in all publications are solely those of the individual author(s) and contributor(s) and not of MDPI and/or the editor(s). MDPI and/or the editor(s) disclaim responsibility for any injury to people or property resulting from any ideas, methods, instructions or products referred to in the content.

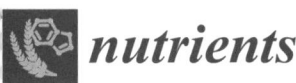

Article

Women's Satisfaction with Breastfeeding and Risk of Exclusive Breastfeeding Interruption

Agnes Meire Branco Leria Bizon [1,*], Camila Giugliani [2,3] and Elsa Regina Justo Giugliani [1,3]

1. Programa de Pós-Graduação em Saúde da Criança e do Adolescente, Faculdade de Medicina, Universidade Federal do Rio Grande do Sul (UFRGS), Porto Alegre 90035-003, RS, Brazil
2. Programa de Pós-Graduação em Epidemiologia, Faculdade de Medicina, Universidade Federal do Rio Grande do Sul (UFRGS), Porto Alegre 90035-003, RS, Brazil; cgiugliani@hcpa.edu.br
3. Hospital de Clínicas de Porto Alegre, Porto Alegre 90035-003, RS, Brazil
* Correspondence: agnesbizon.nutri@gmail.com; Tel.: +55-14991414789

Abstract: This prospective cohort study was conducted to evaluate the association between women's satisfaction with breastfeeding at 1 month post-partum and the risk of exclusive breastfeeding (EBF) interruption before 6 months. 287 mother–infant dyads randomly selected from two maternity hospitals were followed from birth to 24 months of infant's age. Women's satisfaction with breastfeeding was assessed using the Maternal Breastfeeding Evaluation Scale (MBFES) at 1 month. The association between women's satisfaction with breastfeeding and risk of EBF interruption before 6 months was estimated using Cox proportional hazards model. Kaplan–Meier survival curves for EBF were compared between women with lower satisfaction with breastfeeding (MBFES score < median 124) and those with higher satisfaction (MBFES score $\geq$ 124). Median EBF duration in women with higher satisfaction was 120 days (95%CI 109–131), vs. 26 days (95%CI 19–33) in less satisfied women. Each additional point on MBFES promoted a reduction of 2.0% in the risk of EBF interruption. Among women with satisfaction scores < 124, the risk of EBF interruption was 86% higher when compared with those $\geq$ 124 (adjusted hazard ratio 1.86; 95%CI 1.41–2.46). Lower maternal satisfaction with breastfeeding in the first month post-partum is associated with a higher risk of EBF interruption before 6 months.

Keywords: exclusive breastfeeding; maternal and child health; personal satisfaction

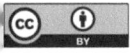

1. Introduction

Despite the large body of evidence supporting the positive impact of breastfeeding on both child and maternal health, this way of feeding a small infant is still too seldom practiced [1]. At the global level, 48% of infants younger than 6 months are exclusively breastfed, 70% are breastfed at 1 year, and 45% at 2 years [2]. In Brazil, these breastfeeding indicators are below the global average: 45.8%, 52.1% and 35.5%, respectively [3]. Both globally and in Brazil, much effort will be needed to achieve the WHO/UNICEF 2030 targets for exclusive breastfeeding (70%), continued breastfeeding up to at least 1 year (80%), and continued breastfeeding up to at least 2 years (60%) [2].

The identification of factors that can influence breastfeeding duration—especially modifiable ones—is paramount for the planning and implementation of interventions, especially in populations which are most vulnerable to early interruption of breastfeeding. Among the modifiable factors that deserve investigation, women's satisfaction with breastfeeding has become increasingly valuable, since it involves aspects that are often neglected by health professionals, such as expectations, desires, and the needs of breastfeeding women and their infants, the bonding between mother and child, as well as the woman's self-confidence as a mother [4–7].

Breastfeeding success is often assessed by researchers and health professionals based on its duration or on the absence of problems. Nevertheless, some studies have shown that, from the woman's point of view, the quality of the breastfeeding experience seems to be as important as or even more important than the duration or exclusivity of breastfeeding [5–10]. Still, women's satisfaction with breastfeeding has been given little value so far.

The first studies on the relationship between maternal satisfaction with breastfeeding and the duration of this practice emerged in the 1990s. Since then, two studies have shown a weak correlation between women's satisfaction with breastfeeding and its duration [8] and one found a strong correlation [10]. Two other studies showed a positive association between them [5,6]. Studies evaluating the influence of women's satisfaction on exclusive breastfeeding duration are scarce [10,11] and none have evaluated the influence of maternal satisfaction with breastfeeding in the first month after birth on the practice of exclusive breastfeeding throughout the first 6 months of the infant's life. Thus, considering the importance of exclusive breastfeeding and the scarcity of studies exploring women's satisfaction with breastfeeding, especially in Brazil, the present study aimed to evaluate the association between women's satisfaction with breastfeeding at 1 month post-partum and the risk of exclusive breastfeeding interruption throughout the first 6 months. These findings might be useful in promoting, protecting and supporting breastfeeding, at both the individual and collective levels, not only to improve indicators, but also to enhance the quality of women's breastfeeding experience.

2. Materials and Methods

In this prospective cohort study conducted in the municipality of Porto Alegre, southern Brazil, mother–infant dyads were followed for 24 months. The sample comprised mothers who gave birth at two large maternity hospitals in the city, one public and one private. In 2016, these two maternity hospitals accounted for 3725 and 4182 deliveries, respectively, of a total of 30,268 [12,13]. In order to be included in the study, mothers and their respective newborns should meet the following criteria: residing in the municipality at the time of delivery; singleton, live full-term newborn (gestational age $\geq$ 37 weeks); mother and infant staying together in the same room (rooming-in) during the hospital stay; and having initiated breastfeeding. Exclusion criteria consisted of any problem observed in the mother or newborn that could significantly affect breastfeeding, e.g., orofacial malformations or any serious illness that required separation between mother and newborn. Dyads residing in areas with high rates of violence (defined as areas where primary health care worker visits were suspended for security reasons) were also excluded in order to preserve the safety of the interviewers.

A sample size of 219 women was calculated for this study's objective, using the WinPepi version 11.43, considering the following parameters: significance level of 5%, power of 80%, 20% of participants lost to follow-up, and a difference of 20 percentage points in the rates of exclusive breastfeeding in infants younger than 6 months between women with higher vs. lower levels of satisfaction, according to data found in the literature [14]. In order to reflect the public vs. private distribution in health service utilization in Brazil (approximately 70% and 30%, respectively [15]), we projected the selection of one woman at a private maternity hospital for every two women at the public facility.

Women were selected daily, also on the weekends, between January and July 2016, at the rooming-in section of the obstetric units. Dyads meeting the inclusion criteria and who had given birth in the past 24 h were considered eligible. Subsequently, the eligible dyads were randomly selected for inclusion using the lottery method. If the initially selected dyad was found to meet an exclusion criterion, or refused to participate, that dyad was replaced by repeating the lottery draw procedure.

The dyads were followed from birth to 24 months of infant's age, or to the age of weaning if before 24 months. For the present study, only the data relating to the infant's 6 months of life were used.

Interviews were conducted by 10 interviewers, all working in the health field and previously trained for the task. The first contact was made at the maternity ward, where women were invited to participate in the study; those who agreed were asked to answer a brief questionnaire covering demographic data and delivery information. Between 31 and 37 days after birth, the first home visit took place. At this occasion, a standardized questionnaire was administered to obtain data on socio-demographic characteristics, woman's health, information on latest pregnancy, delivery and immediate post-partum period, and the first month of life of the infant. Subsequent contacts were made by telephone at 2 and 4 months, and in person during a home visit at 6 months, to obtain updated information on the infant's feeding habits. Dyads who were not found after three telephone contact and one home visit attempts were considered as losses. Whenever dyads were lost to follow-up at some point of the data collection process, attempts were made to interview these women at subsequent data collection points.

Women's satisfaction level with breastfeeding in the first month post-partum was the main variable of interest. The information was obtained via self-application of the Maternal Breastfeeding Evaluation Scale (MBFES) [16] during the first home visit. This instrument assesses maternal perception of the quality of their breastfeeding experience, considering not only maternal factors, but also child factors. The original version of the MBFES [17] is comprised of 30 items, distributed into three subscales: maternal pleasure and role, child satisfaction and growth, and maternal lifestyle and body image. For each item, there are 5 Likert-type answers, ranging from 1 point (totally disagree) to 5 points (totally agree); higher values indicate higher satisfaction levels. The MBFES used in the present study was validated for use in the Brazilian population [16] starting from the version translated and validated into Portuguese by Galvão [6]. The Brazilian version maintained the three subscales of the original instrument, but resulted in 29 items, out of the original 30, due to the low factor loading of one item. Thus, the total possible score could range from 29 to 145. The validation process of the Brazilian version of the MBFES showed that it is a valid and reliable tool to be applied to the Brazilian population (Cronbach's alpha = 0.88, 95%CI 0.86–0.90). More details of the Brazilian Portuguese validation process can be found elsewhere [16].

The outcome of this study was defined as the interruption of exclusive breastfeeding before 6 months of infant's age, measured as days of exclusive breastfeeding. Exclusive breastfeeding was defined according to the WHO criteria, i.e., receiving breast milk, either directly from the mother's breast, extracted from the mother's breast, or human donor breast milk, with no other liquid or solid foods, not even water, except for drops or solutions containing vitamins, oral rehydration salts, mineral supplements or medicine [18].

Statistical analyses were performed using the Statistical Package for the Social Sciences (SPSS) for Windows version 21.0 (IBM, Chicago, IL, USA). Using the chi-square test, the group of women who concluded the study were compared to those who were excluded, to those who refused to participate, and also to those who were lost to follow-up. Results showing $p \leq 0.05$ were considered significant.

Kaplan–Meier survival curves were calculated to illustrate the time to interruption of exclusive breastfeeding among women presenting lower satisfaction with breastfeeding (MBFES score below the median) vs. those with higher satisfaction levels (MBFES score at or above the median). The survival analysis was also used to calculate the median duration of exclusive breastfeeding and to assess the accumulated probability of exclusive breastfeeding duration.

The association between women's satisfaction with breastfeeding and risk of exclusive breastfeeding interruption before 6 months was estimated as hazard ratios and respective 95% confidence intervals (95%CI) using the Cox proportional hazards multivariate regression model. The explanatory variable was used in two different ways: via the MBFES score obtained continuously, and via the median obtained with application of the instrument (124 points).

Variables added to the adjustment model were those reaching $p \leq 0.2$ in the univariate analysis. Categories used as reference were those known to protect exclusive breastfeeding, according to information from the literature. The following variables were explored: sociodemographic characteristics of the woman (age, socio-economic level, schooling level, skin color, parity, and cohabitation with infant's father), infant's sex, data related to hospital care (type of birth and type of hospital (public vs. private)), and breastfeeding problems in the first month post-partum (breast engorgement, pain while breastfeeding, cracked nipples, perceived low milk supply, infant difficulties with latching on/sucking). Socio-economic level was divided in five strata, A (better off) to E, according to criteria proposed by the Brazilian Association of Research Companies [19]. The effect measure was considered to be modified when $p \leq 0.05$.

To control for data quality, answers given to key questions of the questionnaire were checked in approximately 5% of the sample, via telephone contact, concomitantly with data collection, at all data collection stages.

The present study was conducted in line with norms and regulations applicable to research involving humans (Resolution 466/2012 of the Brazilian National Health Council) and was approved by the Ethics Committees of Hospital de Clínicas de Porto Alegre and Hospital Moinhos de Vento (CAAE 49938015.3.0000.5327 and 46775115.0.3002.5330). All women who agreed to participate in the study signed an informed consent form before the start of data collection.

3. Results

Of the 503 women selected for the study using the lottery method, 124 were excluded because they lived in areas with high rates of violence, and 25 (5%) refused to participate in the study. The characteristics of the excluded women did not differ from those of the women who participated in the study with regard to skin color ($p = 0.949$), parity ($p = 0.384$), age ($p = 0.286$) and infant's sex ($p = 0.746$); however, the women excluded showed lower schooling level ($p < 0.001$) and a higher prevalence of vaginal deliveries ($p = 0.01$). Conversely, the profile of the women who refused to participate was similar to that of the women who participated in the study with regard to skin color ($p = 0.125$), parity ($p = 1.00$), and age ($p = 0.279$), but they differed by presenting lower schooling level ($p < 0.001$).

In addition, 67 women could not be located for the first home visit interview. These women showed differences in relation to the women who participated in the study with regard to schooling level and skin color—they showed lower schooling level (none had started college vs. 43.2%; $p < 0.01$) and a higher prevalence of white skin color (87.7% vs. 75.3%; $p = 0.032$). A total of 30 (10.4%) women were lost to follow-up, i.e., interviewed at the end of the first month but not found for the interview at 6 months.

After the losses and excluding women who interrupted breastfeeding before 6 months, the number of mother–infant dyads included in the study at each data collection stage was as follows: 287 at 30 days, 228 at 60 days, 218 at 120 days, and 213 at 180 days.

Maternal age ranged from 16 to 45 years, with a mean of 29 years (standard deviation ± 6.6). Most women had white skin color, lived with the infant's father, and did not have a college degree. The following variables were associated with exclusive breastfeeding duration in the univariate analysis ($p \leq 0.2$) and were therefore included in the multivariate model: maternal age and schooling level, cohabitation with infant's father, and breastfeeding problems in the first 30 days post-partum, namely, cracked nipples, perceived low milk supply, and infant difficulties with latching on/sucking. The socio-economic variable was also associated with the outcome, but was not added to the multivariate analysis due to its strong interaction as a proxy for schooling level (Table 1).

Table 1. Sample characteristics (n = 287). Porto Alegre, Brazil, 2016.

Variable	n = 287	%	Exclusive Breastfeeding Interruption [a] p [b]
Age			
<30 years	142	49.5	0.074
≥30 years [e]	145	50.5	
School level (college)			
Yes [e]	100	34.8	0.016
No	187	65.2	
Socio-economic classification			
A/B [e]	163	56.8	0.233
C/D/E	122	42.5	
Lost	2	0.07	
Skin color			
White	216	75.3	0.554
Black/brown [e]	71	24.7	
Parity			
Primiparous	142	49.5	0.424
Multiparous [e]	145	50.5	
Cohabitation with infant's father			
Yes [e]	248	86.4	0.007
No	39	13.6	
Return to work [c]			
Yes	142	49.5	0.220
No [e]	145	50.5	
Hospital type			
Public [e]	194	67.6	0.706
Private	93	32.4	
Type of delivery			
Vaginal [e]	149	51.9	0.995
C-section	138	48.1	
Newborn sex			
Male [e]	136	47.4	0.814
Female	151	51.6	
Breast engorgement [d]			
Yes	134	46.7	0.860
No [e]	153	53.3	
Pain while breastfeeding [d]			
Yes	182	63.4	0.328
No [e]	105	36.6	

Table 1. Cont.

Variable	n = 287	%	Exclusive Breastfeeding Interruption [a] p [b]
Cracked nipples [d]			
Yes	135	47.0	0.028
No [e]	152	53.0	
Perceived low milk supply [d]			
Yes	84	29.3	<0.001
No [e]	203	70.7	
Difficulties latching on/sucking [d]			
Yes	63	22.0	<0.001
No [e]	224	78.0	

[a] Exclusive breastfeeding interruption before 6 months of infant's age. [b] Cox regression to test variables included in the multivariate model ($p \geq 0.20$). [c] Return to work at any time in the first 6 months post-partum. [d] Breastfeeding problems in the first 30 days post-partum. [e] Reference category.

The median MBFES score in the sample was 124, with an interquartile range of 113 to 131. The median duration of exclusive breastfeeding in the whole sample was 67 days (95%CI 41–93), i.e., 120 days (95%CI 109–131) among women with higher levels of satisfaction (score at or above the median) and 26 days (95%CI 19–33) among the women with lower satisfaction (score below the median). This difference was statistically significant ($p < 0.001$).

Figure 1 shows Kaplan–Meier survival curves calculated for exclusive breastfeeding over the first 6 months of infant's age according to women's satisfaction levels with breastfeeding (higher vs. lower levels) assessed at 30 days of life of the infant.

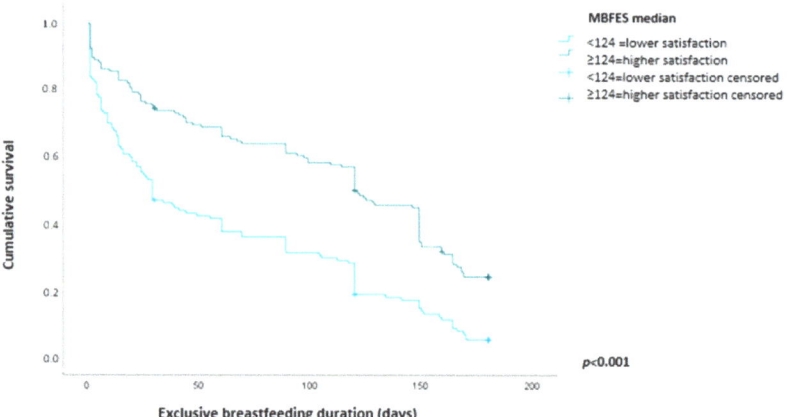

Figure 1. Survival curves for exclusive breastfeeding duration, considering woman's satisfaction with breastfeeding. Porto Alegre, Brazil, 2018. MBFES = Maternal Breastfeeding Evaluation Scale.

A positive association was found between exclusive breastfeeding duration and MBFES score at 30 days: for each additional point in the score, a reduction of 2.0% was observed in the risk of exclusive breastfeeding interruption. Among women with lower levels of satisfaction (score < 124), the risk of exclusive breastfeeding interruption was 86%

higher when compared with women showing higher satisfaction levels (scoring ≥ 124; Table 2).

Table 2. Cox proportional hazards multivariate regression model to test the association between risk of exclusive breastfeeding interruption before 6 months of infant's life and women's satisfaction with breastfeeding in the first month post-partum (n = 287). Porto Alegre, Brazil, 2018.

Model	Univariate Analysis		Multivariate Analysis [a]	
	HR (95%CI)	p	HR (95%CI)	p
Risk of exclusive breastfeeding interruption × MBFES score	0.97 (0.96–0.98)	<0.001	0.98 (0.97–0.99)	<0.001
Risk of exclusive breastfeeding interruption × lower satisfaction with breastfeeding [b]	2.15 (1.66–2.78)	<0.001	1.86 (1.41–2.46)	<0.001

95%CI = 95% confidence interval; HR = hazard ratio; MBFES = Maternal Breastfeeding Evaluation Scale. [a] Adjustment variables: maternal age, maternal schooling level, cohabitation with infant's father, and breastfeeding problems: cracked nipples, perceived low milk supply, and difficulty latching on/sucking. [b] Median MBFES score: 124.

Table 3 presents the accumulated probability of exclusive breastfeeding over the first 6 months of life of the infant, according to maternal satisfaction with breastfeeding. The data show that the risk of breastfeeding interruption among women with lower satisfaction levels increases over time.

Table 3. Cumulative probability of risk of exclusive breastfeeding interruption along the infant's first 6 months of age according to maternal satisfaction with breastfeeding measured at 30 days post-partum. Porto Alegre, Brazil, 2018.

Time	Exclusive Breastfeeding Probability (%) [a]			Exclusive Breastfeeding Interruption before 6 Months, HR [b] (95%CI) [c]	p
	Total Id	MBFES < 124 Id	MBFES ≥ 124 Id		
30 days	58.9	43.6	73.5	1.68 (1.09–2.57)	0.018
60 days	50.4	34.9	65.2	1.64 (1.11–2.43)	0.013
90 days	45.1	29.0	60.3	1.76 (1.24–2.51)	0.002
120 days	33.7	17.4	49.2	1.73 (1.23–2.44)	0.002
150 days	22.8	12.7	32.6	1.73 (1.29–2.32)	<0.001
180 days	14.5	4.8	23.7	1.86 (1.41–2.46)	<0.001

95%CI = 95% confidence interval; HR = hazard ratio; Id = incidence density; MBFES = Maternal Breastfeeding Evaluation Scale. [a] Percentages were obtained using the Kaplan–Meier method. [b] Adjusted for the following variables: maternal age and schooling level, cohabitation with infant's father, occurrence of cracked nipples, perceived low milk supply, and difficulty latching on/sucking. [c] 95%CIs obtained with Cox proportional hazards multivariate regression model.

4. Discussion

The present study showed that women with lower levels of satisfaction with breastfeeding in the first month of life of the infant, as assessed by the MBFES, were at an increased risk of interrupting exclusive breastfeeding before 6 months. For every additional point in the MBFES score, that risk decreased by 2.0%. The risk of exclusive breastfeeding interruption was 86% higher among women scoring below the median when compared to women with higher scores. Particularly interesting is the fact that, throughout the period assessed, lower levels of satisfaction with breastfeeding in the first month increased the risk of exclusive breastfeeding interruption at all subsequent months, suggesting that maternal satisfaction with breastfeeding in the first month post-partum can be an indicator of risk of exclusive breastfeeding interruption over the first 6 months post-partum.

There are already some studies pointing to an association between women's satisfaction with any breastfeeding and its duration. Among the most significant is the study by Galvão [6], carried out with Portuguese women, which showed a close relationship between satisfaction with breastfeeding measured at different times and the duration of any breastfeeding. Yet studies on breastfeeding satisfaction focusing on exclusive breastfeeding are rare. One of them is a longitudinal, quasi-experimental study, conducted in Australia [10]. That study found a strong positive correlation between maternal perception of breastfeeding success, assessed using MBFES, and exclusive breastfeeding length ($r = 0.63$; $p < 0.001$). The other study, conducted in Poland, assessed maternal satisfaction with breastfeeding at 3 months of the infant's life, using a scale from 0 to 10, with 10 being the best level. The authors concluded that maternal satisfaction with breastfeeding was one of the predictors of exclusive breastfeeding at 6 months (adjusted OR (95%CI) 1.44 [1.01–2.06], $p = 0.04$) [11]. The results of those two studies are in line with the results of the present study, corroborating the conclusion that women with lower breastfeeding satisfaction levels breastfeed exclusively for shorter times.

The association between lower woman satisfaction with breastfeeding and higher risk of exclusive breastfeeding interruption before 6 months found in this study is not surprising—women who are more satisfied with breastfeeding are expected to breastfeed for longer. However, demonstrating that association is very important, as it adds one further element to the discussion when evaluating risk of early exclusive breastfeeding interruption. When low levels of maternal satisfaction with breastfeeding are detected, interventions should be discussed with the woman to improve her satisfaction, not only in an attempt to increase exclusive breastfeeding duration (if wished by the mother), but also to make the unique breastfeeding experience with the child a more enjoyable one.

The level of satisfaction with breastfeeding observed among the women assessed in this study was high (median of 124 points from a maximum of 145). In Australia, the mean scores obtained with MBFES for maternal satisfaction with breastfeeding were 116 at 15 days post-partum and 117 at 45 days [5]. In the present study, women seemed more satisfied than in the Australian study, especially if we take into consideration that the maximum score of the original instrument is 150 (not 145, as in the Brazilian version). Conversely, the median found in Portuguese women assessed at 1 and 6 months of infant's age was 133 [4], higher than the median in the present investigation.

The significant difference observed in the median exclusive breastfeeding duration among women with higher satisfaction when compared to those with lower satisfaction levels, namely, 120 vs. 26 days, stands out. Certainly, a difference of 3 months in exclusive breastfeeding duration will have consequences to the infant's health. A study conducted in the United Kingdom found an estimated reduction of 53% in hospitalizations due to diarrhea and of 27% due to respiratory tract infections for every month of exclusive breastfeeding [20].

Although this study has shown an association between women's level of satisfaction with breastfeeding and duration of exclusive breastfeeding, it did not explore the reasons for more or less satisfaction. It is known that post-partum depression may increase the risk of early interruption of breastfeeding [21]; on the other hand, weaning can induce or worsen depression [22]. It is very likely that maternal satisfaction with breastfeeding is involved in this association. In fact, the interrelationship between satisfaction with breastfeeding and symptoms of post-partum depression has already been demonstrated [23]. Therefore, in addition to assessing the women's satisfaction with breastfeeding, it is important and necessary to obtain information about the mother's psychosocial environment, including information on her support network, and the mental health of her companion and other close relatives.

Among the strengths of this original study, we highlight its methodology: a cohort study with a randomly selected sample, followed for 24 months, rigorously conducted with face to face interviews, use of an instrument validated for the Brazilian population (MBFES) for the assessment of woman satisfaction with breastfeeding, not to mention the quality control on data collected throughout the follow-up period. The frequency of interviews conducted in the first 6 months of infant's age (at 1, 2, 4, and 6 months) virtually eliminated any memory bias with regard to exclusive breastfeeding duration.

Notwithstanding, the study also presents some limitations. One of them is the exclusion of women who resided in more violent areas, which may have affected the external validity of the findings. Still, comparison of those women to those who completed the study showed that both groups were similar in most of the variables analyzed, differing only with regard to schooling level and type of delivery. This limitation was minimized by including schooling level in the multivariate model; type of delivery was not included due to the absence of a significant association with the outcome in the univariate analysis. Another limitation was the number of participants lost to follow-up, but we believe that the statistical model employed has helped minimize that bias as well. The differences between the group of women who were lost to follow-up and those who completed the study (schooling level and skin color) may have interfered with the estimated values, but not with the association found between women's satisfaction with breastfeeding in the first month post-partum and duration of exclusive breastfeeding.

5. Conclusions

The present study confirmed the existence of an association between women's lower satisfaction with breastfeeding at the first month post-partum and an increased risk of exclusive breastfeeding interruption before 6 months of infant's age. Given the importance of exclusive breastfeeding for the mother–infant dyad, in terms of health benefits and well-being, this study makes a relevant contribution by highlighting the central role played by mother's satisfaction with breastfeeding, as well as the need to assess it in clinical practice, especially in the first month post-partum. Once the health professional becomes aware of the low levels of satisfaction reported by a breastfeeding woman, and discusses with her the factors that might be contributing to this, it becomes possible to propose interventions, with the aim not only of postponing weaning, but especially of promoting a more enjoyable experience for the mother–infant dyad. This is an important contribution for the practice of primary health care workers, clinical breastfeeding consultants, and community midwives. At the collective level, this study suggests that interventions to increase maternal satisfaction with breastfeeding could be useful as part of breastfeeding promotion, protection and support actions, with the goal of increasing the rates of exclusive breastfeeding in infants younger than 6 months, keeping in mind the WHO's and UNICEF's goal to reach 70% by 2030 [2]. Further similar studies should be conducted with other populations to confirm the present findings. Likewise, studies looking in more detail at the factors associated with higher or lower satisfaction with breastfeeding, and at the factors involved in this association, are also warranted. Such knowledge could then help health professionals prevent and also better handle maternal dissatisfaction with breastfeeding.

Author Contributions: Design, A.M.B.L.B., C.G. and E.R.J.G. Data collection, A.M.B.L.B. and C.G. Data analysis/interpretation, A.M.B.L.B., C.G. and E.R.J.G. Writing—original draft preparation, A.M.B.L.B. Writing—review and editing, A.M.B.L.B., C.G. and E.R.J.G. Supervision, C.G. and E.R.J.G. All authors have read and agreed to the published version of the manuscript.

Funding: This research was funded by Conselho Nacional de Desenvolvimento Científico e Tecnológico (CNPq), grant numbers 448186/2014-4 and 405968/2016-7, Coordenação de Aperfeiçoamento de Pessoal de Nível Superior (CAPES), and Fundo de Incentivo à Pesquisa (FIPE) of Hospital de Clínicas de Porto Alegre.

Institutional Review Board Statement: This study was conducted in line with norms and regulations applicable to research involving humans (Resolution 466/2012 of the Brazilian National Health Council) and was approved by the Ethics Committees of the institutions involved (CAAE 49938015.3.0000.5327 and 46775115.0.3002.5330).

Informed Consent Statement: Informed consent was obtained from all subjects involved in the study.

Data Availability Statement: The datasets used and analyzed in this study are available from the corresponding author on request.

Conflicts of Interest: The authors declare no conflict of interest.

References

1. Victora, C.G.; Bahl, R.; Barros, A.J.D.; França, G.V.A.; Horton, S.; Krasevec, J.; Murch, S.; Sankar, M.J.; Walker, N.; Rollins, N.C. Breastfeeding in the 21st century: Epidemiology, mechanisms, and lifelong effect. *Lancet* **2016**, *387*, 475–490. [CrossRef] [PubMed]
2. UNICEF; World Health Organization. Global Breastfeeding Scorecard. 2022. Available online: https://www.globalbreastfeeding-collective.org/media/1921/file (accessed on 24 October 2023).
3. Boccolini, C.S.; Lacerda, E.M.d.A.; Bertoni, N.; Oliveira, N.; Alves-Santos, N.H.; Farias, D.R.; Crispim, S.P.; Carneiro, L.B.V.; Schincaglia, R.M.; Giugliani, E.R.J.; et al. Trends of breastfeeding indicators in Brazil from 1996 to 2019 and the gaps to achieve the WHO/UNICEF 2030 targets. *BMJ Glob. Health* **2023**, *8*, e012529. [CrossRef] [PubMed]
4. Graça, L. Contributos da Intervenção de Enfermagem na Promoção da Transição Para a Maternidade e do Aleitamento Materno. Ph.D. Thesis, Escola Superior de Enfermagem de Lisboa, Universidade de Lisboa, Lisboa, Portugal, 2010. Available online: http://hdl.handle.net/10451/3710 (accessed on 24 October 2023).
5. Cooke, M.; Sheehan, A.; Schimied, V. A description of the relationship between breastfeeding experiences, breastfeeding satisfaction, and weaning in the first 3 months after birth. *J. Hum. Lact.* **2003**, *19*, 145–156. [CrossRef]
6. Galvão, D.M.P.G. Amamentação bem Sucedida: Alguns Factores Determinantes. Ph.D. Thesis, Instituto de Ciências Biomédicas de Abel Salazar, Universidade do Porto, Porto, Portugal, 2002. Available online: https://hdl.handle.net/10216/64575 (accessed on 24 October 2023).
7. Edwards, R. An exploration of maternal satisfaction with breastfeeding as a clinically relevant measure of breastfeeding success. *J. Hum. Lact.* **2018**, *34*, 93–96. [CrossRef]
8. Leff, E.; Gagne, M.; Jefferis, S. Maternal perceptions of successful breastfeeding. *J. Hum. Lact.* **1994**, *10*, 99–104. [CrossRef] [PubMed]
9. Riordan, J.; Woodley, R.; Heaton, K. Testing validity and reliability of an instrument which measures maternal evaluation of breastfeeding. *J. Hum. Lact.* **1994**, *10*, 231–235. [CrossRef] [PubMed]
10. Sheehan, A. A comparison of two methods of antenatal breast-feeding education. *Midwifery* **1999**, *5*, 274–282. [CrossRef]
11. Maliszewska, K.M.; Bidzan, M.; Świątkowska-Freund, M.; Preis, K. Socio-demographic and psychological determinants of exclusive breastfeeding after six months postpartum—A Polish case-cohort study. *Ginekol. Pol.* **2018**, *89*, 153–159. [CrossRef] [PubMed]
12. Hospital de Clínicas de Porto Alegre. Relatório de Gestão e Contas do Exercício de 2017. 2017. Available online: https://www.hcpa.edu.br/downloads/ccom/inst_gestao_publicacoes/relatorio_de_2016.pdf (accessed on 26 October 2023).
13. Hospital Moinhos De Vento. Relatório Anual. 2017. Available online: https://site-hmv-prod.s3.amazonaws.com/72015312-d35f-417c-95ee-44d341bd5a4c.pdf (accessed on 26 October 2023).
14. Conde, R.G.; Guimarães, C.M.S.; Gomes-Sponholz, F.A.; Oria, M.O.; Monteiro, J.C.S. Autoeficácia na amamentação e duração do aleitamento materno exclusivo entre mães adolescentes. *Acta Paul. Enferm.* **2017**, *30*, 383–389. [CrossRef]
15. Barbat, M.M. Frequências de partos normais e cesarianos. Brasil, região Sul, RS, Porto Alegre. Períodos: 2005, 2011, e 2017. [Completion of Course Work]. Faculdade de Medicina, Universidade Federal do Rio Grande do Sul: Porto Alegre, 2018. Available online: https://lume.ufrgs.br/handle/10183/184286 (accessed on 26 October 2023).
16. Senna, A.F.K.; Giugliani, C.; Lago, J.C.A.; Bizon, A.M.B.L.; Martins, A.C.M.; Oliveira, C.A.V.; Giugliani, E.R.J. Validation of a tool to evaluate women's satisfaction with breastfeeding for the Brazilian population. *J. Pediatr.* **2020**, *96*, 84–91. [CrossRef]
17. Leff, E.; Jefferis, S.; Gagne, M. The Development of the Maternal Breastfeeding Evaluation Scale. *J. Hum. Lact.* **1994**, *10*, 105–111. [CrossRef] [PubMed]
18. World Health Organization; The United Nations Children's Fund. Indicators for Assessing Infant and Young Child Feeding Practices: Definitions and Measurement Methods. 2021. Available online: https://www.who.int/publications/i/item/9789240018389 (accessed on 24 October 2023).
19. ABEP. Associação Brasileira de Empresas de Pesquisa. Critério Brasil 2015 e Atualização da Distribuição de Classes Para 2016. 2015. Available online: http://www.abep.org/Servicos/Download.aspx?id=12 (accessed on 24 October 2023).
20. Quigley, M.A.; Kelly, Y.J.; Sacker, A. Breastfeeding and hospitalization for diarrheal and respiratory infection in the United Kingdom Millennium Cohort Study. *Pediatrics* **2007**, *119*, e837–e842. [CrossRef] [PubMed]
21. Dias, C.C.; Figueiredo, B. Breastfeeding and depression: A systematic review of the literature. *J. Affect. Disord.* **2015**, *171*, 142–154. [CrossRef] [PubMed]
22. Borra, C.; Iacovou, M.; Sevilla, A. New evidence on breastfeeding and postpartum depression: The importance of understanding women's intentions. *Matern. Child Health J.* **2015**, *19*, 897–907. [CrossRef] [PubMed]
23. Avilla, J.C.; Giugliani, C.; Bizon, A.M.B.L.; Martins, A.C.M.; Senna, A.F.K.; Giugliani, E.R.J. Association between maternal satisfaction with breastfeeding and postpartum depression symptoms. *PLoS ONE* **2020**, *15*, e0242333. [CrossRef] [PubMed]

Disclaimer/Publisher's Note: The statements, opinions and data contained in all publications are solely those of the individual author(s) and contributor(s) and not of MDPI and/or the editor(s). MDPI and/or the editor(s) disclaim responsibility for any injury to people or property resulting from any ideas, methods, instructions or products referred to in the content.

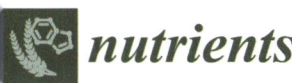 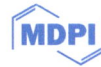

Article

Previous High-Intensity Breastfeeding Lowers the Risk of an Abnormal Fasting Glucose in a Subsequent Pregnancy Oral Glucose Tolerance Test

Sarah J. Melov [1,2,*], James Elhindi [1], Lisa White [3], Justin McNab [1,4], Vincent W. Lee [4,5], Kelly Donnolley [6], Thushari I. Alahakoon [2,4], Suja Padmanabhan [7], N. Wah Cheung [4,7] and Dharmintra Pasupathy [1,2]

1. Reproduction and Perinatal Centre, Faculty of Medicine and Health, The University of Sydney, Sydney, NSW 2006, Australia; james.elhindi@sydney.edu.au (J.E.); justin.mcnab@sydney.edu.au (J.M.); dharmintra.pasupathy@sydney.edu.au (D.P.)
2. Westmead Institute for Maternal and Fetal Medicine, Women's and Newborn Health, Westmead Hospital, Westmead, Sydney, NSW 2145, Australia; indika.alahakoon@health.nsw.gov.au
3. Women's Health Maternity, Blacktown and Mt Druitt Hospitals, Blacktown, NSW 2148, Australia; lisa.white@health.nsw.gov.au
4. Faculty of Medicine and Health, The University of Sydney, Sydney, NSW 2006, Australia; vincent_lee@wmi.usyd.edu.au (V.W.L.); wah.cheung@sydney.edu.au (N.W.C.)
5. Department of Renal Medicine, Westmead Hospital, Westmead, Sydney, NSW 2145, Australia
6. Consumer Representative, Western Sydney Local Health District, Sydney, NSW 2151, Australia
7. Department of Diabetes and Endocrinology, Westmead Hospital, Westmead, Sydney, NSW 2145, Australia; suja.padmanabhan@sydney.edu.au
* Correspondence: sarah.melov@health.nsw.gov.au

Abstract: Breastfeeding is associated with reduced lifetime cardiometabolic risk, but little is known regarding the metabolic benefit in a subsequent pregnancy. The primary aim of this study was to investigate the association between breastfeeding duration and intensity and next pregnancy oral glucose tolerance test (OGTT) results. A retrospective cohort study was conducted from March 2020 to October 2022. All multiparous women who met inclusion criteria and gave birth during the study period were eligible for inclusion. Analysis was stratified by risk for gestational diabetes (GDM). High GDM risk criteria included previous GDM and BMI > 35 kg/m^2. The association between breastfeeding duration and high-intensity breastfeeding (HIBF) and subsequent pregnancy OGTT were assessed with multivariate logistic models adjusted for statistically and clinically relevant covariables. There were 5374 multiparous participants who met the inclusion criteria for analysis. Of these, 61.7% had previously breastfed for >6 months, and 43.4% were at high risk for GDM. HIBF was associated with 47% reduced odds of an abnormal fasting glucose in a subsequent pregnancy OGTT (aOR 0.53; 95%CI 0.38–0.75; $p < 0.01$). There was no association between HIBF and other glucose results on the OGTT. Women who smoked were least likely to breastfeed at high intensity (aOR 0.31; 95%CI 0.21–0.47; $p < 0.01$). South Asian women had 65% higher odds of HIBF than women who identified as White/European (aOR 1.65; 1.36–2.00; $p < 0.01$). This study highlights the importance of exclusive breastfeeding to potentially reduce the prevalence of GDM and may also translate into long-term reduction of cardiometabolic risk.

Keywords: breastfeeding; cardiovascular disease; diabetes; gestational diabetes mellitus; lactation; pregnancy; type 2 diabetes mellitus

Citation: Melov, S.J.; Elhindi, J.; White, L.; McNab, J.; Lee, V.W.; Donnolley, K.; Alahakoon, T.I.; Padmanabhan, S.; Cheung, N.W.; Pasupathy, D. Previous High-Intensity Breastfeeding Lowers the Risk of an Abnormal Fasting Glucose in a Subsequent Pregnancy Oral Glucose Tolerance Test. *Nutrients* **2024**, *16*, 28. https://doi.org/10.3390/nu16010028

Academic Editor: Robert D. Roghair

Received: 26 November 2023
Revised: 16 December 2023
Accepted: 18 December 2023
Published: 21 December 2023

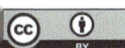

Copyright: © 2023 by the authors. Licensee MDPI, Basel, Switzerland. This article is an open access article distributed under the terms and conditions of the Creative Commons Attribution (CC BY) license (https://creativecommons.org/licenses/by/4.0/).

1. Introduction

Women who breastfeed for a greater duration and more exclusively have a reduced lifetime risk of type 2 diabetes as well as an improved cardiometabolic profile [1–3]. Breastfeeding is supported by groups such as the World Health Organization (WHO), who recommends exclusive breastfeeding as critical for infant health for the first six months of life and continued breastfeeding to age two and beyond [4]. Further to the well-established infant health advantages of breastfeeding, there are globally recognized economic savings linked to the reduction in maternal and infant mortality and morbidity as well as environmental benefits associated with breastfeeding [5,6]. However, exclusive breastfeeding rates remain obstinately low, with little chance that the WHO global target of 70% exclusive breastfeeding during the first six months will be met by the target year of 2030 [7].

Gestational diabetes (GDM) rates vary depending on diagnostic criteria and population; estimates are between 4% and 28%, with a documented rising prevalence [8,9]. Women with GDM have a lifetime twofold increased risk of cardiovascular disease (CVD) and an estimated six- to tenfold maternal future risk of type 2 diabetes [10,11]. The rise in global mortality from non-communicable diseases (NCDs) is a global health crisis, recognized by the United Nations' Sustainable Development Goals to reduce NCD-preventable mortality by one-third by 2030 [12]. To help meet these targets, urgent preventive measures are required to reduce the incidence of GDM and thus maternal and infant type 2 diabetes risk. Various strategies have been adopted, aimed at lowering the prevalence of GDM and type 2 diabetes, focusing principally on lifestyle intervention, with inconsistent findings [13,14]. However, breastfeeding as a type 2 diabetes prevention measure has been inadequately supported despite evidence of reducing the relative risk of type 2 diabetes risk by 50% [15]. The impact of previous breastfeeding on GDM risk in the next pregnancy is largely unknown. Breastfeeding studies investigating diabetes risk have concentrated on changes in postpartum cardiometabolic markers, such as lipids or OGTT results during the early postpartum period and ongoing type 2 diabetes incidence [16,17]. We are not aware of any studies that have investigated breastfeeding and next pregnancy glycaemic metabolism except our pilot study [18]. The pilot study was undertaken in a selected high-risk population (previous GDM) and found that both duration and exclusivity of breastfeeding were associated with improved glucose levels on a subsequent pregnancy OGTT [18].

For multiparous women, it is important to understand previous breastfeeding history to assess cardiometabolic risk and provide an opportunity for lactation support interventions. In recognition of the importance of breastfeeding for both infant and maternal health, the Sydney BLISS check was introduced to improve antenatal breastfeeding support in our health district. The BLISS tool was developed as part of our pilot study [18] and is now used in routine antenatal clinical care to assess breastfeeding during the first 12 weeks postpartum ('fourth trimester') after a woman's previous pregnancy [19].

In this study, we aimed to build on the findings of our pilot study to investigate the association between previous pregnancy breastfeeding intensity and duration and OGTT results in a subsequent pregnancy for an unselected population. The secondary aim was to understand breastfeeding patterns to identify specific groups of women at risk for suboptimal breastfeeding, who may then be at increased risk for cardiometabolic disease.

2. Materials and Methods

We conducted a retrospective cohort study of women booked to give birth in the Western Sydney Local Health District (WSLHD), Sydney, Australia between March 2020 and October 2022. The study period was determined from the implementation into routine clinical care of the antenatal breastfeeding history and the triaging assessment tool, the Sydney BLISS check, which was introduced to improve breastfeeding support.

The population is culturally and linguistically diverse, with approximately 58% of women who give birth in the district born in a non-English speaking country [20]. The WSLHD has three maternity care hospitals, with approximately 10,000 births per year [20]. Hospitals in the district were included in the study cohort after >50% of multiparous women at the hospital received midwifery breastfeeding assessment by the BLISS check at booking. The study period for the health district hospitals were Hospital 1: 1 March 2020–31 October 2022; Hospital 2 and 3: 1 January 2022–31 October 2022 (see Supplementary File S1: Figure S1). All women with a singleton pregnancy $\geq$ 20 weeks' gestation and who had had a previous live birth were included in the study. Exclusion criteria included multiple pregnancy, no BLISS check or OGTT result available, or previous diagnosis of type 1 or type 2 diabetes (Figure 1). Incomplete OGTT results were reviewed; reasons included inadequate documentation, patient unable to tolerate glucose drink and patient declined testing (Figure 1).

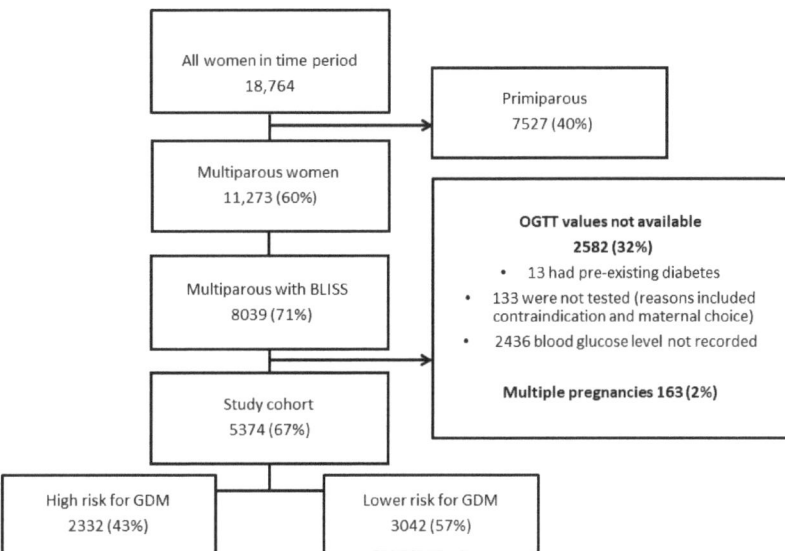

Figure 1. Flow Chart.

2.1. Measures and Data Source

The data source was the electronic maternity database eMaternity, providing routinely collected information during pregnancy, including medical and obstetric history. eMaternity in WSLHD includes Sydney BLISS check data.

2.2. Breastfeeding Measures

The Sydney BLISS tool was embedded into eMaternity WSLHD on 1 March 2020. COVID-19 interrupted the implementation of the assessment tool at the two smaller of the three district hospitals until 2022. The BLISS check was designed by a panel of lactation experts and assesses breastfeeding intensity (exclusivity) in the first three months after a woman's last pregnancy [18]. Intensity is the ratio of breastfeeding to infant formula feeding, with high-intensity breastfeeding (HIBF) being mostly or exclusively breastfeeding. The BLISS assessment aims to identify a history of breastfeeding issues via a standardized scoring system to triage women for antenatal lactation support. The score is auto-generated as part of routine booking electronic data collection and care. The BLISS check also collects information on total duration of any breastfeeding and the reasons for stopping breastfeeding. Women at booking are routinely offered a telehealth antenatal lactation clinic referral for a low BLISS score or if other breastfeeding issues are identified. HIBF is determined as a BLISS score of ≥ 19 as optimal maternal breastfeeding intensity and equates to approximately >70% breastfeeding to formula in the first three months postpartum [18]. Lower intensity breastfeeding (LIBF) reflects less optimal breastfeeding and a BLISS score of <19 [18]. The Sydney BLISS assessment tool is administered by the booking midwife (see Supplementary File S2: Sydney BLISS check). We dichotomized breastfeeding analysis to ≤ 6 months and >6, as this is the recommended time to exclusively breastfeed prior to introduction of family foods [4]. Six months is also a recognized population benchmark time period for assessing any breastfeeding [21].

2.3. Gestational Diabetes Measures

At the study hospitals all women are routinely screened for GDM via a one-step OGTT at 24–28 weeks' gestation, or earlier when clinically indicated. The 24–28 weeks' gestation results in this study were used for analysis if an early test was administered and repeated at 24–28 weeks' gestation. The early gestation results were used if no other OGTT was administered. Pathology results are routinely reviewed by the treating clinician and results entered in electronic records. Diagnosis of GDM in this study used the International Association of Diabetes and Pregnancy Study Group (IADPSG) criteria [22]. IADPSG thresholds were as follows: one or more values $\geq$ thresholds of fasting plasma glucose of 5.1 mmol/L, 1 h 10.0 mmol/L and/or a 2 h plasma glucose level of 8.5 mmol/L following a 75 g OGTT. High risk for GDM for the study cohort was defined as per the Australian Diabetes in Pregnancy Society v2 2014 criteria: previous GDM, maternal age $\geq$ 40 years, family history of diabetes, BMI >35 kg/m^2, previous baby with birth weight >4500 g or >90th centile, polycystic ovarian syndrome and current use of corticosteroids or antipsychotics [23].

2.4. Body Mass Index Measure (BMI)

The BMI variable is a perinatal data collection (PDC) data point collected for all women who birth in the state of New South Wales to assess pregnancy BMI trends [20]. In our health district, it is collected in the eMaternity database. The height is collected by the midwife at first pregnancy hospital booking visit, and the weight is a pre-pregnancy weight provided by the patient. This weight is 'sense-checked' by a current weight taken by the midwife at booking visit. Fidelity of data collection is ensured by frequent review by the data custodian.

2.5. Demographic Measures

Socioeconomic status (SES) is defined by place (suburb) of residence estimate and derived from information provided during the Australian census (2016), which informs the Index of Relative Socioeconomic Disadvantage (IRSD) [24]. Age was calculated at the time of booking for the current pregnancy. Ethnicity was self-assigned by women at booking and does not equate to migrant status. We acknowledge that ethnicity may be also described as race; however, women are asked to self-identify their ethnicity at hospital admission, therefore we are reporting this variable as ethnicity. Women who are migrants provide details of years lived in Australia and are of varied ethnicities.

2.6. Statistical Analysis

Statistical analyses were completed in Stata SE Version 14.2 and R Studio Version 4. Hypotheses were conducted at a significance level of 0.05 with a two-sided alternative.

Breastfeeding intensity and breastfeeding duration were considered co-primary exposures of interest. Breastfeeding duration was considered a linear continuous variable. Our models were adjusted for baseline variables measured at pregnancy booking; maternal age, ethnicity, migrancy, SES, BMI, parity, history of mental illness, history of hypertension, history of GDM and smoking during pregnancy. GDM diagnosis was assessed with a logistic regression model. Abnormal glucose tolerance via routine OGTT is a set of up to three binary outcomes (fasting, one-hour and two-hour) from repeated measurements from the same woman. Therefore, a generalized estimating equation (GEE) model, equipped with a logistic link function and first-order autoregressive correlation structure for within woman covariance, was implemented. Odds ratios, 95% confidence intervals and p values were reported.

To address the secondary aim of our study, maternal characteristics associated with breastfeeding intensity and duration were assessed. In each case, a logistic regression model was implemented. As an outcome, breastfeeding duration was dichotomized to breastfeeding >6 months versus $\leq$6 months. A priori variables were decided on as possible confounders for each exposure of interest and reported individually (see Supplementary File S3) [25]. Fasting blood glucose results were further investigated, grouped by Hyperglycaemia and Adverse Pregnancy Outcomes (HAPO) study blood glucose septiles and divided into HIBF or lower intensity breastfeeding plots with separation of curves analysed for significance [22]. Odds ratios, 95% confidence intervals and p values were reported.

No imputation was made for missing data, as missingness of the primary independent variable was plausibly missing not at random. We comment on the extent of characteristic differences that reflect hypothesized associations with mechanisms of missingness in Supplementary File S4.

3. Results

3.1. Cohort Characteristics and Exposure

During the study period, there were 11,273 multiparous women booked at the study hospitals. There were 5374 (67%) participants who met the inclusion criteria (Figure 1). The mean age was 32.4 (SD 6.8) years, and there were 981 patients (18.3%) diagnosed with GDM. Of all participants, 4074 (75.8%) were documented to be HIBF, 3558 (66.2%) had exclusively breastfed at 3 months, and 3222 (61.7%) of the total cohort breastfed for >6 months. The median duration of breastfeeding was 9 months (IQR 4–16).

Women classified in the HIBF group via the Sydney BLISS check breastfed for a median duration of 12 months (IQR 6–18, n = 4074, 75.8%) compared to those in the lower intensity group, who had a median duration of 3 months (IQR 1–7 months, n = 1300, 24.2%; p <0.01) (see Supplementary file S5: Figure S2). There were 2332 (43%) of the total cohort who were at high risk for GDM (Figure 1). There was no difference in the breastfeeding duration or intensity for women in either the high- or low-risk groupings for GDM (Table 1).

Table 1. Cohort characteristics by exposure of breastfeeding duration and intensity (N = 5374).

Maternal Characteristics	Duration of Breastfeeding Median Months (IQR)	p Value	High-Intensity Breastfeeding (n = 4074, 75.8%)	Low-Intensity Breastfeeding (n = 1300, 24.2%)	p Value
Maternal age		<0.001			<0.001
<25	6 (2–13)		69.46% (232)	30.54% (102)	
25–34	8 (4–15)		74.30% (1772)	25.70% (613)	
35–39	11 (6–18)		77.96% (1765)	22.04% (499)	
>39	12 (6–18)		78.01% (305)	21.99% (86)	
Ethnicity		<0.001			<0.001
South Asian	12 (6–18)		81.73% (1302)	18.27% (291)	
Southeast Asian	10 (5–14)		74.35% (661)	25.65% (228)	
White/European	9 (4–14)		73.09% (690)	26.91% (254)	
Middle Eastern	7 (3–14)		71.73% (789)	28.27% (311)	
Aboriginal and Torres Strait Islander	4 (2–9)		58.14% (50)	41.86% (36)	
Other	8 (4–14)		76.38% (582)	23.62% (180)	
Migrant status		<0.001			<0.001
<5 years	12 (6–18)		78.68% (1011)	21.32% (274)	
5–10 years	12 (6–18)		78.57% (759)	21.43% (207)	
>10 years	9 (4–15)		75.64% (798)	24.36% (267)	
Australian-born	7 (3–14)		71.31% (1213)	28.59% (488)	
Socioeconomic status		<0.001			<0.001
Least advantaged Q1	8 (3–15)		71.28% (1184)	28.72% (477)	
Q2	9 (4–14)		75.83% (549)	24.17% (175)	
Q3	11 (6–18)		77.56% (923)	22.44% (267)	
Q4	10 (5–17)		80.09% (531)	19.91% (132)	
Most advantaged Q5	11 (5–16)		78.06% (715)	21.94% (201)	
Parity		0.006			0.024
1	10 (4–17)		74.63% (2544)	25.37% (865)	
2–3	8 (4–15)		78.10% (1323)	21.90% (371)	
≥4	8 (4–18)		76.38% (207)	23.62% (64)	

Table 1. Cont.

Maternal Characteristics	Duration of Breastfeeding Median Months (IQR)	p Value	High-Intensity Breastfeeding (n = 4074, 75.8%)	Low-Intensity Breastfeeding (n = 1300, 24.2%)	p Value
Current pregnancy					
High risk of GDM *	9 (4–16)	0.859	74.61% (1740)	25.39% (592)	0.073
Lower risk of GDM	10 (4–16)		76.73% (2334)	23.27% (708)	
Smoking	4 (2–12)	<0.001	47.06% (48)	52.94% (54)	<0.001
No smoking	10 (5–17)		76.80% (2655)	23.20% (802)	
Comorbidities					
Polycystic ovary syndrome	8 (4–16)	0.23	73.11% (223)	26.89% (82)	0.26
No polycystic ovary syndrome	10 (4–16)		75.97% (3850)	24.03% (1218)	
History of mental health issue	7 (3–14)	<0.001	68.39% (541)	31.61% (250)	<0.001
No history of mental health issue	10 (4–18)		77.08% (3532)	22.92% (1050)	
History of hypertension	8 (4–14)	0.071	71.53% (206)	28.47% (82)	0.081
No history of hypertension	10 (4–16)		76.05% (3867)	23.95% (1218)	
BMI kg/m^2		<0.001			<0.001
<18.5	8 (4–14)		82.94% (141)	17.06% (29)	
18.5–24.9	11 (5–17)		77.77% (1907)	22.23% (545)	
25.0–29.9	9 (4–17)		77.04% (1258)	22.96% (375)	
≥30.0	7 (3–15)		68.63% (768)	31.37% (351)	
Previous pregnancy complications					
History of GDM	9 (4–16)	0.635	74.96% (518)	25.04% (173)	0.578
No history of GDM	9 (4–16)		75.93% (3556)	24.07% (1127)	
Previous birth: caesarean section	9 (4–18)	0.851	72.94% (949)	27.06% (352)	0.006
Previous birth: vaginal	9 (4–16)		76.72% (3125)	23.28% (948)	
Previous birth: preterm	7 (4–14)	0.003	67.89% (258)	32.11% (122)	<0.001
Previous birth term	10 (4–17)		76.41% (3816)	23.59% (1178)	

GDM, gestational diabetes mellitus. * High-risk GDM criteria: previous GDM, age > 40, family history of diabetes, BMI > 35, previous large for gestation baby, polycystic ovary disease, corticosteroid medication use.

There was a graduated decline in the median breastfeeding duration associated with lower age groupings (Table 1). Women <25 years old had the lowest median duration of breastfeeding (6 months: IQR 2–13) compared to the other age groups; women aged >39 years had the longest median duration (12 months; IQR 6–18). This graduated decline with younger age groups was also evident for HIBF (Table 1).

Australian-born women had a lower median duration of breastfeeding (7 months; IQR 3–14) compared to all migrants. Participants who had lived in Australia >10 years breastfed for a shorter duration than newer migrants (9 versus 12 months) (Table 1). Two factors were associated with the lowest median duration of breastfeeding: current smoking status (4 months; IQR 2–12) and women who identified as Aboriginal or Torres Strait Islander (4 months; IQR 2–9) (Table 1). For previous pregnancy complications, preterm birth was the only factor associated with shorter duration of breastfeeding (7 versus 10 months; $p = 0.003$), and this also was a factor for less intensity (67.9% versus 76.4%; $p < 0.001$) (Table 1). Other factors associated with duration and HIBF are detailed in Table 1.

3.2. Primary Aim: Association between Breastfeeding and OGTT Results in a Subsequent Pregnancy

Compared to women who breastfed at a lower intensity, women who had breastfed at high intensity in the first three months after their previous birth had a 47% reduced odds of an abnormal fasting blood glucose on the OGTT in their subsequent pregnancy (aOR 0.53; 95%CI 0.38–0.75; $p < 0.01$). The association between HIBF and improved fasting glucose was greater in women at a lower risk of GDM, with a 52% reduced odds of abnormal fasting blood glucose (aOR 0.48; 95%CI 0.27–0.86, $p = 0.01$) and 45% reduced odds for the women in the high-risk group (aOR 0.55; CI 0.36–0.83, $p = 0.01$) (Table 2). There were no associations between the OGTT results at one and two hours with HIBF or duration of breastfeeding (Table 2).

Table 2. Association between breastfeeding (BF) in a previous pregnancy and odds ratio (OR) of a gestational diabetes (GDM) diagnosis and/or of an abnormal elevated oral glucose tolerance test (OGTT) blood glucose result in current pregnancy. Total cohort n = 5374. High-intensity breastfeeding n = 4074.

		(a). High-Intensity Breastfeeding (HIBF)–Mostly or Exclusively Breastfeeding.					
Outcome	Cohort	HIBF % (n)	LIBF % (n)	Unadjusted OR (95%CI)	p	Adjusted OR (95%CI)	p
Elevated Fasting OGTT	Total Cohort	5.99% (243)	8.02% (104)	0.53 (0.38, 0.73)	<0.01	0.53 (0.38, 0.75)	<0.01
	High Risk	8.93% (154)	12.24% (72)	0.56 (0.38, 0.83)	0.01	0.55 (0.36, 0.83)	0.01
	Low Risk	3.81% (89)	4.52% (32)	0.47 (0.27, 0.83)	0.01	0.48 (0.27, 0.86)	0.01
Elevated 1 h OGTT	Total Cohort	10.72% (376)	8.83% (100)	1.14 (0.85, 1.52)	0.37	1.20 (0.89, 1.63)	0.23
	High Risk	16.43% (236)	14.57% (73)	1.04 (0.73, 1.47)	0.84	1.05 (0.72, 1.52)	0.81
	Low Risk	6.75% (140)	4.28% (27)	1.52 (0.90, 2.59)	0.12	1.58 (0.92, 2.71)	0.09
Elevated 2 h OGTT	Total Cohort	10.38% (420)	10.78% (139)	0.96 (0.73, 1.26)	0.77	1.01 (0.76, 1.33)	0.97
	High Risk	16.07% (276)	15.92% (93)	0.91 (0.66, 1.26)	0.57	0.92 (0.65, 1.29)	0.62
	Low Risk	6.18% (144)	6.52% (46)	1.18 (0.73, 1.93)	0.50	1.23 (0.75, 2.01)	0.42
Diagnosed GDM	Total Cohort	18.09% (737)	18.77% (244)	0.87 (0.73, 1.03)	0.11	0.91 (0.75, 1.10)	0.34
	High Risk	26.72% (465)	27.87% (165)	0.86 (0.68, 1.07)	0.18	0.84 (0.65, 1.08)	0.18
	Low Risk	11.65% (272)	11.16% (79)	0.95 (0.71, 1.27)	0.75	1.02 (0.75, 1.37)	0.92
		(b). Breastfeeding duration as a continuous variable and elevated glucose.					
Outcome	Cohort	Normal Glucose BF Months (IQR)	Elevated Glucose BF months (IQR)	Unadjusted OR (95%CI)	p	Adjusted OR (95%CI)	p
Fasting OGTT	Total Cohort	9 (4–16)	11 (4–18)	1.03 (1.01, 1.04)	<0.01	1.02 (1.00, 1.04)	0.04
	High Risk	9 (4–16)	9 (4–18)	1.02 (1.00, 1.04)	0.02	1.02 (0.99, 1.04)	0.15
	Low Risk	9 (4–16)	12 (6–19)	1.04 (1.01, 1.07)	0.01	1.03 (0.99, 1.06)	0.06
1 h OGTT	Total Cohort	9 (4–16)	12 (6–18)	1.02 (1.00, 1.03)	0.01	1.01 (0.99, 1.02)	0.34
	High Risk	9 (4–15)	11.5 (6–18)	1.02 (1.00, 1.04)	0.02	1.05 (0.72, 1.52)	0.81
	Low Risk	9 (4–16)	12 (6–18)	1.01 (0.99, 1.04)	0.23	1.00 (0.98, 1.03)	0.84
2 h OGTT	Total Cohort	9 (4–16)	11 (5–18)	1.01 (1.00, 1.02)	0.12	1.00 (0.99, 1.02)	0.86
	High Risk	9 (4–15)	11 (5–18)	1.02 (1.00, 1.04)	0.01	1.01 (0.99, 1.03)	0.62
	Low Risk	9 (4–16)	11 (5–18)	0.99 (0.97, 1.02)	0.50	0.98 (0.96, 1.01)	0.14
GDM	Total Cohort	9 (4–16)	11 (5–18)	1.02 (1.01, 1.02)	<0.01	1.01 (0.99, 1.02)	0.06
	High Risk	9 (4–16)	11 (5–18)	1.02 (1.00, 1.03)	0.01	1.01 (0.99, 1.02)	0.15
	Low Risk	9 (4–16)	12 (5–18)	1.02 (1.00, 1.03)	0.03	1.01 (0.99, 1.02)	0.21

High risk = high risk for GDM; previous GDM, maternal age ≥ 40 years, family history diabetes, BMI >35 kg/m^2, previous baby with birth weight >4500 g or >90th centile, polycystic ovarian syndrome and current use of corticosteroids or antipsychotics. Adjusted covariables: maternal age, ethnicity, migrancy, socioeconomic status, BMI, parity, history of mental illness, history of hypertension, history of GDM and smoking during pregnancy. GDM, gestational diabetes diagnosis AIDPSG criteria, one or more values ≥ thresholds of fasting plasma glucose of 5.1 mmol/L and/or a 2 h plasma glucose level of 8.5 mmol/L following a 75 g OGTT. HIBF, high-intensity breastfeeding; LIBF, lower intensity breastfeeding.

HIBF was not associated with diagnosis of GDM in all women (aOR 0.91; 95%CI 0.75–1.10, p = 0.34); women at reduced risk of GDM diagnosis (aOR 1.02; 95%CI 0.75–1.37, p = 0.92) or at high risk of GDM (aOR 0.84; 95%CI 0.65–1.08, p = 0.18) (Table 2). Breastfeeding duration was not associated with risk for GDM diagnosis overall (aOR 1.01; 95%CI 0.99–1.02, p = 0.06) or in the different risk categories (Table 2).

When fasting blood glucose results were viewed as a continuous graph for the two groups of HIBF and lower intensity, separation of groups occurred at the AIDPSG blood glucose cut-off 5.1 mmol/L, displaying HIBF participants with lower fasting blood glucose (p = 0.01) (see Supplementary File S6: Figure S3).

3.3. Secondary Aim: Factors Associated with Both Reduced High-Intensity Breastfeeding Postpartum and Breastfeeding >6 Months

There were six factors that negatively impacted both HIBF and breastfeeding >6 months: Aboriginal/Torres Strait Islander ethnicity, previous birth caesarean section, previous preterm birth, smoking, obesity and a history of mental health illness (Table 3). Smoking conferred the greatest reduction in odds of HIBF (aOR 0.31; 95%CI 0.21–0.47) and being of Aboriginal/Torres Strait ethnicity the most reduced odds of breastfeeding >6 months when compared to White/European ethnicity (aOR 0.31; 95%CI 0.19–0.50) (Table 3).

Table 3. Factors Associated with High-intensity Breastfeeding and Breastfeeding Duration >6 Months by Maternal Characteristics. Total cohort N = 5374. High-intensity breastfeeding n = 4074. Breastfeeding >6 months n = 3222.

Characteristic	High-Intensity Breastfeeding				Breastfeeding Duration > 6 Months			
	Unadjusted OR (95%CI)	p	aOR (95%CI)	p	Unadjusted OR (95%CI)	p	aOR (95%CI)	p
Maternal age								
<25	0.79 (0.61, 1.01)	ns	0.95 (0.73, 1.23)	ns	0.62 (0.49, 0.78)	<0.01	0.74 (0.58, 0.94)	0.01
25–34	Ref	-	-	-	Ref	-	-	-
35–39	1.22 (1.07, 1.40)	0.01	1.10 (0.96, 1.27)	ns	1.40 (1.24, 1.58)	<0.01	1.25 (1.10, 1.42)	<0.01
40+	1.23 (0.95, 1.59)	ns	1.17 (0.89, 1.53)	ns	1.53 (1.22, 1.93)	<0.01	1.52 (1.20, 1.94)	<0.01
Ethnicity								
South Asian	1.65 (1.36, 2.00)	<0.01	1.65 (1.36, 2.00)	<0.01	1.81 (1.52, 2.15)	<0.01	1.81 (1.52, 2.15)	<0.01
South-East Asian	1.07 (0.87, 1.31)	ns	1.07 (0.87, 1.31)	ns	1.27 (1.04, 1.54)	0.02	1.27 (1.04, 1.54)	0.02
White/European	Ref	-	-	-	Ref	-	-	-
Middle Eastern	0.93 (0.77, 1.13)	ns	0.93 (0.77, 1.13)	ns	0.79 (0.66, 0.94)	0.01	0.79 (0.66, 0.94)	0.01
Aboriginal/Torres Strait Islander	0.51 (0.33, 0.80)	0.01	0.51 (0.33, 0.80)	0.01	0.31 (0.19, 0.50)	<0.01	0.31 (0.19, 0.50)	<0.01
Other	1.19 (0.95, 1.48)	ns	1.19 (0.95, 1.48)	ns	0.97 (0.79, 1.18)	ns	0.97 (0.79, 1.18)	ns
Migrant status								
<5 years	1.48 (1.25, 1.76)	<0.01	1.20 (0.97, 1.48)	ns	1.94 (1.66, 2.26)	<0.01	1.60 (1.32, 1.94)	<0.01
5–10 years	1.48 (1.22, 1.78)	<0.01	1.18 (0.94, 1.47)	ns	1.95 (1.65, 2.31)	<0.01	1.56 (1.27, 1.91)	<0.01
>10 years	1.25 (1.05, 1.49)	0.01	1.10 (0.90, 1.35)	ns	1.51 (1.29, 1.77)	<0.01	1.32 (1.09, 1.59)	0.01
Australian-born	Ref	-	-	-	Ref	-	-	-
Previous complications								
History of GDM	0.95 (0.79, 1.14)	ns	0.92 (0.76, 1.11)	ns	1.05 (0.88, 1.24)	ns	0.97 (0.82, 1.15)	ns
History of hypertension	0.79 (0.61, 1.03)	ns	0.88 (0.68, 1.15)	ns	0.90 (0.70, 1.14)	ns	1.03 (0.80, 1.33)	ns
Previous birth caesarean section	0.82 (0.71, 0.94)	0.01	0.78 (0.67, 0.91)	<0.01	0.93 (0.82, 1.06)	ns	0.85 (0.74, 0.97)	0.02
Previous birth preterm	0.65 (0.52, 0.82)	<0.01	0.61 (0.48, 0.77)	<0.01	0.73 (0.59, 0.91)	0.01	0.76 (0.60, 0.95)	0.02
Current pregnancy								
Smoking	0.27 (0.18, 0.40)	<0.01	0.31 (0.21, 0.47)	<0.01	0.33 (0.22, 0.49)	<0.01	0.44 (0.29, 0.67)	<0.01
BMI kg/m^2								
<18.5	1.39 (0.92, 2.10)	ns	1.53 (1.01, 2.32)	ns	0.87 (0.63, 1.21)	ns	0.96 (0.69, 1.33)	ns
18.5–24.9	Ref	-	-	-	Ref	-	-	-
25.0–29.9	0.96 (0.83, 1.11)	ns	0.89 (0.77, 1.04)	ns	0.87 (0.76, 0.99)	0.04	0.86 (0.75, 0.99)	0.04
≥30.0	0.63 (0.53, 0.73)	<0.01	0.62 (0.52, 0.73)	<0.01	0.59 (0.51, 0.68)	<0.01	0.69 (0.57, 0.78)	<0.01
History of mental health issue	0.64 (0.55, 0.76)	<0.01	0.69 (0.58, 0.83)	<0.01	0.67 (0.57, 0.78)	<0.01	0.78 (0.65, 0.91)	<0.01

GDM = gestational diabetes. ns = not statistically significant. Ref = reference. Multivariate model may adjusted for: age, ethnicity, time in Australia, SES, BMI, parity, history of mental illness, history of hypertension, history of GDM, history of caesarean section, history of preterm birth, unplanned pregnancy, smoking.

Women who had a caesarean section birth had 22% reduced odds to breastfeed at high intensity (aOR 0.78; 95%CI 0.67–0.91; $p < 0.01$) and they were less likely to breastfeed >6 months (aOR 0.85; 95%CI 0.74–0.97, $p = 0.02$). A history of preterm birth was associated with 39% reduced odds of HIBF (aOR 0.61; 95%CI 0.48–0.77, $p < 0.01$) (Table 2) and reduced odds of breastfeeding >6 months (aOR 0.76; 95%CI 0.60–0.95, $p = 0.02$).

Compared to women with a healthy BMI (18.5–24.9 kg/m^2), a high BMI $\geq$ 30 kg/m^2 negatively impacted breastfeeding, with 38% reduced odds of HIBF (aOR 0.62; 95%CI 0.52–0.73 $p < 0.01$) and 31% reduced odds of breastfeeding >6 months (aOR 0.69; 95%CI 0.57–0.78, $p < 0.01$). The other previous pregnancy characteristic to negatively impact breastfeeding was a history of mental illness, with lower odds of both HIBF (aOR 0.69; 95%CI 0.58–0.83, $p < 0.01$) and breastfeeding >6 months (aOR 0.78; 95%CI 0.65–0.91, $p < 0.01$).

South Asian ethnicity was the only factor positively associated with both improved HIBF and breastfeeding >6 months. Compared to White/European ethnicity, women who identified as South Asian had 65% increased odds of HIBF (aOR 1.65; 95%CI 1.36–2.00, $p < 0.01$) and greater odds of breastfeeding >6 months (aOR 1.81; 95%CI 1.52–2.15, $p < 0.01$).

3.4. Factors Only Associated with Breastfeeding >6 Months

Three characteristics were negatively associated with duration of breastfeeding but not intensity; age <25 years compared to the 25–34 age grouping (0.74 aOR; 95%CI 0.58–0.94, $p = 0.01$), Middle Eastern ethnicity compared to White/European ethnic groupings (aOR 0.79; 95%CI 0.66–0.94, $p = 0.01$) and a BMI in an overweight range compared to a healthy BMI (aOR 0.86; 95%CI 0.75–0.99, $p = 0.04$). Other positively associated factors only identified for breastfeeding duration >6 months but not HIBF were for participants over 35 years age (1.25 95%CI 1.10–1.42, $p < 0.01$) or >40 years (1.52 95%CI 1.20–1.94, $p < 0.01$) compared to 25–34-year-old age groupings. Women who identified as South-East Asian ethnicity were also more likely to breastfeed >6 months (aOR 1.27; 95%CI 1.04–1.54, $p = 0.02$) compared to White/European participants. Compared to Australian-born status, migrant status had no association with HIBF; however, migrant status was positively associated with breastfeeding >6 months. Compared to Australian-born women, new migrants who had lived in Australia <5 years had 60% increased odds of breastfeeding >6 months (aOR 1.60; 95%CI 1.32–1.94, $p < 0.01$). All other associations are detailed in Table 3.

4. Discussion

This is the first study we are aware of that has found that optimal breastfeeding patterns can have direct metabolic benefits in a subsequent pregnancy. Potentially, this may reduce both maternal and infant morbidity. In a large, ethnically diverse population, our study has found that women who breastfed at a high intensity (exclusive or mostly breastfeeding) had improved odds of a normal fasting glucose in their subsequent pregnancy. We identified maternal characteristics that differed with length and intensity of breastfeeding, providing a more comprehensive understanding of women's postpartum breastfeeding behaviour. Targeting factors to improve breastfeeding intensity may be one key to improved cardiometabolic health in subsequent pregnancies. Specific groups in this study who were vulnerable to suboptimal breastfeeding intensity and duration include women with a history of preterm birth, women with a high BMI, those who had a history of a mental health illness, women who identify as Aboriginal/Torres Strait Islander and smokers.

Women who do not meet the criteria for a diagnosis of GDM may still have some degree of dysglycaemia or gestational glucose intolerance (GGI) that places them at greater risk of type 2 diabetes [26]. Berekowsky et al. and others have found that an abnormal fasting OGTT was the value most correlated with a future risk of type 2 diabetes compared to OGTT results at one and two hours [27,28]. Other research has also found an abnormal fasting OGTT result alone predicts increased risk of a large for gestational age baby and other adverse pregnancy outcomes [29,30]. Supporting HIBF for all women may therefore reduce their risk for both adverse perinatal outcomes in a subsequent pregnancy and improve maternal long-term cardiometabolic risk.

Postpartum HIBF has been described as potentially an essential part of an endocrine reset process after a pregnancy-induced insulin resistant state [31]. Other research has found that compared to mixed or mostly formula infant feeding, it is HIBF that confers the most benefit for improved postpartum insulin resistance and lipid profiles and may underpin the long-term improved risk for metabolic disorders associated with breastfeeding [32]. The global burden of cardiometabolic disease requires a united and multi-faceted approach to complex drivers. This research identifies women with known risk factors for cardiometabolic disease, such as obesity, smoking and preterm birth, as also vulnerable to suboptimal breastfeeding intensity and duration and subsequent higher odds of failing their fasting pregnancy OGTT. The cumulative impact of existing cardiometabolic risk and poor breastfeeding needs addressing as one of the many drivers for global cardiometabolic disease burden [1–3]. Our study provides further evidence of the importance that early exclusive or mostly breastfeeding may be vital for long-term cardiometabolic health and crucial for an endocrine 'reset' postpartum. Routinely collected breastfeeding data inclusive of intensity information via tools such as the Sydney BLISS check will assist in uncovering drivers for optimal health outcomes for women.

Breastfeeding support programs are effective to improve breastfeeding and generally acceptable to women [33]. However, minimal research has integrated lifestyle programs with breastfeeding support interventions aimed at reducing type 2 diabetes risk [34]. A recent Cochrane Review found that at least 4–8 postpartum lactation support contacts were required to improve breastfeeding rates. Targeted support such as this is particularly important for populations found in this research [33]. If the WHO Sustainable Development Goal to reduce global NCD is to be met, all health promotion avenues should be pursued. Supporting breastfeeding must be included. Understanding the metabolic impact during pregnancy of previous breastfeeding duration and exclusivity, as well as identifying groups at risk for suboptimal breastfeeding, will assist in designing targeted interventions to improve lifetime cardiometabolic risk.

A limitation of this study is that there was no available information on some factors that may influence both breastfeeding and dysglycaemia. These factors include lack of available information in routine data on education level, exercise, diet, interpregnancy weight gain, time period between pregnancies or important baseline metabolic risk factors including lipid levels. The only available weight was for the current pregnancy. Potentially, there are factors such as exercise that participants who breastfeed for a greater duration are less likely to engage in.

Another limitation was the missing BLISS and OGTT values in the routine data. The COVID-19 pandemic may have influenced women attending to routine OGTT investigations. Local research found that some women who were pregnant experienced fear of public places due to the COVID-19 pandemic, and this, as well as lockdowns, may have contributed to reduced attendance for pregnancy OGTTs [35]. However, noncompliance with testing has been documented in various populations to be from 10–50% of women; therefore our missing OGTT data is consistent with other population-level data [36]. The missing BLISS should not be biased by patient selection, but was impacted by slow implementation due to staff shortages and lack of time to complete the new breastfeeding triage tool. Women who had chosen to formula feed in their previous pregnancy and did not breastfeed at all were often not given a BLISS score, and therefore our results do not fully capture the lowest intensity of no breastfeeding.

A strength of this cohort was the diversity of ethnicity, and therefore the results are potentially more applicable to other culturally mixed populations. The use of routine clinical data of both duration and intensity of breastfeeding for the entire health district was also a strength resulting in a large sample size. The Sydney BLISS check is applied to a non-selected clinical care population that is reflective and generalizable, as the participants were not a motivated breastfeeding research cohort.

The high-intensity BLISS check scoring is affirmed as a valid cut-off score via the association with greater duration of breastfeeding [37]. In this study, when compared to the LIBF group, we found HIBF in the first three months postpartum was associated with a 9-month greater median breastfeeding duration. Further highlighting that the fourth trimester postpartum period is crucial to provide breastfeeding support to optimise greater duration of breastfeeding and associated benefits to women and babies.

Another strength of the Sydney BLISS is the validation of the HAPO cut-off value of 5.1 mmol/L for fasting glucose in our ethnically diverse population. When our results were disaggregated by low and high intensity and glucose levels along a continuum, HIBF participants clearly diverged from the LIBF group at the IADPSG fasting normal cut-off point [38]. Higher IADPSG cut-off values are associated with increased obstetric morbidity, HIBF therefore may potentially be association with lower obstetric morbidity that will need further investigation.

In Australia, nearly 40% of women who do not breastfeed state 'unsuccessful' previous experience as the reason [39]. Successful implementation of the antenatal Sydney BLISS check in the study health district assists in addressing this issue for multiparous women, as they are given the opportunity for antenatal referral to a new telehealth lactation consultant clinic. Promoting and protecting breastfeeding for short- and long-term metabolic health, as well as infant health, requires population-level data to underpin appropriate support that the Sydney BLISS check can provide.

5. Conclusions

The objectives of this study were to understand, in an unselected culturally diverse population, if breastfeeding duration and intensity was associated with improved OGTT results in a subsequent pregnancy and identify specific groups of women who may be susceptible to suboptimal breastfeeding. This study provides information not only on the important gains of optimal breastfeeding for next pregnancy glycaemic control, but also identifies vulnerable breastfeeding populations to drive targeted intervention programs. During the pandemic era with constraints on health budgets and staffing, it has been difficult to provide evidence-based lactation support. Breastfeeding duration is vital for infant and maternal health, but this study has found the importance of mostly or exclusively breastfeeding as a public health issue to reduce GDM risk in a subsequent pregnancy and potentially improve long-term health.

Supplementary Materials: The following supporting information can be downloaded at: https://www.mdpi.com/article/10.3390/nu16010028/s1, File S1. Sydney BLISS check uptake by site; File S2. The Sydney BLISS check; File S3. Statistical notes confounding factors; File S4. Statistical notes missingness; File S5. Correlation breastfeeding length and intensity; File S6. Breastfeeding intensity and OGTT. References [25,40,41] are cited in supplementary file.

Author Contributions: S.J.M. and D.P. conceptualization of the study, analysis plan, methodology, analysis, wrote the original draft and reviewed and edited the manuscript. J.E. provided statistical support, contributed to methodology, analysis, discussion and reviewed and edited the manuscript. L.W., J.M., V.W.L., K.D., T.I.A., S.P. and N.W.C. contributed to methodology, analysis, discussion and reviewed and edited the manuscript. All authors have read and agreed to the published version of the manuscript.

Funding: This research was partially funded by the Westmead Hospital Charitable Trust.

Institutional Review Board Statement: The study was conducted in accordance with the Declaration of Helsinki and approved by the Western Sydney Local Health District Human Research Ethics Committee approved this study and waived the informed consent requirement (WSLHD HREC approval 2022/ETH00604, and the approval date was 6 June 2022).

Informed Consent Statement: Institutional review board (WSLHD HREC) granted patient waiver of consent as the study met the criteria set by the Australian National Statement on Ethical Conduct in Human Research including the study was low risk and it is impracticable to obtain consent due to the quantity of the records.

Data Availability Statement: The dataset generated during the current study are not publicly available due to institutional restrictions on patient data but are available from the corresponding author upon reasonable request and institutional approval.

Conflicts of Interest: The authors declare no conflict of interest. The funders had no role in the design of the study; in the collection, analyses, or interpretation of data; in the writing of the manuscript; or in the decision to publish the results.

References

1. Gunderson, E.P.; Jacobs Jr, D.R.; Chiang, V.; Lewis, C.E.; Feng, J.; Quesenberry, C.P., Jr.; Sidney, S. Duration of lactation and incidence of the metabolic syndrome in women of reproductive age according to gestational diabetes mellitus status: A 20-Year prospective study in CARDIA (Coronary Artery Risk Development in Young Adults). *Diabetes* **2010**, *59*, 495–504. [CrossRef] [PubMed]
2. Tschiderer, L.; Seekircher, L.; Kunutsor, S.K.; Peters, S.A.E.; O'Keeffe, L.M.; Willeit, P. Breastfeeding Is Associated with a Reduced Maternal Cardiovascular Risk: Systematic Review and Meta-Analysis Involving Data From 8 Studies and 1 192 700 Parous Women. *J. Am. Heart Assoc.* **2022**, *11*, e022746. [CrossRef] [PubMed]
3. Victora, C.G.; Bahl, R.; Barros, A.J.; França, G.V.; Horton, S.; Krasevec, J.; Murch, S.; Sankar, M.J.; Walker, N.; Rollins, N.C. Breastfeeding in the 21st century: Epidemiology, mechanisms, and lifelong effect. *Lancet* **2016**, *387*, 475–490. [CrossRef] [PubMed]
4. World Health Organization Guideline. *Protecting, Promoting and Supporting Breastfeeding in Facilities Providing Maternity and Newborn Services*; World Health Organization: Geneva, Switzerland, 2017.
5. Smith, J.P. "Lost milk?": Counting the economic value of breast milk in gross domestic product. *J. Hum. Lact.* **2013**, *29*, 537–546. [CrossRef] [PubMed]
6. Walters, D.D.; Phan, L.T.H.; Mathisen, R. The cost of not breastfeeding: Global results from a new tool. *Health Policy Plan.* **2019**, *34*, 407–417. [CrossRef] [PubMed]
7. Neves, P.A.; Vaz, J.S.; Maia, F.S.; Baker, P.; Gatica-Domínguez, G.; Piwoz, E.; Rollins, N.; Victora, C.G. Rates and time trends in the consumption of breastmilk, formula, and animal milk by children younger than 2 years from 2000 to 2019: Analysis of 113 countries. *Lancet Child Adolesc. Health* **2021**, *5*, 619–630. [CrossRef] [PubMed]
8. Cheung, N.W.; Jiang, S.; Athayde, N. Impact of the IADPSG criteria for gestational diabetes, and of obesity, on pregnancy outcomes. *Aust. N. Z. J. Obstet. Gynaecol.* **2018**, *58*, 553–559. [CrossRef] [PubMed]
9. Behboudi-Gandevani, S.; Amiri, M.; Bidhendi Yarandi, R.; Ramezani Tehrani, F. The impact of diagnostic criteria for gestational diabetes on its prevalence: A systematic review and meta-analysis. *Diabetol. Metab. Syndr.* **2019**, *11*, 11. [CrossRef]
10. Kramer, C.K.; Campbell, S.; Retnakaran, R. Gestational diabetes and the risk of cardiovascular disease in women: A systematic review and meta-analysis. *Diabetologia* **2019**, *62*, 905–914. [CrossRef]
11. Vounzoulaki, E.; Khunti, K.; Abner, S.C.; Tan, B.K.; Davies, M.J.; Gillies, C.L. Progression to type 2 diabetes in women with a known history of gestational diabetes: Systematic review and meta-analysis. *BMJ* **2020**, *369*, m1361. [CrossRef]
12. Publications UN. *The Sustainable Development Goals Report 2021*; Jensen, L., Ed.; Department of Economic and Social Affairs: New York, NY, USA, 2021.
13. Fu, J.; Retnakaran, R. The life course perspective of gestational diabetes: An opportunity for the prevention of diabetes and heart disease in women. *EClinicalMedicine* **2022**, *45*, 101294. [CrossRef] [PubMed]
14. Retnakaran, M.; Viana, L.V.; Kramer, C.K. Lifestyle intervention for the prevention of type 2 diabetes in women with prior gestational diabetes: A systematic review and meta-analysis. *Diabetes Obes. Metab.* **2023**, *25*, 1196–1202. [CrossRef] [PubMed]
15. Gunderson, E.P.; Lewis, C.E.; Lin, Y.; Sorel, M.; Gross, M.; Sidney, S.; Jacobs, D.R.; Shikany, J.M.; Quesenberry, C.P. Lactation Duration and Progression to Diabetes in Women Across the Childbearing Years: The 30-Year CARDIA Study. *JAMA Intern. Med.* **2018**, *178*, 328–337. [CrossRef] [PubMed]
16. Gunderson, E.P.; Hedderson, M.M.; Chiang, V.; Crites, Y.; Walton, D.; Azevedo, R.A.; Fox, G.; Elmasian, C.; Young, S.; Salvador, N.; et al. Lactation intensity and postpartum maternal glucose tolerance and insulin resistance in women with recent GDM: The SWIFT cohort. *Diabetes Care* **2012**, *35*, 50–56. [CrossRef] [PubMed]
17. Shen, Y.; Leng, J.; Li, W.; Zhang, S.; Liu, H.; Shao, P.; Wang, P.; Wang, L.; Tian, H.; Zhang, C.; et al. Lactation intensity and duration to postpartum diabetes and prediabetes risk in women with gestational diabetes. *Diabetes Metab. Res. Rev.* **2019**, *35*, e3115. [CrossRef]
18. Melov, S.J.; White, L.; Simmons, M.; Kirby, A.; Stulz, V.; Padmanabhan, S.; Alahakoon, T.I.; Pasupathy, D.; Cheung, N.W. The BLIiNG study—Breastfeeding length and intensity in gestational diabetes and metabolic effects in a subsequent pregnancy: A cohort study. *Midwifery* **2022**, *107*, 103262. [CrossRef] [PubMed]
19. Tully, K.P.; Stuebe, A.M.; Verbiest, S.B. The fourth trimester: A critical transition period with unmet maternal health needs. *Am. J. Obstet. Gynecol.* **2017**, *217*, 37–41. [CrossRef]
20. Centre for Epidemiology and Evidence. *New South Wales Mothers and Babies 2020*; Ministry of Health: Sydney, Australia, 2021.
21. Breastfeeding Report Card United States. 2022. Available online: https://www.cdc.gov/breastfeeding/data/reportcard.htm (accessed on 27 March 2023).

22. International Association of Diabetes and Pregnancy Study Groups Consensus Panel; Metzger, B.E.; Gabbe, S.G.; Persson, B.; Buchanan, T.A.; Catalano, P.A.; Damm, P.; Dyer, A.R.; Leiva, A.d.; Hod, M.; et al. International association of diabetes and pregnancy study groups recommendations on the diagnosis and classification of hyperglycemia in pregnancy. *Diabetes Care* **2010**, *33*, 676–682. [CrossRef]
23. ADIPS. Consensus Guidelines for the Testing and Diagnosis of Hyperglycaemia in Pregnancy in Australia and New Zealand. Available online: https://www.adips.org/downloads/2014ADIPSGDMGuidelinesV18.11.2014.pdf (accessed on 4 April 2022).
24. Census of Population and Housing: Socio-Economic Indexes for Areas (SEIFA), Australia. 2016. Available online: https://www.abs.gov.au/ausstats/abs@.nsf/Lookup/by%20Subject/2033.0.55.001~2016~Main%20Features~IRSD~19 (accessed on 4 April 2022).
25. Bandoli, G.; Palmsten, K.; Chambers, C.D.; Jelliffe-Pawlowski, L.L.; Baer, R.J.; Thompson, C.A. Revisiting the Table 2 fallacy: A motivating example examining preeclampsia and preterm birth. *Paediatr. Perinat. Epidemiol.* **2018**, *32*, 390–397. [CrossRef]
26. Selen, D.J.; Thaweethai, T.; Schulte, C.C.; Hsu, S.; He, W.; James, K.; Kaimal, A.; Meigs, J.B.; Powe, C.E. Gestational Glucose Intolerance and Risk of Future Diabetes. *Diabetes Care* **2023**, *46*, 83–91. [CrossRef]
27. Berezowsky, A.; Raban, O.; Aviram, A.; Zafrir-Danieli, H.; Krispin, E.; Hadar, E. Glucose tolerance test with a single abnormal value in pregnancy and the risk of type-2 diabetes mellitus. *Arch. Gynecol. Obstet.* **2022**, *305*, 869–875. [CrossRef] [PubMed]
28. Cheung, N.W.; Helmink, D. Gestational diabetes: The significance of persistent fasting hyperglycemia for the subsequent development of diabetes mellitus. *J. Diabetes Complicat.* **2006**, *20*, 21–25. [CrossRef] [PubMed]
29. Roeckner, J.T.; Sanchez-Ramos, L.; Jijon-Knupp, R.; Kaunitz, A.M. Single abnormal value on 3-hour oral glucose tolerance test during pregnancy is associated with adverse maternal and neonatal outcomes: A systematic review and metaanalysis. *Am. J. Obstet. Gynecol.* **2016**, *215*, 287–297. [CrossRef] [PubMed]
30. Shen, S.; Lu, J.; Zhang, L.; He, J.; Li, W.; Chen, N.; Wen, X.; Xiao, W.; Yuan, M.; Qiu, L.; et al. Single Fasting Plasma Glucose Versus 75-g Oral Glucose-Tolerance Test in Prediction of Adverse Perinatal Outcomes: A Cohort Study. *eBioMedicine* **2017**, *16*, 284–291. [CrossRef] [PubMed]
31. Stuebe, A.M.; Rich-Edwards, J.W. The reset hypothesis: Lactation and maternal metabolism. *Am. J. Perinatol.* **2009**, *26*, 81–88. [CrossRef] [PubMed]
32. Zhang, Z.; Lai, M.; Piro, A.L.; Alexeeff, S.E.; Allalou, A.; Röst, H.L.; Dai, F.F.; Wheeler, M.B.; Gunderson, E.P. Intensive lactation among women with recent gestational diabetes significantly alters the early postpartum circulating lipid profile: The SWIFT study. *BMC Med.* **2021**, *19*, 241. [CrossRef] [PubMed]
33. Gavine, A.; Shinwell, S.C.; Buchanan, P.; Farre, A.; Wade, A.; Lynn, F.; Marshall, J.; Cumming, S.E.; Dare, S.; McFadden, A. Support for healthy breastfeeding mothers with healthy term babies. *Cochrane Database Syst. Rev.* **2022**, *10*, Cd001141. [PubMed]
34. Marschner, S.; Chow, C.; Thiagalingam, A.; Simmons, D.; McClean, M.; Pasupathy, D.; Smith, B.J.; Flood, V.; Padmanabhan, S.; Melov, S.; et al. Effectiveness of a customised mobile phone text messaging intervention supported by data from activity monitors for improving lifestyle factors related to the risk of type 2 diabetes among women after gestational diabetes: Protocol for a multicentre randomised controlled trial (SMART MUMS with smart phones 2). *BMJ Open* **2021**, *11*, e054756.
35. Melov, S.J.; Galas, N.; Swain, J.; Alahakoon, T.I.; Lee, V.; Cheung, N.W.; McGee, T.; Pasupathy, D.; McNab, J. Women's experience of perinatal support in a high migrant Australian population during the COVID-19 pandemic: A mixed methods study. *BMC Pregnancy Childbirth* **2023**, *23*, 429. [CrossRef]
36. Lachmann, E.H.; Fox, R.A.; Dennison, R.A.; Usher-Smith, J.A.; Meek, C.L.; Aiken, C.E. Barriers to completing oral glucose tolerance testing in women at risk of gestational diabetes. *Diabet. Med.* **2020**, *37*, 1482–1489. [CrossRef]
37. Piper, S.; Parks, P.L. Use of an intensity ratio to describe breastfeeding exclusivity in a national sample. *J. Hum. Lact.* **2001**, *17*, 227–232. [CrossRef] [PubMed]
38. HAPO Study Cooperative Research Group; Metzger, B.E.; Lowe, L.P.; Dyer, A.R.; Trimble, E.R.; Chaovarindr, U.; Coustan, D.R.; Hadden, D.R.; McCance, D.R.; Hod, M.; et al. Hyperglycemia and adverse pregnancy outcomes. *N. Engl. J. Med.* **2008**, *358*, 1991–2002. [PubMed]
39. Australian Institute of Health Welfare. *2010 Australian National Infant Feeding Survey: Indicator Results*; Australian Institute of Health Welfare: Canberra, Australia, 2011.
40. Westreich, D.; Greenland, S. The Table 2 Fallacy: Presenting and Interpreting Confounder and Modifier Coefficients. *Am. J. Epidemiol.* **2013**, *177*, 292–298. [CrossRef] [PubMed]
41. Jakobsen, J.C.; Gluud, C.; Wetterslev, J.; Winkel, P. When and how should multiple imputation be used for handling missing data in randomised clinical trials—A practical guide with flowcharts. *BMC Med. Res. Methodol.* **2017**, *17*, 162. [CrossRef]

Disclaimer/Publisher's Note: The statements, opinions and data contained in all publications are solely those of the individual author(s) and contributor(s) and not of MDPI and/or the editor(s). MDPI and/or the editor(s) disclaim responsibility for any injury to people or property resulting from any ideas, methods, instructions or products referred to in the content.

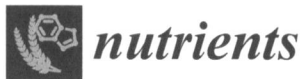

Article

Evaluation of the Impact of a Midwife-Led Breastfeeding Group Intervention on Prevention of Postpartum Depression: A Multicentre Randomised Clinical Trial

Isabel Rodríguez-Gallego [1,2], Rafael Vila-Candel [3,4,5,*], Isabel Corrales-Gutierrez [6,7,*], Diego Gomez-Baya [8] and Fatima Leon-Larios [9]

[1] Foetal Medicine, Genetics and Reproduction Unit, Virgen del Rocío University Hospital, 41009 Seville, Spain; isroga@cruzroja.es
[2] Red Cross Nursing University Centre, University of Seville, 41013 Seville, Spain
[3] Faculty of Health Sciences, Universidad Internacional de Valencia (VIU), 46002 Valencia, Spain
[4] La Ribera Primary Health Department, 46600 Alzira, Spain
[5] Foundation for the Promotion of Health and Biomedical Research in the Valencian Region (FISABIO), 46020 Valencia, Spain
[6] Surgery Department, Faculty of Medicine, University of Seville, 41009 Seville, Spain
[7] Foetal Medicine Unit, Virgen Macarena University Hospital, 41009 Seville, Spain
[8] Department of Social, Developmental and Educational Psychology, Universidad de Huelva, 21007 Huelva, Spain; diego.gomez@dpee.uhu.es
[9] Nursing Department, School of Nursing, Physiotherapy and Podiatry, University of Seville, 41009 Seville, Spain; fatimaleon@us.es
* Correspondence: rafael.vila@professor.universidadviu.com (R.V.-C.); icorrales@us.es (I.C.-G.)

Abstract: Postpartum depression is a significant health issue affecting both mothers and newborns during the postpartum period. Group support interventions during this period have proven effective in helping women cope with depression and improving breastfeeding rates. This study aimed to assess the effectiveness of a midwife-led breastfeeding support group intervention on breastfeeding rates, postpartum depression and general self-efficacy. This was a multicentric cluster randomised controlled trial with control and intervention groups and was not blinded. It was conducted in Andalusia (southern Spain) from October 2021 to May 2023. A total of 382 women participated in the study. The results showed a significant difference in exclusive breastfeeding rates at 4 months postpartum between the groups (control 50% vs. intervention 69.9%; $p < 0.001$). Additionally, there was a lower mean score on the Edinburgh Postnatal Depression Scale in the intervention group (12.49 ± 3.6 vs. 13.39 ± 4.0; $p = 0.044$). Similarly, higher scores of general self-efficacy were observed among breastfeeding women at 2 and 4 months postpartum (77.73 ± 14.81; $p = 0.002$ and 76.46 ± 15.26; $p < 0.001$, respectively). In conclusion, midwife-led breastfeeding support groups enhanced self-efficacy, prolonged breastfeeding and reduced postpartum depression 4 months after giving birth.

Keywords: breastfeeding; support group; lactation; self-help group; postpartum depression; general self-efficacy; women's mental health

1. Introduction

The postpartum period entails significant physical, psychosocial and social changes for women as they adapt to a new situation. Therefore, it is known as a period of special vulnerability related to maternal mental health [1]. Approximately 9.6% to 19.2% of mothers experience a major or minor depressive episode during the first 12 months after childbirth [2]. Thus, one of the main complications during the postpartum period is postpartum depression (PPD) [3,4].

Globally, one in five women is estimated to develop PPD. However, the prevalence of PPD varies significantly between geographic areas and cultures. Southern Africa has the highest reported prevalence (39.96%), eastern Europe (16.62%) and southern Europe (16.34%) show intermediate prevalence and Oceania (11.11%) has some of the lowest reported figures [5–7]. Furthermore, countries with higher income and developed countries have a significantly lower prevalence than lower income or developing countries [5]. However, these figures may underestimate the true extent of the problem due to barriers to detection and the stigma associated with mental illnesses in the perinatal context. Some estimates suggest that more than 50% of women with PPD are not diagnosed [6]. PPD generally occurs within 4 weeks after delivery and can last 6 months or longer after delivery, although some authors indicate that it could last up to 2 years after delivery [4,8–10].

Breastfeeding provides multiple demonstrated benefits on the physical, cognitive and social levels for both the mother and the newborn [11–13]. However, the psychological benefits, especially those concerning PPD, are still largely unknown. There is a complex physiological relationship between breastfeeding and PPD. During pregnancy, lactation begins with an increase in progesterone and estrogens that prepares the breast ducts as part of the stimulation process, but in the first days after delivery, there is a rapid decrease in both that signals the start of milk production. This rapid drop in progesterone and estrogen is a potential catalyst for the onset of mood lability and therefore PPD [14]. Progesterone derivatives (pregnenolone and allopregnanolone) target their effect in regions of the brain related to processing emotions. Establishing the exact role of these progesterone derivatives in the development of PPD treatment may enlighten a new perspective on the general pathophysiology of mood disorders because allopregnanolone interacts with GABA-A receptors and has significant anti-depressant, anti-stress, sedative and anxiolytic effects [15]. Some studies indicate that depression during pregnancy and postpartum is one of the factors that can contribute to breastfeeding failure. Other studies also suggest an association between breastfeeding and PPD, suggesting that PPD can reduce breastfeeding rates and that breastfeeding can decrease the risk of PPD. Additionally, there is evidence that breastfeeding can prevent PPD or help symptoms to recede more quickly. However, the direction of this association is still uncertain [16,17].

Due to all these reasons, PPD has become a significant health issue that affects not only women's health by increasing maternal morbidity and mortality but also a newborn's feeding patterns and, consequently, behavioural, emotional and cognitive development during early childhood [5,18].

Group interventions during the postpartum period, during which women share a safe space of mutual acceptance and understanding, have proven effective in improving depressive symptoms and empowering women to cope with their situation [19]. Additionally, there are also encouraging results demonstrating that group interventions are effective at maintaining breastfeeding during the postpartum period, especially when this peer support is combined with the leadership of a healthcare professional or an International Board Certified Lactation Consultant (IBCLC) [20]. Likewise, there is evidence of the positive impact that breastfeeding has on women's mental health by enhancing their well-being, increasing perceived self-efficacy and promoting interaction with the newborn [21,22].

At the individual level, affective characteristics, or the "qualities that represent the typical ways of feeling of individuals", are particularly important determinants of breastfeeding practices [23]. One of these key affective characteristics is self-efficacy, defined by Bandura [24] as "the belief in one's capabilities to organise and execute the courses of action required to produce certain achievements or results". In contrast, low levels of self-efficacy have been shown in previous studies to be a risk factor for the development of PPD [25].

Thus, the mental health of the mother constitutes a significant underlying factor linked to barriers and reduced rates of intention, initiation and maintenance of breastfeeding. Given the evidence of a bidirectional association between maternal mental health and breastfeeding, it is essential to consider both aspects when evaluating the effectiveness of interventions aimed at improving these outcomes [16–27].

The principal aim of this study was to assess the effectiveness of a midwife-led breastfeeding support group intervention on the maintenance of breastfeeding, the prevention of

PPD and on general self-efficacy. Additionally, the study aimed to explore the relationship between maternal depression and breastfeeding success.

2. Materials and Methods

2.1. Study Design

This was a multicentric cluster randomised controlled trial with a control group (CG) and an intervention group (IG) and was not blinded. This study was conducted according to the latest Consolidated Standards of Reporting Trials 2010 guidelines for reporting randomised controlled trials [28] and was completed as described in our published protocol [29]. Prior to the start of the trial, it was registered in the International Standard Registered Clinical/Social Study Number registry (Trial ID: ISRCTN17263529; date recorded: 17 June 2020).

2.2. Participants and Study Area

Women who met the eligibility criteria were enrolled as participants from primary health centres in Andalusia, Spain. Andalusia is an autonomous community with a birth rate of 7.72 per 1000 inhabitants (2021) [30] and 4,328,407 women of reproductive age [31] with the average age at which the first child is born being 32.7 years [32]. The study involved populations from the provinces of Seville, Cadiz, Huelva, Granada and Jaen.

2.3. Inclusion and Exclusion Criteria

The inclusion criteria included the following:

- Healthy women performing exclusive or partial breastfeeding 10 days after birth and who attended antenatal lessons at the primary health center;
- Women over 18 years of age;
- Women who accepted and signed the informed consent form.

Exclusion criteria included the following:

- Human immunodeficiency virus-positive;
- Cancer;
- Tuberculosis infection;
- No intention to breastfeed;
- Impossibility or contraindication to breastfeed due to medical conditions;
- Premature and/or complicated labour or newborn in a neonatal intensive care unit during the first month of life;
- Communication difficulties due to language barriers.

2.4. Sample Size

According to 2021 data from the National Statistical Institute of Spain, there were a total of 65,650 births in Andalusia. Specifically, the provinces of Seville (15,655 births), Granada (7083), Huelva (4227), Jaen (4499) and Cadiz (8904) accounted for 40,368 births, constituting 61.79% of the total births in the region [33]. The rate of exclusive breastfeeding (EBF) at 6 months in Andalusia is 39% [34], which was considered the baseline value in the CG. An anticipated increase of 10%, as suggested by previous research [35,36], in the rate of EBF at 6 months was established. To achieve this difference between the two groups, a two-tailed hypothesis was posed, with a power of 80% and allowing for a type I error of 5%. The necessary sample size amounted to 371 women distributed between the two study groups.

2.5. Randomisation and Recruitment

Primary health centres were randomly assigned to either the IG or the CG (receiving usual care), considering whether any form of group breastfeeding support intervention was already available. The allocation of health centres into these groups was performed by a research technician, who was independent of the researchers responsible for participant recruitment, using a random sequence [37]. The technician provided random unique identifiers to the health centres, distinguishing between those belonging to the CG and IG.

Subsequently, the women were again randomised following a simple strategy (1:1) at 35–37 weeks of gestation by the collaborating primary health centre midwives. Finally, each participant received an identification code based on the group to which she was assigned.

2.6. Intervention

Participants in the CG received standard care in terms of maternal education and postpartum visits, following the guidelines outlined in the Protocol for Care during Pregnancy, Childbirth and Puerperium by the Andalusian Health and Social Welfare Council [38], similar to the women in the IG. Within the initial 10 days after giving birth, they underwent a one-on-one visit with the midwife to address individual concerns. Additionally, women had the opportunity to request individual postpartum consultations with the designated midwife at their health centre as needed.

Women in the IG received the usual prenatal and postpartum care, just like those in the CG. Subsequently, they engaged in monthly 2 h in-person and/or virtual group sessions known as breastfeeding support groups, during which the midwife assumed the roles of leader and moderator. These sessions encompassed an educational element, featuring theoretical and practical presentations related to breastfeeding and aligned with the recommendations of the Baby-Friendly Hospital Initiative [39]. They also included motivational and social or peer support components established within the group. Consequently, on a monthly basis, women received support from an organised and proactive professional. In addition to these monthly gatherings, participants had the opportunity to interact with each other, connect with other breastfeeding women and communicate with the designated midwife through a Facebook™ and/or WhatsApp™ group specifically created for this purpose. This strengthened peer support, and queries regarding the topic were addressed using information and communication technologies [40]. Similarly, participating women retained the option to request individual consultations with the designated midwife on demand, similar to those receiving standard care.

2.7. Assessment

Sociodemographic and obstetric clinical data were collected by a questionnaire designed for this purpose via a web application. Incorrect or incomplete data were corrected via direct consultation with participants or were collected from their medical records with their consent. The data collected included the following:

- Sociodemographic variables: maternal age, country of origin, civil status (single, married, separated, widow), educational level (none, primary school, secondary school, university), employment status (self-employed, employed, unemployed);
- Obstetric variables: parity (primiparous, multiparous), gestational age, labour onset (induction, spontaneous), type of birth (eutocic, instrumental, elective caesarean section, emergent caesarean section), newborn sex, birth weight.

The type of breastfeeding was recorded at hospital discharge, as well as at three established follow-up time points: 10 days postpartum (T1), 2 months postpartum (T2) and 4 months postpartum (T3). Distinctions were made between EBF, breastfeeding with occasional supplementation of formula, mixed feeding and formula feeding.

PPD was measured using the Edinburgh Postnatal Depression Scale (EPDS) designed by Cox et al. [41] in 1987 and validated for the Spanish population by García-Esteve et al. [42] in 2003. This is a 10-item self-reported scale in which women indicate how they felt in the last 7 days. The scale is structured into three factors: anhedonia (items 1, 2 and 10), anxiety (items 3–6) and depressive symptomatology (items 7–9) [43]. The minimum possible score is 0, and the maximum is 30. The best cut-off of the Spanish validation of the EPDS was 10/11 for combined major and minor depression, the sensitivity was 79% and the specificity was 95.5%, with a positive predictive value of 63.2% and a negative predictive value of 97.7%. At this cut-off, all cases of major depression were detected. The area under the receiver operating characteristic curve was 0.976 ($p = 0.001$) with an asymptotic 95% confidence interval between 0.968 and 0.984 [42].

General self-efficacy was measured using the General Self-efficacy Scale (GSE) designed by Baessler and Schwarcer [44] in 1996. It was validated for the Spanish population by Sanjuán et al. [45]. This scale assesses the enduring sense of personal competence to effectively handle a wide variety of stressful situations. It is a unidimensional scale with 10 Likert-type questions [44]. A change in the original response form (10-point Likert-type scale instead of a 4-point scale) was introduced in order to adapt the scale to other research instruments. The reliability of the Spanish version of the GSE, as measured by the Cronbach alpha coefficient, was 0.87 [45].

The main control and outcome variables were measured before the start of the intervention (baseline) and at 2- and 4-month follow-ups.

2.8. Data Collection

The enrolment of participants commenced in October 2021 and concluded in May 2023. This process was performed by the midwives overseeing each health centre. These midwives underwent prior training for the project and received guidance from a research technician midwife associated with the project but not directly involved in the intervention. The designated midwife at the health centre, during consultations with eligible women, provided information about the study's nature and objectives, as well as details regarding the follow-up procedures. Once participants provided information via the project's web application, they agreed to participate and signed the informed consent form in duplicate. The web application automatically sent them reminder messages and emails at the three evaluation time points established in the study.

The data relating to electronic follow-up were coded and safeguarded by the research team. All data were stored in an electronic database accessible only to members of the research team.

2.9. Data Analysis

Descriptive data analyses were conducted to characterise the variables. Baseline characteristics were compared between the group experiencing potential losses during follow-up and the group completing follow-up using cross-tabulation analysis. Means were compared using Fisher's exact or *t*-tests, as appropriate. Associations between baseline and childbirth variables and EBF maintenance at 10 days, 2 months and 4 months postpartum were examined using cross-tabulation analysis.

A per-protocol analysis was performed. Chi-square or Fisher's exact tests and ANOVA or *t*-tests, as appropriate, were employed for mean comparisons. To assess the effect of the intervention on EBF maintenance at various postpartum time points, cross-tabulation analysis and chi-square tests were utilised. Additionally, a multivariate logistic model was employed to calculate adjusted odds ratios and their 95% confidence intervals for each time point.

The assumption that variables were normally distributed was checked using the Kolmogorov–Smirnov test. Group homogeneity analyses based on baseline and childbirth variables were conducted using cross-tabulation analysis, utilising chi-square or Fisher's exact tests as needed. ANOVA and *t*-tests were employed for mean comparisons.

Data analysis was conducted using SPSS v. 28.1 for Windows (IBM Corp. 2018, Armonk, NY, USA) and R (R Project 2019, version 4.0.2). The threshold for statistical significance was set at $p < 0.05$.

2.10. Ethical Considerations

Before beginning the study, it was approved by the Research Ethics Committees of the Virgen Macarena and Virgen del Rocío hospitals (Seville, Spain) on 13 March 2021 (Code 2722-N-20).

Participation in the project was voluntary, as was the participation request. Verbal and written informed consent information was provided to every participant in the study. The study was designed according to Spanish Law No. 14/2007 of 3 July regarding biomedical research and complied with the study suitability requirements and with the procedure regarding the study objectives. The data were anonymously handled according to the Spanish Organic Law on Protection of Personal Data and Guarantee of Digital Rights (Spanish Organic Law 3/2018).

3. Results

3.1. Characteristics of the Sample

A total of 512 participants were initially selected, with 130 (25.4%) excluded from randomisation for the following reasons: 73 (56.2%) were not breastfeeding their newborns and 57 (43.8%) declined follow-up in the first 10 days postpartum.

The analysis focused on a total sample of 382 mother–child dyads, randomly distributed, with 151 (39.5%) in the CG and 231 (60.5%) in the IG. There were 51 (13.35%) dropouts between T1 and T2 ($n = 331$), 27 (7.06%) of them due to discontinuation of breastfeeding. In addition, 28 participants (7.32%) dropped out between T2 and T3 ($n = 303$), motivated by discontinuation of breastfeeding, resulting in a total of 79 participants who did not continue responding to surveys (Figure 1).

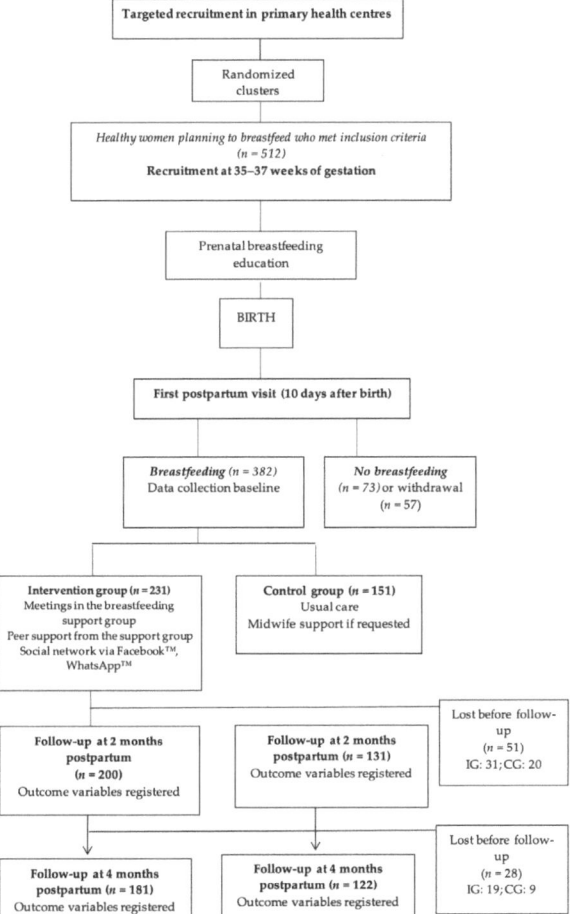

Figure 1. Participant selection flowchart.

We compared baseline characteristics between the dropout group ($n = 79$ [CG: 29; IG: 50]) and the final analysed group ($n = 303$). Fisher's exact and t-tests were used, as appropriate for variable types, to compare the groups. We observed that only those women in the IG dropout group had a lower rate of university education compared to the follow-up group (52.0% vs. 66.9%); this difference was statistically significant ($p = 0.038$). Thus, despite these losses, group homogeneity was maintained, indicating their random origin.

3.2. Sociodemographic and Obstetric–Neonatal Variables

The participants had a mean age of 33.4 ± 4.7 years, with 93.5% (357/382) born in Spain. The majority had a university education (64.4%), were married (55.0%) and had gainful employment (61.5%). The mean gestational age at birth was 39.5 ± 1.2 weeks, and 53.9% (206/382) of participants were primiparous, with 60.7% (232/382) experiencing a spontaneous onset of labour culminating in vaginal delivery (61.8%). The average birth weight was 3271 ± 434.3 g.

The relative rate of breastfeeding experience was 38.4% (58/151) in the CG and 44.6% (103/231) in the IG. We did not find statistically significant differences between the sociodemographic or obstetric–neonatal characteristics of the two groups, except for early skin-to-skin contact ($p = 0.028$) and feeding type at 4 months ($p < 0.001$; Table 1).

Table 1. Distributions of baseline variables in control and intervention groups ($n = 382$).

		Control Group $n = 151$ (39.5%)		Intervention Group $n = 231$ (60.5%)		p-Value *
		n	%	n	%	
Country of origin	Spain	142	94	215	93.1	0.709
	Foreign	9	6	16	6.9	
Civil status	Single	73	48.3	95	41.1	0.326
	Married	76	50.3	134	58	
	Separate	2	1.3	2	0.9	
	Widow	0	0	0	0	
Educational level	None	0	0	1	0.4	0.846
	Primary school	5	3.3	9	3.9	
	Secondary school	47	31.1	74	32	
	University	99	65.6	147	63.6	
Employment status	Self-employed	11	7.3	27	11.7	0.353
	Employed	97	64.2	138	59.7	
	Unemployed	43	28.5	66	28.6	
Parity	Primiparous	87	57.6	119	51.5	0.242
	Multiparous	64	42.4	112	48.5	
Previous BF experience	No	93	61.6	128	55.4	0.232
	Yes	58	38.4	103	44.6	
Labour onset	Induction	61	40.4	89	38.5	0.715
	Spontaneous	90	59.6	142	61.5	
Type of birth	Eutocic	96	63.6	140	60.6	0.411
	Instrumental	26	17.2	51	22.1	
	Elective CS	5	3.3	12	5.2	
	Emergent CS	24	15.9	28	12.1	
E-SSC	No	25	16.6	21	9.1	0.028
	Yes	126	83.4	210	90.9	
Newborn sex	Male	79	52.3	116	50.2	0.688
	Female	72	47.7	115	49.8	

Table 1. Cont.

		Control Group n = 151 (39.5%)		Intervention Group n = 231 (60.5%)		p-Value *
		n	%	n	%	
Type of feeding at discharge (n = 382)	EBF	121	80.1	178	77.1	0.841
	BF with OH	17	11.3	32	13.8	
	Mixed	13	8.6	21	9.1	
	Formula	-	-	-	-	
Type of feeding T1 (n = 382)	EBF	118	78.1	180	77.9	0.960
	BF with OH	20	13.3	31	13.4	
	Mixed	13	8.6	20	8.7	
	Formula	-	-	-	-	
Type of feeding T2 (n = 331)	EBF	84	64.1	146	73	0.335
	BF with OH	14	10.7	18	9	
	Mixed	19	14.5	23	11.5	
	Formula	14	10.7	13	6.5	
Type of feeding T3 (n = 303)	EBF	61	50	128	69.9	<0.001
	BF with OH	13	10.7	21	11.60	
	Mixed	22	18	12	6.62	
	Formula	26	21.3	20	10.9	
Quantitative Variables	Group	n		Mean	SD	p-value **
Maternal age (year)	CG	151		33.28	5.03	0.063
	IG	231		33.50	4.41	
Gestational age (week)	CG	151		39.46	1.38	0.820
	IG	231		39.45	1.14	
Birth weight (gram)	CG	151		3299	430	0.819
	IG	230		3253	437	
EPDS T1 (n = 382)	CG	151		12.65	3.68	0.090
	IG	231		12.11	3.26	
EPDS T2 (n = 331)	CG	131		12.50	3.66	0.487
	IG	200		12.62	3.70	
EPDS T3 (n = 303)	CG	122		13.39	4.00	0.116
	IG	181		12.49	3.63	
GSE T1 (n = 382)	CG	151		78.59	14.36	0.699
	IG	231		79.58	13.87	
GSE T2 (n = 331)	CG	131		75.65	14.39	0.607
	IG	200		77.73	14.81	
GSE T3 (n = 303)	CG	122		75.36	15.17	0.881
	IG	181		76.46	15.26	

* Chi-squared test; ** ANOVA; BF: breastfeeding; CS: caesarean section; E-SSC: early skin-to-skin contact; EBF: exclusive breastfeeding; BF with OH: breastfeeding with occasional help; T1: 10 days postpartum; T2: 2 months postpartum; T3: 4 months postpartum; SD: standard deviation; EPDS: Edinburg Postnatal Depression Scale; GSE: General Self-efficacy Scale; CG: control group; IG: intervention group.

During the follow-up period, we observed a gradual reduction in the breastfeeding rate from 78.0% (298/382) at 10 days to 69.5% (230/331) at 2 months and 62.4% (189/303) at 4 months postpartum. Statistically significant differences were found between the rates of breastfeeding in the CG (50.0%) and the IG (70.7%) at 4 months postpartum ($p < 0.001$; Table 2).

Table 2. Analysis of the between-group differences in the maintenance of exclusive breastfeeding.

				Group		Total	p-Value *
				CG	IG		
EBF T1 (n = 382)	No	n		33	51	84	0.959
		%		21.90	22.10	22.00	
	Yes	n		118	180	298	
		%		78.10	77.90	78.00	
EBF T2 (n = 331)	No	n		47	54	101	0.086
		%		35.90	27.00	30.50	
	Yes	n		84	146	230	
		%		64.10	73.00	69.50	
EBF T3 (n = 303)	No	n		61	53	114	<0.001
		%		50.00	29.28	37.62	
	Yes	n		61	128	189	
		%		50.00	70.72	62.38	

* Chi-square test; CG: control group; IG: intervention group; EBF: exclusive breastfeeding; T1: 10 days postpartum; T2: 2 months postpartum; T3: 4 months postpartum.

Statistically significant differences between the groups were observed in PPD at 4 months postpartum, with a lower mean score on the EPDS in the IG than the CG (12.49 ± 3.6 vs. 13.39 ± 4.0; $p = 0.044$; Table 3).

Table 3. Effectiveness of the intervention at reducing postpartum depression, as evidenced by between-group differences.

		n	Mean	SD	95% CI Upper Limit	95% CI Lower Limit	Minimum	Maximum	F	p-Value *
EPDS T1	CG	151	12.65	3.686	12.06	13.24	6	23	2.258	0.134
	IG	231	12.11	3.268	11.68	12.53	6	23		
	Total	382	12.32	3.445	11.98	12.67	6	23		
EPDS T2	CG	131	12.50	3.666	11.87	13.14	6	24	0.072	0.789
	IG	200	12.62	3.702	12.10	13.13	6	22		
	Total	331	12.57	3.683	12.17	12.97	6	24		
EPDS T3	CG	122	13.39	4.001	12.67	14.10	6	23	4.077	0.044
	IG	181	12.49	3.636	11.96	13.02	6	24		
	Total	303	12.85	3.805	12.42	13.28	6	24		

* ANOVA; SD: standard deviation; CI: confidence interval; EPDS: Edinburg Postnatal Depression Scale; T1: 10 days postpartum; T2: 2 months postpartum; T3: 4 months postpartum; CG: control group; IG: intervention group.

We examined the relationships between the maintenance of EBF and both EPDS and GSE scores during the study period. We observed statistically significant differences in the GSE scores of women who did and did not perform EBF only at T2 and T3, with women performing EBF obtaining higher scores (78.1 ± 14.3 vs. 74.3 ± 15.2 at T2 [$p = 0.014$]; 78.3 ± 14.4 vs. 72.4 ± 15.9 at T3 [$p < 0.001$]; Table 4). Statistically significant differences were observed in the EPDS scores of women who did and did not perform EBF only at T2 and T3, with lower mean scores in women performing EBF (12.2 ± 3.5 vs. 13.5 ± 3.9 at T2 [$p = 0.002$]; 12.1 ± 3.6 vs. 14.1 ± 3.8 at T3 [$p < 0.001$]; Table 4).

Table 4. Relationships between the maintenance of EBF and both EPDS and GSE scores during the study period.

			n	Mean	SD	Standard Error of the Mean	Levene's Test for Equality of Variances		t-Test for Equality of Means					95% CI	
									Significance						
							F	p-Value	t	df	One-Way p-Value	Two-Way p-Value	Mean Difference	Standard Error of Difference	Lower	Upper
EBF T1	EPDS T1	No	84	12.4	3.1	0.3	1.006	0.317	0.285	380	0.388	0.776	0.121	0.426	−0.716	0.959
		Yes	298	12.3	3.5	0.2										
	GSE T1	No	84	80.2	12.1	1.3	1.799	0.181	0.744	380	0.229	0.457	1.293	1.738	−2.123	4.709
		Yes	298	78.9	14.6	0.8										
EBF T2	EPDS T2	No	101	13.5	3.9	0.4	2.180	0.141	3.165	329	0.001	0.002	1.373	0.434	0.519	2.226
		Yes	230	12.2	3.5	0.2										
	GSE T2	No	101	74.3	15.2	1.5	0.281	0.596	−2.202	329	0.014	0.028	−3.831	1.740	−7.253	−0.408
		Yes	230	78.1	14.3	0.9										
EBF T3	EPDS T3	No	116	14.1	3.7	0.3	0.023	0.880	4.656	303	<0.001	<0.001	2.015	0.433	1.163	2.867
		Yes	187	12.1	3.6	0.3										
	GSE T3	No	116	72.4	15.9	1.5	1.121	0.291	−3.318	303	<0.001	<0.001	−5.587	1.809	−9.331	−2.384
		Yes	187	78.3	14.4	1.0										

EBF: Exclusive breastfeeding; T1: 10 days postpartum; T2: 2 months postpartum; T3: 4 months postpartum; EPDS: Edinburg Postnatal Depression Scale; GSE: General Self-efficacy Scale.

Table 5 presents the factors associated with the maintenance of EBF across the three distinct postpartum periods. Logistic regression analysis results revealed significant associations between various variables and the likelihood of sustaining EBF during each period. At T1, the absence of early skin-to-skin contact was significantly associated with a decrease in the likelihood of maintaining EBF (OR = 0.432, p = 0.014). At T2, EPDS scores were significantly associated with the likelihood of maintaining EBF. Specifically, an increase in EPDS T2 scores was linked to a significant decrease in the likelihood of sustaining EBF (OR = 0.915, p = 0.012). This finding suggests that higher levels of depressive symptoms during the second postpartum period were associated with a reduction in the likelihood of maintaining EBF. Similarly, at T3, EPDS scores were significantly associated with the probability of maintaining EBF, with an increase in score linked to a significant decrease in the likelihood of sustaining EBF (OR = 0.887, p = 0.002). Finally, the absence of intervention was related to a significant decrease in the probability of maintaining EBF at T3 (OR = 0.474, p = 0.003).

Table 5. Multivariate logistic regression models of factors favouring exclusive breastfeeding during the study period.

		β	Standard Error	Wald	df	p-Value	Exp (β)	95% CI	
								Lower	Upper
T1	E-SSC (No)	−0.839	0.341	6.047	1.000	0.014	0.432	0.221	0.843
	Gestational age	0.164	0.097	2.866	1.000	0.090	1.178	0.975	1.424
	EPDS T1	−0.011	0.036	0.085	1.000	0.770	0.989	0.921	1.063
	GSE T1	−0.007	0.009	0.591	1.000	0.442	0.993	0.975	1.011
	Intervention (No)	0.083	0.259	0.102	1.000	0.749	1.086	0.653	1.807
	Constant	−4.392	3.924	1.252	1.000	0.263	0.012		
T2	E-SSC (No)	−0.333	0.376	0.781	1.000	0.377	0.717	0.343	1.499
	Gestational age	0.043	0.101	0.177	1.000	0.674	1.044	0.856	1.273
	EPDS T2	−0.089	0.035	6.315	1.000	0.012	0.915	0.853	0.981
	GSE T2	0.009	0.009	1.028	1.000	0.311	1.009	0.992	1.026
	Intervention (No)	−0.403	0.249	2.612	1.000	0.106	0.668	0.410	1.090
	Constant	−0.187	4.044	0.002	1.000	0.963	0.829		

Table 5. Cont.

		β	Standard Error	Wald	df	p-Value	Exp (β)	95% CI	
								Lower	Upper
T3	E-SSC (No)	−0.737	0.397	3.438	1.000	0.064	0.479	0.220	1.043
	Gestational age	0.069	0.105	0.430	1.000	0.512	1.072	0.872	1.317
	EPDS T3	−0.120	0.039	9.406	1.000	0.002	0.887	0.822	0.958
	GSE T3	0.011	0.010	1.189	1.000	0.275	1.011	0.992	1.030
	Intervention (No)	−0.746	0.255	8.566	1.000	0.003	0.474	0.288	0.782
	Constant	−1.076	4.292	0.063	1.000	0.802	0.341		

Adjusted R^2 for T1: 0.219; adjusted R^2 for T2: 0.472; adjusted R^2 for T3: 0.37; Exp (β): odds ratio; T1: 10 days postpartum; T2: 2 months postpartum; T3: 4 months postpartum; E-SSC: early skin-to-skin contact; EPDS: Edinburg Postnatal Depression Scale; GSE: General Self-efficacy Scale.

4. Discussion

The purpose of this study was to assess the effect of midwife-led breastfeeding support groups on the maintenance of breastfeeding, the prevalence of PPD and the perceived general self-efficacy of the participants.

In our study, one of the most important factors related to the initiation of breastfeeding was early skin-to-skin contact after delivery. This result aligns with findings from a Cochrane review indicating that this intimate contact between the newborn and the mother provides a unique environment that meets basic biological needs, according to mammalian neuroscience, and programs future behaviours that aid in the maintenance of EBF [46]. Breastfeeding is considered a protective factor against PPD because it causes the release of oxytocin, which contributes to the well-being of the woman [47].

Another factor in our study related to the initiation of breastfeeding was greater gestational age at birth, indicating that these newborns had greater biological maturity that allowed for a more satisfactory initiation of breastfeeding and better adaptation to extrauterine life. Conversely, early term infants (born between weeks 37 + 0 and 38 + 6) are more likely to experience adverse neonatal outcomes that necessitate medical interventions, thereby complicating the initiation of breastfeeding [48,49]. This could not be analysed in our study, as participants with preterm pregnancies were not included.

The maintenance of breastfeeding during the first 6 months plays a crucial role in the health and well-being of the mother–infant dyad. According to our data on postpartum depressive symptoms, as measured by the EPDS, higher levels of depressive symptoms were associated with a reduction in the maintenance of EBF at 2 months (T2) and 4 months (T3). However, we must clarify that the direction of the association is unknown, as we do not know whether women who report fewer signs and symptoms of PPD have better breastfeeding experiences or whether those who continue breastfeeding for a longer period adapt more effectively postpartum and therefore have lower PPD scores. This challenge has already been identified by other authors who reported that women who breastfed for a longer duration had a statistically significantly lower EPDS risk score for PPD [50]. A study by Bascom et al. [51] suggested that, when depressive symptoms appear in postpartum women prematurely, difficulties with breastfeeding often lead to its early cessation.

Another key factor for the maintenance of breastfeeding is education and support through breastfeeding support groups. Our findings align with those of other studies, which have shown that interventions for promoting breastfeeding based on a combination of social support from peers and leadership by IBCLCs yield better results in maintaining breastfeeding during the first 6 months postpartum [29]. In our study, we did not observe differences at 2 months postpartum, when the first breastfeeding challenge occurs [52], but we did observe differences at 4 months postpartum, when women return to work, as indicated by other studies in which interventions were effective at 4 and 6 months postpartum [53]. The national regulation for maternity leave in Spain in relation to the workers' statute and public employees is 16 weeks with the following distribution: 6 mandatory interrupted weeks that must be enjoyed full-time immediately after giving birth and 10 more weeks that can be enjoyed on a full- or part-time basis [54]. This period of time aligns with the return to work.

General self-efficacy in breastfeeding, which is based on confidence, helps to improve breastfeeding rates [55]. In our study, it was linked to breastfeeding and PPD. Women who demonstrated higher general self-efficacy showed higher levels of breastfeeding [56] and lower levels of PPD. Additionally, those who participated in breastfeeding support groups had better outcomes for the aforementioned parameters. This aligns with the findings of Tsen et al. [57] in their randomised controlled trial, which indicate that previous breastfeeding experiences (performance accomplishments), along with observing successful breastfeeding in peers (vicarious experience) and verbal encouragement from a leader promoting breastfeeding (verbal persuasion), lead to breastfeeding success. The stress and anxiety reduction provided by these support groups increases self-efficacy and, consequently, breastfeeding [57]. Additionally, our study showed that women who were part of midwife-led breastfeeding support groups maintained breastfeeding for a longer duration and experienced less PPD. Hence, multiple findings suggest that support groups have numerous benefits as a health promotion strategy and coping mechanism for illnesses through informative support, shared experiences and opportunities to learn from others [58,59].

We must acknowledge some limitations of our study. Firstly, in the control group, no intervention unrelated to breastfeeding was carried out, but it did include psychosocial care. The reason was that in this study, we compared the standard care that women receive during this period [38] with an additional intervention designed primarily to improve breastfeeding rates. However, we also presumed that it could potentially enhance maternal mental health. Furthermore, since the direction of the association between breastfeeding and postpartum depression is uncertain, implementing an emotional support intervention in the control group could indirectly improve breastfeeding rates and confound the results. Nevertheless, women in the control group had access to on-demand consultations with the midwife for assistance or advice if needed. Secondly, only healthy women and newborns were included, thereby limiting the variability of observed physiological parameters and potentially simplifying their interpretation. Data related to breastfeeding type were self-reported, which could introduce a memory bias, even though data collection was conducted chronologically over time. Additionally, pregnant women might have misclassified types of breastfeeding (EBF, breastfeeding with other foods, etc.), which could also be related to memory bias. However, maternal recall for reporting these data has been shown to be a valid and reliable estimate of breastfeeding [60]. Furthermore, no data were collected on informal support or on the partners of the participants (age, gender, education, occupation...). Thirdly, we lacked a baseline assessment prior to pregnancy of women's rates of depression. We cannot determine if women who experienced PPD had previously suffered from depression or showed signs of being at risk. Another limitation was the withdrawal of patients from both the CG and the IG throughout the period of data collection. Finally, follow-up was conducted only until 4 months postpartum, as it is reported to be a significant period for early discontinuation of breastfeeding, particularly due to work-related reasons. In subsequent studies, it would be relevant to address up to 6 months postpartum, as per the World Health Organization's recommendation for breastfeeding.

We would like to highlight several strengths of our study, such as the prospective, consecutive and randomised inclusion of patients in five provinces of Andalusia, a southern region of Spain, allowing the findings to be applicable in routine clinical practice. The training provided by the research team to the midwives recruiting pregnant women ensured that the CG and IG samples were as homogeneous as possible. Another significant strength of this study was the use of multivariate logistic regression to determine the factors favouring breastfeeding at different data collection time points (from T1 to T3), a statistical approach not implemented in previous studies.

5. Conclusions

Women participating in midwife-led breastfeeding support groups exhibited higher levels of general self-efficacy, maintained breastfeeding for a longer duration and showed less PPD at 4 months after childbirth compared to women in the CG. These findings suggest the need for healthcare providers (midwives) to develop intervention strategies that address factors supporting the initiation and maintenance of breastfeeding by enhancing self-efficacy to reduce the occurrence of PPD, as these have been identified as promising interventions, although further research is needed.

Author Contributions: Conceptualisation and methodology: F.L.-L. and I.R.-G.; analysis of data: R.V.-C.; writing—original draft preparation, writing—review and editing: F.L.-L., I.R.-G., R.V.-C., I.C.-G. and D.G.-B. All authors have read and agreed to the published version of the manuscript.

Funding: This is a project document that has received a public grant for its development in the call for Research, Development, and Innovation on Biomedicine and Health Sciences in Andalusia of the Health and Family Council (Consejería de Salud y Familias), Spain (Code PI-0008-2019). The funders had no role in the design of this study nor in its execution, analyses, data interpretation, or presentation of results.

Institutional Review Board Statement: The study was conducted in accordance with the Declaration of Helsinki, and approved by the Research Ethics Committees of the Virgen Macarena and Virgen del Rocío hospitals (Seville, Spain) on 13 March 2021 (Code 2722-N-20), for studies involving humans.

Informed Consent Statement: Informed consent was obtained from all subjects involved in the study. Written informed consent has been obtained from the patients to publish this paper.

Data Availability Statement: The data presented in this study are available on request from the corresponding author. The data are not publicly available due to confidentiality issues.

Acknowledgments: We would like to thank all the mothers who agreed to take part in the study.

Conflicts of Interest: The authors declare no conflict of interest. The funders had no role in the design of the study; in the collection, analyses, or interpretation of data; in the writing of the manuscript; or in the decision to publish the results.

References

1. Zhao, X.H.; Zhang, Z.H. Risk factors for postpartum depression: An evidence-based systematic review of systematic reviews and meta-analyses. *Asian J. Psychiatry* **2020**, *53*, 102353. [CrossRef] [PubMed]
2. Banti, S.; Mauri, M.; Oppo, A.; Borri, C.; Rambelli, C.; Ramacciotti, D.; Montagnani, M.S.; Camilleri, V.; Cortopassi, S.; Rucci, P.; et al. From the third month of pregnancy to 1 year postpartum. Prevalence, incidence, recurrence, and new onset of depression. Results from the perinatal depression-research & screening unit study. *Compr. Psychiatry* **2011**, *52*, 343–351. [CrossRef] [PubMed]
3. Wang, J.; Wu, X.; Lai, W.; Long, E.; Zhang, X.; Li, W.; Zhu, Y.; Chen, C.; Zhong, X.; Liu, Z.; et al. Prevalence of depression and depressive symptoms among outpatients: A systematic review and meta-analysis. *BMJ Open* **2017**, *7*, e017173. [CrossRef] [PubMed]
4. American Psychiatric Association. *Diagnostic and Statistical Manual of Mental Disorders*, 5th ed.; American Psychiatric Association: Arlington, TX, USA, 2014; pp. 123–125.
5. Wang, Z.; Liu, J.; Shuai, H.; Cai, Z.; Fu, X.; Liu, Y.; Xiao, X.; Zhang, W.; Krabbendam, E.; Liu, S.; et al. Mapping global prevalence of depression among postpartum women. *Transl. Psychiatry* **2021**, *11*, 543; Erratum in *Transl. Psychiatry* **2021**, *11*, 640. [CrossRef] [PubMed]
6. Payn, J.L.; Maguire, J. Pathophysiological mechanisms implicated in postpartum depression. *Front. Neuroendocrinol.* **2019**, *52*, 165–180. [CrossRef] [PubMed]
7. De la Fe Rodríguez-Muñoz, M.; Le, H.N.; de la Cruz, I.V.; Crespo, M.E.O.; Méndez, N.I. Feasibility of screening and prevalence of prenatal depression in an obstetric setting in Spain. *Eur. J. Obstet. Gynecol. Reprod. Biol.* **2017**, *215*, 101–105. [CrossRef] [PubMed]
8. O'Hara, M.W.; Wisner, K.L. Perinatal mental illness: Definition, description and aetiology. *Best Pract. Res. Clin. Obstet. Gynaecol.* **2014**, *28*, 3–12. [CrossRef]
9. Bruist, A. Perinatal mental health: A guide to the Edinburgh Postnatal Depression Scale. *Arch. Women's Ment. Health* **2004**, *7*, 96.
10. Mayberry, L.J.; Horowitz, J.A.; Declercq, E. Depression symptom prevalence and demographic risk factors among U.S. women during the first 2 years postpartum. *J. Obstet. Gynecol. Neonatal Nurs.* **2007**, *36*, 542–549. [CrossRef]
11. Department of Health and Human Service Office on Women's Health. Benefits of breastfeeding. *Nutr. Clin. Care* **2003**, *3*, 125–131.
12. Binns, C.; Lee, M.; Low, W.Y. The Long-Term Public Health Benefits of Breastfeeding. *Asia Pac. J. Public Health* **2016**, *1*, 7–14. [CrossRef] [PubMed]

13. Chowdhury, R.; Sinha, B.; Sankar, M.J.; Taneja, S.; Bhandari, N.; Rollins, N.; Bahl, R.; Martines, J. Breastfeeding and maternal health outcomes: A systematic review and meta-analysis. *Acta Paediatry* **2015**, *467*, 96–113. [CrossRef]
14. Pang, W.W.; Hartmann, P.E. Initiation of human lactation: Secretory differentiation and secretory activation. *J. Mammary Gland Biol. Neoplasia* **2007**, *12*, 211–221. [CrossRef] [PubMed]
15. Stefaniak, M.; Dmoch-Gajzlerska, E.; Jankowska, K.; Rogowski, A.; Kajdy, A.; Maksym, R.B. Progesterone and Its Metabolites Play a Beneficial Role in Affect Regulation in the Female Brain. *Pharmaceuticals* **2023**, *16*, 520. [CrossRef] [PubMed]
16. Figueiredo, B.; Dias, C.C.; Brandão, S.; Canário, C.; Nunes-Costa, R. Breastfeeding and postpartum depression: State of the art review. *J. Pediatr.* **2013**, *89*, 332–338. [CrossRef]
17. Xia, M.; Luo, J.; Wang, J.; Liang, Y. Association between breastfeeding and postpartum depression: A meta-analysis. *J. Affect. Disord.* **2022**, *308*, 512–519. [CrossRef] [PubMed]
18. Dennis, C.L.; Boyce, P. Further psychometric testing of a brief personality scale to measure vulnerability to postpartum depression. *J. Psychosom. Obstet. Gynaecol.* **2004**, *25*, 305–311. [CrossRef] [PubMed]
19. Gillis, B.D.; Parish, A.L. Group-based interventions for postpartum depression: An integrative review and conceptual model. *Arch. Psychiatry Nurs.* **2019**, *33*, 290–298. [CrossRef]
20. Rodríguez-Gallego, I.; Leon-Larios, F.; Corrales-Gutierrez, I.; González-Sanz, J.D. Impact and Effectiveness of Group Strategies for Supporting Breastfeeding after Birth: A Systematic Review. *Int. J. Environ. Res. Public Health* **2021**, *18*, 2550. [CrossRef]
21. Nishioka, E.; Haruna, M.; Ota, E.; Matsuzaki, M.; Murayama, R.; Yoshimura, K.; Murashima, S. A prospective study of the relationship between breastfeeding and postpartum depressive symptoms appearing at 1–5 months after delivery. *J. Affect. Disord.* **2011**, *133*, 553–559. [CrossRef]
22. Pope, C.J.; Mazmanian, D. Breastfeeding and Postpartum Depression: An Overview and Methodological Recommendations for Future Research. *Depress. Res. Treat.* **2016**, *2016*, 4765310. [CrossRef] [PubMed]
23. McCoach, D.B.; Gable, R.K.; Madura, J.P. *Instrument Development in the Affective Domain. School and Corporate Applications*, 3rd ed.; Springer: New York, NY, USA, 2013.
24. Bandura, A. Self-efficacy: Toward a unifying theory of behavioral change. *Psychol. Rev.* **1977**, *2*, 191–215. [CrossRef]
25. Han, L.; Zhang, J.; Yang, J.; Yang, X.; Bai, H. Between Personality Traits and Postpartum Depression: The Mediated Role of Maternal Self-Efficacy. *Neuropsychiatr. Dis. Treat.* **2022**, *18*, 597–609. [CrossRef] [PubMed]
26. Henshaw, E.J. Breastfeeding and Postpartum Depression: A Review of Relationships and Potential Mechanisms. *Curr. Psychiatry Rep.* **2023**, *31*, 803–808. [CrossRef] [PubMed]
27. Pezley, L.; Cares, K.; Duffecy, J.; Koenig, M.D.; Maki, P.; Odoms-Young, A.; Clark Withington, M.H.; Lima Oliveira, M.; Loiacono, B.; Prough, J.; et al. Efficacy of behavioral interventions to improve maternal mental health and breastfeeding outcomes: A systematic review. *Int. Breastfeed J.* **2022**, *17*, 67. [CrossRef] [PubMed]
28. Moher, D.; Hopewell, S.; Schulz, K.F.; Montori, V.; Gøtzsche, P.C.; Devereaux, P.; Elbourne, D.; Egger, M.; Altman, D.G. CONSORT 2010 explanation and elaboration: Updated guidelines for reporting parallel group randomised trials. *BMJ* **2010**, *340*, c869. [CrossRef]
29. Rodríguez-Gallego, I.; Leon-Larios, F.; Ruiz-Ferrón, C.; Lomas-Campos, M.D. Evaluation of the impact of breastfeeding support groups in primary health CENTRES in Andalusia, Spain: A study protocol for a cluster randomized controlled trial (GALMA project). *BMC Public Health* **2020**, *20*, 1129; Erratum in *BMC Public Health* **2020**, *20*, 1445. [CrossRef]
30. Instituto Nacional de Estadística. Oficina Estadística Española. Registro INE 2021. Available online: https://www.ine.es/jaxiT3/Datos.htm?t=1433#!tabs-tabla (accessed on 20 July 2023).
31. Instituto Nacional de Estadística (INE). Series Detalladas Desde 2002. Población Residente por fecha, Sexo, Grupo de edad y Nacionalidad (Agrupación de Países). Oficina Estadística Española. Registro INE 2022. Available online: https://www.ine.es/jaxiT3/Datos.htm?t=9689 (accessed on 20 July 2023).
32. Instituto de Estadística y Cartografía de Andalucía. Movimiento Natural de la Población (MNP) 2022. Available online: https://www.juntadeandalucia.es/institutodeestadisticaycartografia/dega/movimiento-natural-de-la-poblacion-mnp/nota-divulgativa-datos-definitivos-2022 (accessed on 2 January 2024).
33. Instituto Nacional de Estadística (INE). Movimiento Natural de la Población: Nacimientos. Fenómenos Demográficos por Comunidades y Ciudades Autónomas y tipo de Fenómeno Demográfico. Oficina Estadística Española. Registro INE 2021. Available online: https://www.ine.es/jaxiT3/Datos.htm?t=6567 (accessed on 20 July 2023).
34. Ministerio de Sanidad. Encuesta Nacional de Salud de España 2017 (ENSE 2017). Determinantes de Salud. Tipo de Lactancia. Tabla 3.078. Según Sexo y Clase Social Basada en la Ocupación de la Persona de Referencia. Available online: https://www.sanidad.gob.es/estadEstudios/estadisticas/encuestaNacional/encuestaNac2017/ENSE17_MOD3_REL.pdf (accessed on 20 July 2023).
35. Nabulsi, M.; Hamadeh, H.; Tamim, H.; Kabakian, T.; Charafeddine, L.; Yehya, N.; Sinno, D.; Sidani, S. A complex breastfeeding promotion and support intervention in a developing country: Study protocol for a randomized clinical trial. *BMC Public Health* **2014**, *14*, 36. [CrossRef]
36. Rollins, N.C.; Bhandari, N.; Hajeebhoy, N.; Horton, S.; Lutter, C.K.; Martines, J.C.; Piwoz, E.G.; Richter, L.M.; Victora, C.G.; Lancet Breastfeeding Series Group. Why invest, and what it will take to improve breastfeeding practices? *Lancet* **2016**, *387*, 491–504. [CrossRef]

37. Guillaumes, S.; O'Callaghan, C. Versión en español del software gratuito OxMaR para minimización y aleatorización de estudios clínicos. *Gac. Sanit.* **2019**, *33*, 395–397. [CrossRef]
38. Aceituno, L.; Maldonado, J.; Arribas, L.; Caño, A.; Corona, I.; Martín, J.E.; Mora, M.A.; Morales, L.; Ras, J.; Sánchez, T.; et al. *Embarazo, Parto y Puerperio. Proceso Asistencial Integrado*, 3rd ed.; Consejería De Igualdad, Salud y Políticas Sociales: Junta de Andalucía, Spain, 2014; pp. 24–46.
39. World Health Organization; UNICEF. *Protecting, Promoting, and Supporting Breastfeeding in Facilities Providing Maternity and Newborn Services: The Revised Baby-Friendly Hospital Initiative 2018*; Implementation guidance; WHO: Geneva, Switzerland, 2018.
40. Robinson, A.; Lauckner, C.; Davis, M.; Hall, J.; Anderson, A.K. Facebook support for breastfeeding mothers: A comparison to offline support and associations with breastfeeding outcomes. *Digit. Health* **2019**, *5*, 2055207619853397. [CrossRef] [PubMed]
41. Cox, J.L.; Holden, J.M.; Sagovsky, R. Detection of postnatal depression. Development of the 10-item Edinburgh Postnatal Depression Scale. *Br. J. Psychiatry* **1987**, *150*, 782–786. [CrossRef] [PubMed]
42. Garcia-Esteve, L.; Ascaso, C.; Ojuel, J.; Navarro, P. Validation of the Edinburgh Postnatal Depression Scale (EPDS) in Spanish mothers. *J. Affect. Disord.* **2003**, *75*, 71–76. [CrossRef] [PubMed]
43. Gutierrez-Zotes, A.; Gallardo-Pujol, D.; Labad, J.; Martín-Santos, R.; García-Esteve, L.; Gelabert, E.; Jover, M.; Guillamat, R.; Mayoral, F.; Gornemann, I.; et al. Factor Structure of the Spanish Version of the Edinburgh Postnatal Depression Scale. *Actas Esp. Psiquiatr.* **2018**, *46*, 174–182. [PubMed]
44. Baessler, J.; Schwarcer, R. Evaluación de la autoeficacia: Adaptación española de la escala de Autoeficacia General. *Actas Esp. Psiquiatr.* **1996**, *2*, 174–182.
45. Sanjuán, P.; Pérez, A.M.; Bermúdez, J. Escala de autoeficacia general: Datos psicométricos de la adaptación para población española. *Psicothema* **2000**, *12*, 509–513.
46. Moore, E.R.; Bergman, N.; Anderson, G.C.; Medley, N. Early skin-to-skin contact for mothers and their healthy newborn infants. *Cochrane Database Syst. Rev.* **2016**, *11*, CD003519. [CrossRef] [PubMed]
47. Niwayama, R.; Nishitani, S.; Takamura, T.; Shinohara, K.; Honda, S.; Miyamura, T.; Nakao, Y.; Oishi, K.; Araki-Nagahashi, M. Oxytocin Mediates a Calming Effect on Postpartum Mood in Primiparous Mothers. *Breastfeed Med.* **2017**, *12*, 103–109. [CrossRef]
48. Nejsum, F.M.; Måstrup, R.; Torp-Pedersen, C.; Løkkegaard, E.C.L.; Wiingreen, R.; Hansen, B.M. Exclusive breastfeeding: Relation to gestational age, birth weight, and early neonatal ward admission. A nationwide cohort study of children born after 35 weeks of gestation. *PLoS ONE* **2023**, *18*, e0285476. [CrossRef]
49. Fan, H.S.L.; Wong, J.Y.H.; Fong, D.Y.T.; Lok, K.Y.W.; Tarrant, M. Association between early-term birth and breastfeeding initiation, duration, and exclusivity: A systematic review. *Birth* **2019**, *46*, 24–34. [CrossRef]
50. Toledo, C.; Cianelli, R.; Villegas Rodriguez, N.; De Oliveira, G.; Gattamorta, K.; Wojnar, D.; Ojukwu, E. The significance of breastfeeding practices on postpartum depression risk. *Public Health Nurs.* **2022**, *39*, 15–23. [CrossRef] [PubMed]
51. Bascom, E.M.E.; Napolitano, M.A. Breastfeeding Duration and Primary Reasons for Breastfeeding Cessation among Women with Postpartum Depressive Symptoms. *J. Hum. Lact.* **2016**, *32*, 282–291. [CrossRef] [PubMed]
52. Franco-Antonio, C.; Santano-Mogena, E.; Sánchez-García, P.; Chimento-Díaz, S.; Cordovilla-Guardia, S. Effect of a brief motivational intervention in the immediate postpartum period on breastfeeding self-efficacy: Randomized controlled trial. *Res. Nurs. Health* **2021**, *44*, 295–307. [CrossRef] [PubMed]
53. Franco-Antonio, C.; Calderón-García, J.F.; Santano-Mogena, E.; Rico-Martín, S.; Cordovilla-Guardia, S. Effectiveness of a brief motivational intervention to increase the breastfeeding duration in the first 6 months postpartum: Randomized controlled trial. *J. Adv. Nurs.* **2020**, *76*, 888–902. [CrossRef] [PubMed]
54. Leon-Larios, F.; Pinero-Pinto, E.; Arnedillo-Sanchez, S.; Ruiz-Ferron, C.; Casado-Mejia, R.; Benitez-Lugo, M. Female employees' perception of breastfeeding-friendly support in a public university in Spain. *Public Health Nurs.* **2019**, *36*, 370–378. [CrossRef]
55. Oliver-Roig, A.; d'Anglade-González, M.L.; García-García, B.; Silva-Tubio, J.R.; Richart-Martínez, M.; Dennis, C.L. The Spanish version of the Breastfeeding Self-Efficacy Scale-Short Form: Reliability and validity assessment. *Int. J. Nurs. Study* **2012**, *49*, 169–173. [CrossRef] [PubMed]
56. Nilsson, I.M.S.; Kronborg, H.; Rahbek, K.; Strandberg-Larsen, K. The significance of early breastfeeding experiences on breastfeeding self-efficacy one week postpartum. *Matern. Child Nutr.* **2020**, *16*, e12986. [CrossRef]
57. Tseng, J.F.; Chen, S.R.; Au, H.K.; Chipojola, R.; Lee, G.T.; Lee, P.H.; Shyu, M.L.; Kuo, S.Y. Effectiveness of an integrated breastfeeding education program to improve self-efficacy and exclusive breastfeeding rate: A single-blind, randomised controlled study. *Int. J. Nurs. Study* **2020**, *111*, 103770. [CrossRef]
58. Jablotschkin, M.; Binkowski, L.; Markovits Hoopii, R.; Weis, J. Benefits and challenges of cancer peer support groups: A systematic review of qualitative studies. *Eur. J. Cancer Care* **2022**, *31*, e13700. [CrossRef]
59. Grubesic, T.H.; Durbin, K.M. Geodemographies of Breastfeeding Support. *J. Hum. Lact.* **2021**, *37*, 301–313. [CrossRef]
60. Li, R.; Scanlon, K.S.; Serdula, M.K. The validity and reliability of maternal recall of breastfeeding practice. *Nutr. Rev.* **2005**, *63*, 103–110. [CrossRef] [PubMed]

Disclaimer/Publisher's Note: The statements, opinions and data contained in all publications are solely those of the individual author(s) and contributor(s) and not of MDPI and/or the editor(s). MDPI and/or the editor(s) disclaim responsibility for any injury to people or property resulting from any ideas, methods, instructions or products referred to in the content.

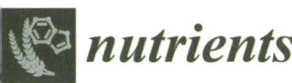

Article

Factors Influencing Duration of Breastfeeding: Insights from a Prospective Study of Maternal Health Literacy and Obstetric Practices

Rafael Vila-Candel [1,2,3], Francisco Javier Soriano-Vidal [3,4,5,*], Cristina Franco-Antonio [6,*], Oscar Garcia-Algar [7], Vicente Andreu-Fernandez [8] and Desirée Mena-Tudela [9]

[1] Faculty of Health Sciences, Universidad Internecinal de Valencia (VIU), 46002 Valencia, Spain; rafael.vila@professor.universidadviu.com
[2] La Ribera Primary Health Department, 46600 Alzira, Spain; vila_rafcan@gva.es
[3] Foundation for the Promotion of Health and Biomedical Research in the Valencian Region (FISABIO), 46020 Valencia, Spain
[4] Department of Obstetrics and Gynecology, Xàtiva-Oninyent Health Department, 46800 Xàtiva, Spain
[5] Department of Nursing, Universitat de València, 46007 Valencia, Spain
[6] Department of Nursing, Universidad de Extremadura, 10003 Cáceres, Spain
[7] Neonatology Unit, ICGON, Hospital Clínic-Maternitat, BCNatal, 08028 Barcelona, Spain; ogarciaa@clinic.cat
[8] Instituto de Investigaciones Biosanitarias, Universidad Internacional de Valencia (VIU), 46002 Valencia, Spain; vicente.andreu@professor.universidadviu.com
[9] Department of Nursing, Instituto Universitario de Estudios Feministas y de Género Purificación Escribano, Universitat Jaume I, 12071 Castellón de la Plana, Spain; dmena@uji.es
* Correspondence: francisco.j.soriano@uv.es (F.J.S.-V.); cfrancox@unex.es (C.F.-A.)

Citation: Vila-Candel, R.; Soriano-Vidal, F.J.; Franco-Antonio, C.; Garcia-Algar, O.; Andreu-Fernandez, V.; Mena-Tudela, D. Factors Influencing Duration of Breastfeeding: Insights from a Prospective Study of Maternal Health Literacy and Obstetric Practices. *Nutrients* **2024**, *16*, 690. https://doi.org/10.3390/nu16050690

Academic Editor: Andrea Vania

Received: 8 February 2024
Revised: 25 February 2024
Accepted: 26 February 2024
Published: 28 February 2024

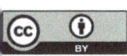

Copyright: © 2024 by the authors. Licensee MDPI, Basel, Switzerland. This article is an open access article distributed under the terms and conditions of the Creative Commons Attribution (CC BY) license (https://creativecommons.org/licenses/by/4.0/).

Abstract: Numerous factors concerning early breastfeeding abandonment have been described, including health literacy (HL). This study's objective was to analyze factors related to early breastfeeding abandonment (<6 months). This prospective multicentric study examined the duration of breastfeeding at 6 months postpartum and was conducted in four different regions of Spain from January 2021 to January 2023. A total of 275 women participated in this study, which focused on maternal HL and obstetric practices. A decrease in the breastfeeding rate was observed from hospital discharge (n = 224, 81.5%) to the sixth month postpartum (n = 117, 42.5%). A Cox regression analysis revealed that inadequate HL levels, lack of mobilization during labour, and induced labour were significantly associated with early breastfeeding cessation (p = 0.022, p = 0.019, and p = 0.010, respectively). The results highlight that women with adequate HL had a 32% lower risk of early breastfeeding abandonment. In comparison, mobilization during labour and induction of labour were linked to a 32.4% reduction and a 53.8% increase in this risk, respectively. These findings emphasize the importance of considering obstetric and HL factors when addressing the breastfeeding duration, indicating opportunities for educational and perinatal care interventions.

Keywords: breastfeeding; health literacy; abandonment; nursing

1. Introduction

Breastfeeding (BF) is a health-promoting behaviour [1]. Furthermore, the associated relationship between mother and baby goes beyond mere nourishment [2]. Despite its notable and numerous physical, emotional, and psychological benefits and the significant role that BF plays in maternal and infant health in the short, medium, and long term, BF rates remain improvable.

International organizations, such as the World Health Organization (WHO) and the United Nations International Children's Emergency Fund (UNICEF), recommend maintaining exclusive breastfeeding (EBF) for at least the first six months of infants' lives. However, according to data, it is estimated that globally, 43.8% of infants under 6 months are exclusively breastfed [3]. In Europe, this figure rises to 60%, but it is unknown whether it pertains to EBF or any other form of breastfeeding [4]. It is also important to note significant variability in the data depending on the European country of origin. In Spain, the national health survey in 2017 showed that the percentage of EBF at 6 months was 39% [5]. However, other studies have reported significant variability between cities and autonomous communities. For example, the reported EBF rate in Madrid was 25.4% [6], 16.8% in Catalonia [7], and 21.6% in the Vasque Country [8]. The latest multicentre study that reported figures in Spain indicates that 57.3% of women maintained breastfeeding, including EBF and mixed feeding, up to 6 months postpartum [9]. In order to contribute to improving these figures, it is relevant to understand the factors that influence the duration of breastfeeding to promote optimal practices.

Health literacy (HL) has been defined as "The ability of an individual to obtain and translate knowledge and information in order to maintain and improve health in a way that is appropriate to the individual and system contexts" [10]. Furthermore, HL is understood to be a continuous learning process that requires the ability to access, comprehend, critically evaluate, and apply health-related information [10,11]. Among the many published articles, in 2001, Kaufman [12] was the first to establish a correlation between HL and the maintenance of BF. Subsequent studies, however, have presented diverse outcomes, with the anticipated link between HL and BF maintenance not uniformly affirmed in all instances. This variability may stem from the specific characteristics of the study population, or the nuances of the screening tools employed, which are often adapted from languages other than the one under investigation. Consequently, this underscores the imperative for meticulously scrutinizing contextual and methodological elements in deciphering the association between HL and BF duration.

The limited comparability with other studies emanates from incongruent definitions of BF outcomes and the myriad methods utilized to assess HL. Researchers [12–14] employed questionnaires, such as the Short Test of Functional Health Literacy in Adults or Rapid Estimates of Adult Literacy in Medicine, to measure HL. Despite the divergent HL assessment approaches, a consistent finding emerged, which revealed positive correlations between HL and BF behaviour. Nevertheless, the distinct criteria used to assess BF outcomes introduce additional intricacies into direct comparisons. Conversely, other authors [15,16] have reported no statistically significant association between functional HL, as evaluated using the Newest Vital Sign screening tool, and EBF for more than 4 months. Considering the observed variability in results, our study is positioned as a valuable addition to the existing body of evidence. However, recognizing that maternal HL levels may influence the understanding and adherence to BF recommendations, further research is warranted.

Historically, it has been observed that the medicalization of childbirth significantly impacted BF rates. At the beginning of the 20th century, most births occurred at home, and a breastfeeding culture was well-established, with knowledge transmitted effectively between women; this context resulted in high breastfeeding rates [17]. In contrast to this, the model of care centred on medical authority led to barriers in breastfeeding related to obstetric practices, such as the separation of the mother–child dyad during the clinical postpartum period [17,18]. Currently, we know that mother–baby separation after birth, the excessive use of medical interventions during childbirth, or a lack of support during the clinical postpartum period are practices that do not favour the establishment and maintenance of breastfeeding. On the other hand, despite high levels of intervention, as in a surgical procedure, like a Caesarean section, it is known that respecting dyad practices, such as early skin-to-skin contact or early and spontaneous breastfeeding initiation, favour the establishment and long-term maintenance of breastfeeding [19–21].

As breastfeeding practices significantly contribute to infant health and development, unravelling the intricate relationship between maternal HL, obstetric practices, and BF duration holds the potential to guide evidence-based approaches for promoting and sustaining optimal breastfeeding practices. Therefore, this study aimed to analyze factors related to early breastfeeding discontinuation (<6 months).

2. Materials and Methods

2.1. Study Design

This multicentre prospective study was conducted in four public hospitals across Spain from January 2021 to January 2023.

2.2. Participants and Study Area

Women meeting the eligibility criteria were enrolled in primary health centres between 24 and 37 weeks of pregnancy. This study strategically chose four hospitals that were geographically dispersed—three in the east and one in the west of Spain—to ensure a diverse analysis. This inclusive approach facilitated result generalization while mitigating biases. Specifically, the eastern region included the General Hospital of Castellón (northeast (H3)), Hospital de la Ribera (H1), and Hospital Lluis Alcanyis (southeast (H2)), with comparable annual deliveries. The General Hospital of Cáceres (H4) in the west of Spain offers maternity care to women with distinct characteristics. All four hospitals share similarities in birth rates, treated prematurity, and participation in the IHAN program for maternity healthcare quality. Collectively serving 500,000 people, they witness approximately 5000 births annually, with pregnant women recruited during their third trimester from primary care clinics managed by affiliated midwives.

2.3. Inclusion and Exclusion Criteria

Participants were enrolled during the third trimester of pregnancy in the midwifery-led primary care consultations in each participating centre. The inclusion criteria were women who accepted and signed the informed consent form, had Internet access, and intended to breastfeed.

This study's exclusion criteria were females under 16 years of age; individuals with cognitive impairments, language barriers, or illiteracy (unable to read in Spanish); newborns with congenital malformations; and multi-child pregnancies.

2.4. Sample Size

We estimated the necessary sample size based on an annual population of 5000 births across the 4 participating hospitals, assuming a 65% discontinuation rate of breastfeeding at 6 months, with a significance level of 0.05% and a power of 90%, along with an estimated 10% loss to follow-up. The total sample size calculated was 261 participants.

2.5. Baseline Variables

The baseline data collection encompassed the following variables:

- Sociodemographic variables: maternal age, country of origin (Spain/foreign), level of education (primary to secondary school/university), employment status (professional to employee/unemployed/student), civil status (married/others), economic status (<EUR 1000 per month/>EUR 1000 per month), and financial status (bad–regular/good–very good).
- Health-literacy-related variables: HLS-EU-Q16, which assesses the population's HL through a Likert scale with 16 items according to "very easy (1 point)", "easy (1 point)", "difficult (0 points)", and "very difficult (0 points)". This unifactorial scale exhibits good internal consistency, with a McDonald's omega value of 0.982 in the Spanish population [22]. Level of HL: adequate (>12 points) or inadequate ($\leq$12 points) (Supplementary Table S1).
- Obstetric–neonatal variables: gestational age at birth, parity (nulliparous/multiparous), type of onset of labour (spontaneous or elective Caesarean section/induced), type of rupture of membranes (spontaneous/artificial), group B streptococcus status (positive/negative), intrapartum antibiotic use (yes/no), intrapartum analgesia (inhalatory/local/epidural/none), Kristeller manoeuvre (yes/no), completion of birth (spontaneous vaginal/instrumental (vacuum, spatulas, forceps)/Caesarean section), episiotomy (yes/no), perineal condition following birth (intact/grade 1/grade 2/

grade 3/grade 4) [23], newborn gender (female/male), newborn weight (grams), early skin-to-skin contact [(within 30 min and lasting for at least 2 continuous hours) (yes/no/with father)], early start of breastfeeding (within 2 h/after more than 2 h), drinking allowed during labour (yes/no), accompaniment of maternal choice allowed (yes/no), mobilization allowed during labour (yes/no), and positioning at the moment of birth (vertical/lying down—lithotomy position/lateral decubitus).
- Response variable: type of nursing (BF/supplementary feeding (SF)/mixed feeding (MF)) at 6 months postpartum, assessing the newborn and infant feeding practices. The response variable "Suspension of BF at 6 months" (yes/no) considered whether the infant was receiving SF ("yes") or continued with BF or MF ("no") at 6 months.
- Variables related to previous breastfeeding education: information/training in breastfeeding (none/previous information received from relatives; friends; or health professionals, such as midwives, pediatric nurses, obstetricians, and paediatricians); consultation of texts; participation in birth preparation groups, nursing groups, or postpartum groups; and the use of digital tools.

2.6. Data Collection

A web platform was developed for study monitoring in each of the four cohorts in Spain: Hospital de la Ribera (H1), Hospital Lluis Alcanyis (H2), General Hospital of Castellón (H3), and General Hospital of Cáceres (H4), all of which had comparable annual birth rates. After recruitment and electronic acceptance of the informed consent form, the participants received a survey via email based on the expected due date. In the initial baseline survey, all sociodemographic data and health literacy levels were collected using the screening tool HLS-EU-Q16. After childbirth, each participant received surveys at 15 days, 6 weeks, 3 months, and 6 months postpartum. Collaborating researchers from each health department of the 4 regions (H1, H2, H3, and H4) were given secure access to the platform to record birth data and the number of visits made by various healthcare professionals during the study period. The collected information was entered into an electronic database while ensuring compliance with current regulations and guaranteeing confidentiality and anonymity. Losses and dropouts during this study and their causes were recorded. However, researchers were not authorized to view the planned surveys that the participants completed during the study follow-up. Finally, the data manager was responsible for matching the participants' survey responses with their birth dates and the follow-ups performed by various healthcare professionals for up to 6 months. This approach ensured confidentiality and complied with data protection regulations. Our methodology prioritized user anonymity and data security, which allowed for accurate matching while safeguarding participants' privacy rights.

2.7. Data Analysis

The dataset underwent comprehensive descriptive analyses, which involved examining the distinctive features of each variable. Statistical tests, such as Fisher's test or t-test, were selectively applied to compare means. Bivariate comparisons scrutinized the early breastfeeding abandonment (<6 months) (yes/no) at multiple time points, including at discharge, 15 days, 6 weeks, 3 months, and 6 months, while considering sociodemographic, health literacy, and obstetric–neonatal variables through the chi-square test. Additionally, survival analysis using the Kaplan–Meier method gauged the statistical significance of variables related to early breastfeeding abandonment over 6 months. A Cox regression model was formulated and incorporated statistically significant variables.

The statistical analysis was performed using SPSS v. 28.1 for Windows (IBM Corp. 2018, Armonk, NY, USA), with a significance threshold set at $p < 0.05$.

3. Results

Out of a total of 280 women, 5 were excluded for the following reasons: 2 perinatal deaths and 3 lost to follow-up. The total analyzed sample consisted of 275 participants.

A total of 44.7% (123/275) of the births were attended at H1, 27.3% (75/275) at H4, 15.6% (43/275) at H3, and 12.4% (34/275) at H2. Table 1 presents a chi-square analysis to assess the associations between various variables and early BF abandonment. The chi-square test was applied by comparing each category's observed and expected frequencies, with results stratified by the responses (no or yes) regarding early BF abandonment. The associated p-values indicate the statistical significance of these associations. Notably, the comparisons were made by analyzing the table's columns.

Table 1. Sociodemographic and obstetric–neonatal characteristics of the sample (N = 275).

		Early BF Abandonment in the Previous 6 Months				
		No $n = 117$ (42.5%)		Yes $n = 158$ (57.5%)		
		n	%	n	%	p-Value *
Country of origin	Spain	108	92.3	140	88.6	0.308
	Foreign	9	7.7	18	11.4	
Education level	Primary to secondary school	54	46.2	73	46.2	0.994
	University	63	53.8	85	53.8	
Civil status	Others	37	31.6	55	34.8	0.994
	Married	80	68.4	103	65.2	
Employment status	Unemployed or student	38	32.5	59	37.3	0.994
	Employee or professional	79	67.5	99	62.7	
Economic status	<EUR 1000/month	50	42.7	74	46.8	0.499
	>EUR 1000/month	67	57.3	84	53.2	
Financial stability level	Bad or medium	51	43.6	83	52.5	0.142
	Good or very good	66	56.4	75	47.5	
Desired type of breastfeeding	Exclusive	110	94	138	87.3	0.177
	Mixed	5	4.3	13	8.2	
	Not desired yet	2	1.7	7	4.4	
Previous breastfeeding information	No information	4	3.4	10	6.3	0.093
	Family or friend	21	17.9	47	29.7	
	Healthcare professional	34	29.1	36	22.8	
	Books	10	8.5	5	3.2	
	Birth preparation	19	16.2	18	11.4	
	Breastfeeding group	1	0.9	1	0.6	
	Digital tools	28	23.9	41	25.9	
Health literacy level by HLS-EU-16Q	Inadequate	28	23.9	56	35.4	0.040
	Adequate	89	76.1	102	64.6	
Parity	Nulliparous	81	69.2	121	76.6	0.172
	Multiparous	36	30.8	37	23.4	

Table 1. Cont.

		Early BF Abandonment in the Previous 6 Months				
		No n = 117 (42.5%)		Yes n = 158 (57.5%)		
		n	%	n	%	p-Value *
Pregnancy risk	Low risk	92	78.6	118	74.7	0.649
	Gestational diabetes	9	7.7	16	10.1	
	Hypothyroidism	4	3.4	5	3.2	
	Preeclampsia/hypertension	2	1.7	2	1.3	
	Infertility	1	0.9	1	0.6	
	Premature birth	0	0	4	2.5	
	Other gestational diseases	8	6.8	8	5.1	
	Chronic condition with medication	1	0.9	4	2.5	
Onset of labour	Spontaneous or elective C-section	95	81.2	100	63.3	0.014
	Induction	22	18.8	58	36.7	
Type of rupture of membranes	Spontaneous	83	70.9	89	56.3	0.013
	Artificial	34	29.1	69	43.7	
Streptococcus Agalactie B	Negative	96	82.1	129	81.6	0.931
	Positive	21	17.9	29	18.4	
Intrapartum use of antibiotic	No	98	83.8	126	79.7	0.397
	Yes	19	16.2	32	20.3	
Type of analgesia	Inhalator	0	0	0	0	0.420
	Local	3	2.6	8	5.1	
	Epidural	92	78.6	123	77.8	
	Without analgesia	9	7.7	16	10.1	
	Spinal	13	11.1	11	7	
Kristeller manoeuvre	No	103	88	145	91.8	0.303
	Yes	14	12	13	8.2	
Drinking allowed during labour	No	28	23.9	57	36.1	0.031
	Yes	89	76.1	101	63.9	
Labour accompaniment	No	8	6.8	6	3.8	0.257
	Yes	109	93.2	152	96.2	
Mobilization allowed during labour	No	27	23.1	57	36.3	0.019
	Yes	90	76.9	100	63.7	
Positioning in birth (n = 218)	Vertical	8	8.4	21	17.1	0.087
	Lithotomy	61	64.2	81	65.9	
	Lateral decubitus	26	27.4	21	17.1	
Type of birth	Spontaneous vaginal	66	56.4	90	57	0.443
	Instrumental vaginal	30	25.6	32	20.3	
	C-section	21	17.9	36	22.8	

Table 1. Cont.

		Early BF Abandonment in the Previous 6 Months				
		No n = 117 (42.5%)		Yes n = 158 (57.5%)		
		n	%	n	%	p-Value *
Type of instrumental birth	Vacuum	26	86.7	24	75	0.472
	Spatulas	2	6.7	5	15.6	
	Forceps	2	6.7	3	9.4	
Episiotomy	No	68	70.8	81	66.4	0.484
	Yes	28	29.2	41	33.6	
Perineum injury	Intact	19	27.9	27	32.5	0.846
	Grade I	28	41.2	29	34.9	
	Grade II	20	29.4	25	30.1	
	Grade III	1	1.5	2	2.4	
Sex of newborn	Female	63	53.8	75	47.5	0.296
	Male	54	46.2	83	52.5	
Early skin-to-skin contact	No	2	1.7	7	4.4	0.288
	Yes	108	92.3	137	86.7	
	Companion	7	6	14	8.9	
Breastfeeding initiation	<2 h	90	76.9	109	69	0.146
	>2 h	27	23.1	49	31	

* Chi-square test; significant p-values < 0.05. C-section: Caesarean section; HLS-EU-16Q: health literacy survey European Union short questionnaire in Spanish.

The mean age of participants was 33.2 ± 4.4 years ($p = 0.977$), with 90.2% (248/275) being Spanish-born women ($p = 0.308$) (Table 1). Most participants had a university education (53.8%, $n = 148/275$; $p = 0.994$), were married (66.5%, $n = 183/275$; $p = 0.994$), were employed (64.7%, $n = 178/275$; $p = 0.994$), had an adequate level of income (54.9%, $n = 151/275$; $p = 0.499$), and perceived good or very good economic stability (51.3%, $n = 141/275$; $p = 0.142$). All women desired to breastfeed, with 90.2% (248/275) aiming for EBF, 6.5% (18/275) opting for MF, and the rest undecided ($p = 0.177$). Information on BF was primarily received from family and friends (24.7%, $n = 68/275$), healthcare professionals (25.5%, $n = 70/275$), and digital tools (25.1%, $n = 69/275$) ($p = 0.093$). Approximately, 76.4% (210/275) of pregnancies were classified as low risk, without differences between groups ($p = 0.649$). The mean gestational age at birth was 39.3 ± 1.2 weeks ($p = 0.475$), 73.4% were primiparous (202/275; $p = 0.172$), and the mean birth weight was 3254 ± 401 g ($p = 0.494$). The induction rate was 29.1% (80/275), with 37.4% (103/275) undergoing artificial rupture of membranes. Women who discontinued breastfeeding early had a higher rate of induced labour and artificial rupture of membranes ($p = 0.014$ and $p = 0.013$, respectively). Most women were negative for group B Streptococcus (81.8%, $n = 225/275$; $p = 0.931$); received epidural analgesia (78.2%, $n = 215/275$; $p = 0.420$); had a spontaneous vaginal birth (56.7%, $n = 156/275$; $p = 0.443$); and had no episiotomy (54.2%, $n = 149/275$; $p = 0.484$), with 16.7% (46/275) having an intact perineum without differences between groups ($p = 0.846$). During labour, 69.1% (190/275) were allowed to drink, their partner accompanied in 94.9% (261/275; $p = 0.257$) of cases, and 69.1% (190/275) could move during dilation, with the lithotomy position used for birth in 51.6% (142/218, excluding C-sections; $p = 0.087$). Statistically significant differences were observed regarding early BF discontinuation, with a higher percentage of women not allowed to drink ($p = 0.031$) and those with restricted mobility ($p = 0.019$). Maternal skin-to-skin contact (SSC) was performed in most cases

(89.1%, n = 245/275; p = 0.288), with early initiation of breastfeeding in 72.4% (199/275; p = 0.146). No statistically significant differences were found between the key variables or with the predictor variables of the model presented according to the women's hospital of origin.

The HL level showed that 69.5% (191/275) of women had an adequate level. Statistically significant differences were observed between the HL level and early breastfeeding discontinuation, with women that had inadequate levels discontinuing breastfeeding at a higher rate at all cutoff points: at discharge (p = 0.031), at 15 days (p = 0.025), at 6 weeks (p = 0.017), at 3 months (p = 0.012), and at 6 months (p = 0.04). No statistically significant differences were observed between the HL level and the different sociodemographic variables, such as country of origin (p = 0.323), educational level (p = 0.400), marital status (p = 0.255), employment status (p = 0.231), economic status (p = 0.178), and financial stability (p = 0.239).

Regarding the type of breastfeeding, we can observe in Figure 1 a reduction from 81.5% (224/275) at discharge to 42.5% (117/275) at 6 months postpartum. The mean time of BF duration was 108.1 ± 72.8 days.

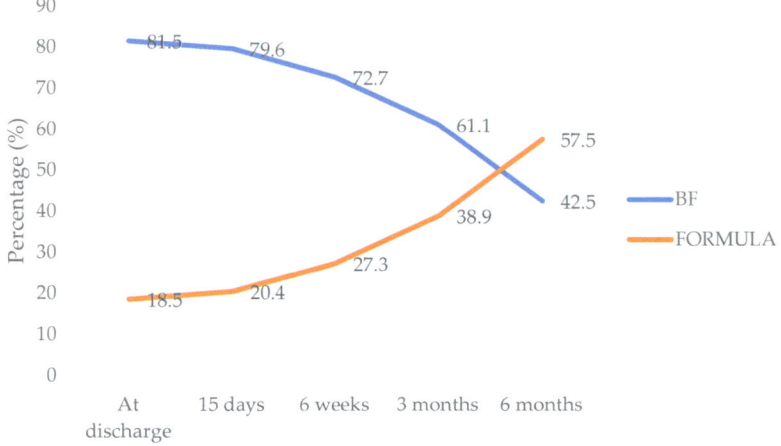

Figure 1. Rates of breastfeeding during the study follow-up (N = 275).

We were interested in analyzing the correlation between the average time until early abandonment of BF and variables that showed statistical significance in the bivariate analysis (Table 2 and Figure 2). Additionally, we present the results of Kaplan–Meier survival models used to analyze the BF duration based on statistical variables in the bivariate analysis. The log-rank test (Mantel–Cox) was applied to assess differences in survival functions between the compared groups and determine the statistical significance of these differences. Significant differences were observed in the mean breastfeeding duration between health literacy levels (p = 0.010), type of onset of labour (p = 0.004), type of rupture of membranes (p = 0.046), fluid intake during labour (p = 0.019), and mobilization during labour (p = 0.009).

Table 2. Kaplan–Meier survival analysis for the duration of breastfeeding (N = 275).

	Mean				Median		Log Rank (Mantel–Cox)		
	Estimation	SE	95% Confidence Interval		Estimation	SE	Chi-Square	df	p-Value
			Lower Limit	Upper Limit					
HL level									
Inadequate	89.17	8.18	73.13	105.2	80	28.41	6.615	1	0.01
Adequate	116.44	5.07	106.5	126.38	132				
Global	108.11	4.38	99.52	116.7	123	7.77			
Onset of labour									
Spontaneous or elective C-section	112.74	5.37	102.22	123.26	145		8.25	1	0.004
Induction	96.83	7.33	82.45	111.2	110	11.72			
Global	108.11	4.38	99.52	116.7	123	7.77			
Type of rupture of membranes									
Spontaneous	111.27	5.75	100	122.53	140		3.979	1	0.046
Artificial	102.83	6.67	89.77	115.9	114	8.46			
Global	108.11	4.38	99.52	116.7	123	7.77			
Drinking allowed during labour									
No	92.4	8.01	76.69	108.11	99	20.49	5.513	1	0.019
Yes	115.14	5.15	105.04	125.24	130				
Global	108.11	4.38	99.52	116.7	123	7.77			
Mobilization allowed during labour									
No	91.42	8.06	75.63	107.2	98	20.62	6.833	1	0.009
Yes	115.43	5.16	105.31	125.54	132				
Global	108.07	4.4	99.44	116.69	123	8.01			

Significant p-values < 0.05.

Survival curves, which were generated using the Kaplan–Meier method, provide visual information about the probability of an event occurring over time. These curves, as shown in Figure 2, show the probability of maintaining BF without early abandonment as time progressed (as represented on the x-axis) from initiation. We observed differences over time, with early abandonment of BF occurring earlier in women with inadequate HL, induced labour, artificial rupture of membranes, inability to drink during labour, and lack of mobility during labour.

Finally, the Cox regression analysis assessed the association between specific variables and the BF duration. We employed a Cox regression model to investigate the multiple factors that influenced the duration of BF, with a particular focus on significant variables in the survival analysis. The results, as presented in Table 3, elucidate the predictive value of the HL level, mobilization during labour, and the type of onset of labour.

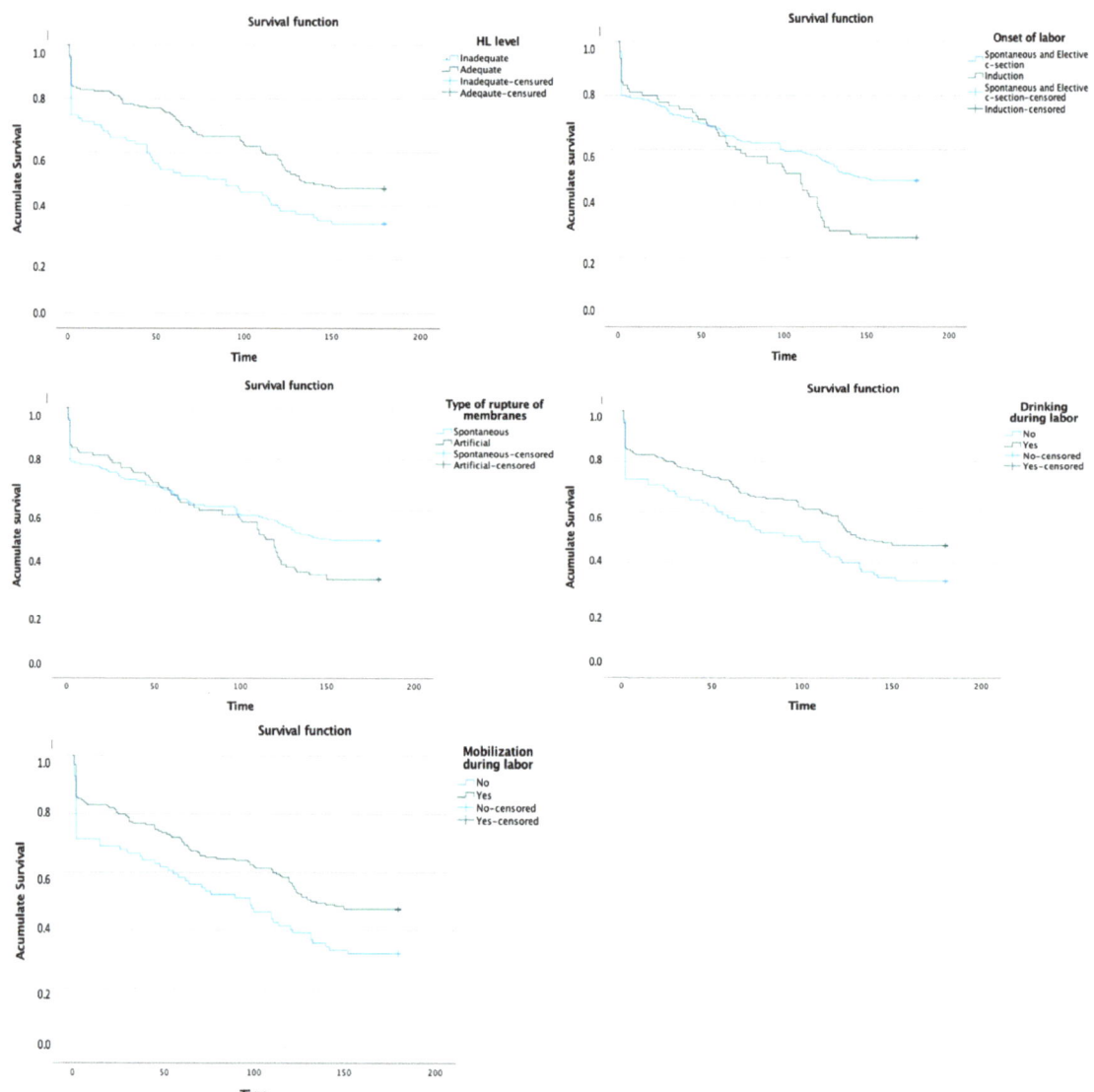

Figure 2. Survival curves for early breastfeeding abandonment based on statistically significant variables. Each curve corresponds to a distinct group within the variable, portraying the cumulative probability of participants within that group continuing to breastfeed over time. The x-axis denotes time, and the y-axis represents the proportion of women maintaining breastfeeding at each time point. Disparities between the curves signify variations in the likelihood of breastfeeding continuation between the compared groups.

The coefficient for the HL level was −0.384 ($p = 0.022$), indicating a statistically significant association. The Exp(B) value of 0.681 suggests that women with an adequate HL level had an approximately 32% lower risk of early BF abandonment compared with the reference group.

Table 3. Cox regression analysis for predicting early breastfeeding abandonment.

	B	SD	Wald	df	p-Value	Exp(B)
HL level	−0.384	0.168	5.257	1	0.022	0.681
Mobilization allowed during labour	−0.392	0.167	5.537	1	0.019	0.676
Type of onset of labour	0.431	0.167	6.640	1	0.010	1.538

SD: standard deviation; df: degrees of freedom; Exp(B): odds ratio; significant p-values < 0.05. The statistical significance and Exp(B) values provide insights into the magnitude and direction of the associations, supporting the relevance of these factors in understanding early BF abandonment.

Mobilization during labour demonstrated significance, with a coefficient of −0.392 (p = 0.019). The corresponding Exp(B) value of 0.676 indicates a 32.4% reduction in the risk of early BF abandonment for women who were allowed mobilization during labour.

The type of onset of labour exhibited significance with a coefficient of 0.431 (p = 0.010). The Exp(B) value of 1.538 suggests a 53.8% increase in the risk of early BF abandonment for induced labour compared with the reference group.

These findings underline the importance of HL, mobilization during labour, and the type of onset of labour as significant predictors of BF duration.

4. Discussion

Our study results suggest the influence of certain variables on breastfeeding practices, highlighting the importance of obstetric and socio-educational considerations in promoting BF, with less abandonment found when women had adequate HL, labour was not induced, membranes were ruptured spontaneously, and the ability to drink and mobilize was present during labour.

As in previous studies in our country [6–8], the rates of BF in the sixth month did not reach those recommended by international organizations, such as the WHO [24], with rates in our sample being lower than those reported by other studies conducted in our country [9]. However, compared with rates in the rest of Europe, Spain obtained similar figures for BF at six months [25]. It is essential to bear in mind that our analysis of the BF rate included both exclusive and mixed breastfeeding. Therefore, the results obtained were lower than the proposed target rates.

In our study, we observed that various factors had a negative impact on the continuation of BF. HL is one of the most significant factors in determining whether BF is continued or abandoned early. This association has been observed by different authors using various screening tools, leading to heterogeneous results [13,16,26]. In our case, we used a validated tool adapted to Spanish with an alpha coefficient of 0.982 [22].

Various variables influencing maternal HL have been described, such as educational level and economic status [27]. No socioeconomic variable was associated with HL level in our study, aligning with different authors [28,29]. In clinical practice, it would be interesting to assess the HL level of each expectant mother to provide tailored information. The standard information we offer to women should be adapted to their level, potentially clarifying vital information to prevent early breastfeeding abandonment [30]. Therefore, including an HL assessment as a healthcare policy could reduce the attrition rate if confirmed by other authors in diverse samples with heterogeneous characteristics [31]. Alternatively, each woman's level of breastfeeding literacy could be assessed on an individualized and personalized basis through specific instruments [32]. Future studies should assess this aspect in more depth.

Another facilitating factor for early BF abandonment that was found in our study was immobilization during labour. At first glance, this relationship was not explored in previous studies. We know that mobilization is positively associated with spontaneous vaginal births, as it can help to facilitate the birthing process; relatedly, immobility is linked to an increase in childbirth interventions, and it is related to worse pain management [33,34]. Therefore, birth interventions and difficulty in pain management may increase the perception of lack of self-control, which may increase stress and decrease self-efficacy and satisfaction after childbirth [35], which could negatively affect the mother's ability or willingness to continue breastfeeding [36]. Regarding other intrapartum variables, we are also aware of aspects that can be directly related to breastfeeding. In particular, it is known that maternal water restriction during labour can be a problem. As stated in the context of the current popularization, no one would think of running a long-distance race without drinking water, but we still apply it to women during labour. It is necessary to add that we are aware and concerned that there are still, in Spain, some intrapartum manoeuvres, such as the Kristeller manoeuvre, that are not being correctly registered [37]. Therefore, other variables may not have been recorded and could have been related to the results obtained. This relationship should be explored in future studies to test this hypothesis.

Finally, labour induction is positively associated with early weaning of BF. Similar to mobilization, induced labour is linked to a higher number of dystocic births and specifically increases the rate of Caesarean sections compared with spontaneous labour [38]. Labour induction often involves the administration of medications and medical procedures to initiate or expedite the birthing process [39]. This may lead to a potentially more intense childbirth experience compared with spontaneous labour. The additional stress and more intense experience could influence the mother's willingness and ability to initiate and maintain breastfeeding. Previous studies suggested that labour induction can negatively affect the emotional well-being of women in the postpartum period [40,41], which is a factor related to the BF duration in the literature [42,43]. Caesarean sections, especially those performed emergently, may be associated with initial difficulties in breastfeeding initiation due to the need for surgical recovery and other potential factors [44]. Thus, the relationship between labour induction and early BF abandonment may result from a combination of factors related to the birthing experience, potential complications, and the influence on natural hormonal processes that support BF.

This study had several limitations. First, the sample selection was not based on probabilistic sampling and was relatively small, and thus, the results may not represent the general population due to the sample size and selection method. However, sample representativeness was achieved as it exceeded the estimated sample size, and despite the non-probabilistic selection, this fact added robustness to the results. While it is true that our research reflected local practices in Spain, we recognize the importance of emphasizing the novelty and unique contributions our study brings to the existing literature in the field. Our study stands out for its comprehensive exploration of the intricate relationship between HL, obstetric practices, and the duration of BF. The prospective and multicentric nature allowed for a broader perspective, capturing diverse experiences and practices within Spanish regions.

Second, the data collection method through electronic surveys implied a limitation inherent to the validity of self-reported responses, as these may be subject to subjective interpretation and participant memory bias. Additionally, the possibility of response bias should be considered, where participants may selectively respond or provide socially desirable answers.

Finally, while our study provides insights into breastfeeding practices, it is essential to acknowledge the potential impact of the COVID-19 pandemic. The pandemic has disrupted healthcare systems and society, therefore affecting maternal well-being. These factors may indirectly influence breastfeeding behaviours [45]. However, due to the nature of our data collection, we could not assess the pandemic's effect on breastfeeding initiation, duration, or exclusivity. Future research should consider prospective designs and explore how pandemic-related stress, isolation, and healthcare access may shape maternal decisions regarding breastfeeding.

5. Conclusions

Our findings underscore the importance of considering obstetric and maternal health literacy factors when addressing breastfeeding duration. The research highlights the crucial role of health literacy; spontaneous rupture of membranes; and supportive labour practices, such as mobilization during dilation, in promoting and sustaining breastfeeding. Given the rates were below the WHO recommendations, the need for personalized health literacy assessments and targeted strategies to bridge the gap between current practices and global health guidelines is evident. These findings emphasize the complexity of factors influencing breastfeeding and advocate for specific interventions to enhance maternal and child health outcomes.

Based on the findings from our study, health stakeholders and policymakers should comprehensively grasp the intricate nature of maternity care. Routine care taken during childbirth can have repercussions beyond the immediate birth; health strategies should be implemented to achieve overall maternal well-being. Healthcare decisions should focus on immediate health outcomes and consider the broader impact on maternity care.

Supplementary Materials: The following supporting information can be downloaded from https://www.mdpi.com/article/10.3390/nu16050690/s1—Table S1: HLS-EU-Q16 questionnaire, Spanish version.

Author Contributions: Conceptualization and methodology, R.V.-C.; formal analysis, R.V.-C.; data curation, R.V.-C., C.F.-A. and F.J.S.-V.; writing—original draft preparation, R.V.-C., F.J.S.-V. and D.M.-T.; writing—review and editing, R.V.-C., F.J.S.-V., D.M.-T., O.G.-A., V.A.-F. and C.F.-A. All authors have read and agreed to the published version of the manuscript.

Funding: This research was funded by Foundation for the Promotion of Health and Biomedical Research in the Valencian Region (FISABIO), Valencia, Spain, in the II Call for Nursing R&D&I Grants 2020; grant number UGP-20-245.

Institutional Review Board Statement: This study was conducted in accordance with the guidelines of the Declaration of Helsinki and approved by the Research Ethics Committee of Hospital Universitario La Ribera with protocol code (HULR2021_0302) approved on 3 February 2021 and by the corresponding committees of the other participating centres: Lluis Alcanyis Hospital protocol code (HLLA20210407) approved on 7 April 2021, General Hospital of Cáceres protocol code 031-2021 approved on 26 March 2021 and General Hospital of Castellón with protocol code HGC-065-2021, approved on 22 February 2021.

Informed Consent Statement: Patient consent was obtained before participating in this study.

Data Availability Statement: Data are available upon reasonable request. All necessary data are supplied and available in the manuscript; however, the corresponding author will provide the dataset upon request.

Acknowledgments: Thanks are due to all the healthcare staff members who participated directly or indirectly in the care of the patients, and to the Institutions of Hospital Universitario de la Ribera, Hospital Lluis Alcanyis, Hospial General de Castellón, and Hospital San Pedro de Alcántara of Cáceres.

Conflicts of Interest: The authors declare no conflicts of interest.

References

1. Louis-Jacques, A.F.; Stuebe, A.M. Enabling Breastfeeding to Support Lifelong Health for Mother and Child. *Obstet. Gynecol. Clin. N. Am.* **2020**, *47*, 363–381. [CrossRef]
2. Linde, K.; Lehnig, F.; Nagl, M.; Kersting, A. The association between breastfeeding and attachment: A systematic review. *Midwifery* **2020**, *81*, 102592. [CrossRef]
3. World Health Organization (WHO); United Nations Children's Fund (UNICEF). *Protecting, Promoting and Supporting Breast-Feeding: The Special Role of Maternity Services/a Joint WHO/UNICEF Statement*; World Health Organization: Geneva, Switzerland, 1989.
4. World Health Organization; European Health Information Gateway. % of Infants Breastfed at Age 6 Months. Available online: https://gateway.euro.who.int/en/indicators/hfa_616-7260-of-infants-breastfed-at-age-6-months/#id=19721 (accessed on 23 January 2024).
5. Instituto Nacional de Estadística (INE). Tipo de Lactancia Según Sexo y Clase Social Basada en la Ocupación de la Persona de Referencia. *Población de 6 Meses a 4 Años. Encuesta Nacional de Salud España.* Available online: https://www.ine.es/jaxi/Tabla.htm?path=/t15/p419/a2017/p06/l0/&file=06001.px&L=0 (accessed on 10 December 2023).

6. Ramiro González, M.D.; Ortiz Marrón, H.; Arana Cañedo-Argüelles, C.; Esparza Olcina, M.J.; Cortés Rico, O.; Terol Claramonte, M.; Ordobás Gavín, M. Prevalence of breastfeeding and factors associated with the start and duration of exclusive breastfeeding in the Community of Madrid among participants in the ELOIN. *An. Pediatr.* **2018**, *89*, 32–43. [CrossRef] [PubMed]
7. Cabedo, R.; Manresa, J.M.; Cambredó, M.V.; Montero, L.; Reyes, A.; Gol, R.; Falguera, G. Tipos de lactancia materna y factores que influyen en su abandono hasta los 6 meses. Estudio LACTEM. *Matronas Profesión* **2019**, *20*, 54–61.
8. López de Aberasturi Ibáñez de Garayo, A.; Santos Ibáñez, N.; Ramos Castro, Y.; García Franco, M.; Artola Gutiérrez, C.; Arara Vidal, I. Prevalence and determinants of breastfeeding: The Zorrotzaurre study. *Nutr. Hosp.* **2020**, *38*, 50–59. [CrossRef] [PubMed]
9. Vila-Candel, R.; Mena-Tudela, D.; Franco-Antonio, C.; Quesada, J.A.; Soriano-Vidal, F.J. Effects of a mobile application on breastfeeding maintenance in the first 6 months after birth: Randomised controlled trial (COMLACT study). *Midwifery* **2024**, *128*, 103874. [CrossRef]
10. Liu, C.; Wang, D.; Liu, C.; Jiang, J.; Wang, X.; Chen, H.; Ju, X.; Zhang, X. What is the meaning of health literacy? A systematic review and qualitative synthesis. *Fam. Med. Community Health* **2020**, *8*, e000351. [CrossRef] [PubMed]
11. Sørensen, K.; Van Den Broucke, S.; Fullam, J.; Doyle, G.; Pelikan, J.; Slonska, Z.; Brand, H. Health literacy and public health: A systematic review and integration of definitions and models. *BMC Public Health* **2012**, *12*, 80. [CrossRef]
12. Kaufman, H.; Skipper, B.; Small, L.; Terry, T.; McGrew, M. Effect of literacy on breast-feeding outcomes. *South. Med. J.* **2001**, *94*, 293–296. [CrossRef]
13. Stafford, J.D.; Goggins, E.R.; Lathrop, E.; Haddad, L.B. Health Literacy and Associated Outcomes in the Postpartum Period at Grady Memorial Hospital. *Matern. Child Health J.* **2021**, *25*, 599–605. [CrossRef]
14. Stafford, J.D.; Lathrop, E.; Haddad, L. Health Literacy and Associated Outcomes in the Postpartum Period at Grady Memorial Hospital [2H]. *Obstet. Gynecol.* **2016**, *127*, 66S–67S. [CrossRef]
15. Mirjalili, N.; Jaberi, A.A.; Jaberi, K.A.; Bonabi, T.N. The role of maternal health literacy in breastfeeding pattern. *J. Nurs. Midwifery Sci.* **2018**, *5*, 53–58. [CrossRef]
16. Graus, T.M.; Brandstetter, S.; Seelbach-Göbel, B.; Melter, M.; Kabesch, M.; Apfelbacher, C.; Fill Malfertheiner, S.; Ambrosch, A.; Arndt, P.; Baessler, A.; et al. Breastfeeding behavior is not associated with health literacy: Evidence from the German KUNO-Kids birth cohort study. *Arch. Gynecol. Obstet.* **2021**, *304*, 1161–1168. [CrossRef] [PubMed]
17. Shannon, T.; O'donnell, M.J.; Skinner, K. Breastfeeding in the 21st Century: Overcoming Barriers to Help Women and Infants. *Nurs. Women's Heal.* **2007**, *11*, 568–575. [CrossRef] [PubMed]
18. Bohren, M.A.; Hofmeyr, G.J.; Sakala, C.; Fukuzawa, R.K.; Cuthbert, A. Continuous support for women during childbirth. *Cochrane Database Syst. Rev.* **2017**, *7*, CD003766. [CrossRef] [PubMed]
19. Finnie, S.; Peréz-Escamilla, R.; Buccini, G. Determinants of early breastfeeding initiation and exclusive breastfeeding in Colombia. *Public Health Nutr.* **2020**, *23*, 496–505. [CrossRef] [PubMed]
20. Sen, K.K.; Mallick, T.S.; Bari, W. Gender inequality in early initiation of breastfeeding in Bangladesh: A trend analysis. *Int. Breastfeed. J.* **2020**, *15*, 18. [CrossRef]
21. John, J.R.; Mistry, S.K.; Kebede, G.; Manohar, N.; Arora, A. Determinants of early initiation of breastfeeding in Ethiopia: A population-based study using the 2016 demographic and health survey data. *BMC Pregnancy Childbirth* **2019**, *19*, 69. [CrossRef]
22. Nolasco, A.; Barona, C.; Tamayo-Fonseca, N.; Irles, M.Á.; Más, R.; Tuells, J.; Pereyra-Zamora, P. Alfabetización en salud: Propiedades psicométricas del cuestionario HLS-EU-Q16. *Gac. Sanit.* 2018, in press. [CrossRef]
23. Alcaraz-Vidal, L.; Leon-Larios, F.; Robleda, G.; Vila-Candel, R. Exploring home births in Catalonia (Spain): A cross-sectional study of women's experiences and influencing factors. *J. Adv. Nurs.* **2023**, 1–16. [CrossRef]
24. World Health Organization; UNICEF. *Global Nutrion Target 2025. Breastfeeding Policy Brief*; World Health Organization: Geneva, Switzerland, 2014.
25. Theurich, M.A.; Davanzo, R.; Busck-Rasmussen, M.; Díaz-Gómez, N.M.; Brennan, C.; Kylberg, E.; Bærug, A.; McHugh, L.; Weikert, C.; Abraham, K.; et al. Breastfeeding rates and programs in europe: A survey of 11 national breastfeeding committees and representatives. *J. Pediatr. Gastroenterol. Nutr.* **2019**, *68*, 400–407. [CrossRef]
26. Gaupšienė, A.; Vainauskaitė, A.; Baglajeva, J.; Stukas, R.; Ramašauskaitė, D.; Paliulytė, V.; Istomina, N. Associations between maternal health literacy, neonatal health and breastfeeding outcomes in the early postpartum period. *Eur. J. Midwifery* **2023**, *7*, 5–10. [CrossRef] [PubMed]
27. Estrela, M.; Semedo, G.; Roque, F.; Ferreira, P.L.; Herdeiro, M.T. Sociodemographic determinants of digital health literacy: A systematic review and meta-analysis. *Int. J. Med. Inform.* **2023**, *177*, 105124. [CrossRef]
28. Vila-Candel, R.; Martínez-Arnau, F.M.; de la Cámara-de Las Heras, J.M.; Castro-Sánchez, E.; Pérez-Ros, P. Interventions to Improve Health among Reproductive-Age Women of Low Health Literacy: A Systematic Review. *Int. J. Environ. Res. Public Health* **2020**, *17*, 7405. [CrossRef] [PubMed]
29. Vila-Candel, R.; Navarro-Illana, E.; Mena-Tudela, D.; Pérez-Ros, P.; Castro-Sánchez, E.; Soriano-Vidal, F.J.; Quesada, J.A. Influence of puerperal health literacy on tobacco use during pregnancy among spanish women: A transversal study. *Int. J. Environ. Res. Public Health* **2020**, *17*, 2910. [CrossRef] [PubMed]
30. Valero-Chillerón, M.J.; Mena-Tudela, D.; Cervera-Gasch, Á.; González-Chordá, V.M.; Soriano-Vidal, F.J.; Quesada, J.A.; Castro-Sánchez, E.; Vila-Candel, R. Influence of Health Literacy on Maintenance of Exclusive Breastfeeding at 6 Months Postpartum: A Multicentre Study. *Int. J. Environ. Res. Public Health* **2022**, *19*, 5411. [CrossRef] [PubMed]

31. Castro-Sánchez, E.; Chang, P.W.S.; Vila-Candel, R.; Escobedo, A.A.; Holmes, A.H. Health literacy and infectious diseases: Why does it matter? *Int. J. Infect. Dis.* **2016**, *43*, 103–110. [CrossRef] [PubMed]
32. Valero-Chillerón, M.J.; Vila-Candel, R.; Mena-Tudela, D.; Soriano-Vidal, F.J.; González-Chordá, V.M.; Andreu-Pejo, L.; Antolí-Forner, A.; Durán-García, L.; Vicent-Ferrandis, M.; Andrés-Alegre, M.E.; et al. Development and Validation of the Breastfeeding Literacy Assessment Instrument (BLAI) for Obstetric Women. *Int. J. Environ. Res. Public Health* **2023**, *20*, 3808. [CrossRef] [PubMed]
33. Berta, M.; Lindgren, H.; Christensson, K.; Mekonnen, S.; Adefris, M. Effect of maternal birth positions on duration of second stage of labor: Systematic review and meta-analysis. *BMC Pregnancy Childbirth* **2019**, *19*, 466. [CrossRef]
34. Gupta, J.K.; Sood, A.; Hofmeyr, G.J.; Vogel, J.P. Position in the second stage of labour for women without epidural anaesthesia. *Cochrane Database Syst. Rev.* **2017**, *2017*, CD002006. [CrossRef]
35. Jafari, E.; Mohebbi, P.; Mazloomzadeh, S. Factors related to women's childbirth satisfaction in physiologic and routine childbirth groups. *Iran. J. Nurs. Midwifery Res.* **2017**, *22*, 219–224. [CrossRef] [PubMed]
36. Fan, H.S.L.; Fong, D.Y.T.; Lok, K.Y.W.; Tarrant, M. The Association Between Breastfeeding Self-Efficacy and Mode of Infant Feeding. *Breastfeed. Med.* **2022**, *17*, 687–697. [CrossRef] [PubMed]
37. Ministry of Health and Social Policy and Equality. *Report on Attention to Delivery and Birth in the National Health System*; Ministry of Health and Social Policy and Equality: Madrid, Spain, 2012. (In Spanish)
38. Rydahl, E.; Eriksen, L.; Juhl, M. Effects of induction of labor prior to post-term in low-risk pregnancies: A systematic review. *JBI Database Syst. Rev. Implement. Rep.* **2019**, *17*, 170–208. [CrossRef] [PubMed]
39. Carlson, N.; Ellis, J.; Page, K.; Dunn Amore, A.; Phillippi, J. Review of Evidence-Based Methods for Successful Labor Induction. *J. Midwifery Women's Heal.* **2021**, *66*, 459–469. [CrossRef]
40. Froeliger, A.; Deneux-Tharaux, C.; Loussert, L.; Bouchghoul, H.; Madar, H.; Sentilhes, L. Prevalence and risk factors for postpartum depression 2 months after a vaginal delivery: A prospective multicenter study. *Am. J. Obstet. Gynecol.* **2023**. [CrossRef] [PubMed]
41. Ponti, L.; Ghinassi, S.; Tani, F. Spontaneous and induced labor: Association with maternal well-being three months after childbirth. *Psychol. Heal. Med.* **2022**, *27*, 896–901. [CrossRef] [PubMed]
42. Slomian, J.; Honvo, G.; Emonts, P.; Reginster, J.Y.; Bruyère, O. Consequences of maternal postpartum depression: A systematic review of maternal and infant outcomes. *Women's Heal.* **2019**, *15*, 1745506519844044. [CrossRef]
43. Gila-Díaz, A.; Carrillo, G.H.; de Pablo, Á.L.L.; Arribas, S.M.; Ramiro-Cortijo, D. Association between maternal postpartum depression, stress, optimism, and breastfeeding pattern in the first six months. *Int. J. Environ. Res. Public Health* **2020**, *17*, 7153. [CrossRef]
44. Vila-Candel, R.; Piquer-Martín, N.; Perdomo-Ugarte, N.; Quesada, J.A.; Escuriet, R.; Martin-Arribas, A. Indications of Induction and Caesarean Sections Performed Using the Robson Classification in a University Hospital in Spain from 2010 to 2021. *Healthcare* **2023**, *11*, 1521. [CrossRef]
45. Turner, S.; McGann, B.; Brockway, M.M. A review of the disruption of breastfeeding supports in response to the COVID-19 pandemic in five Western countries and applications for clinical practice. *Int. Breastfeed. J.* **2022**, *17*, 38. [CrossRef]

Disclaimer/Publisher's Note: The statements, opinions and data contained in all publications are solely those of the individual author(s) and contributor(s) and not of MDPI and/or the editor(s). MDPI and/or the editor(s) disclaim responsibility for any injury to people or property resulting from any ideas, methods, instructions or products referred to in the content.

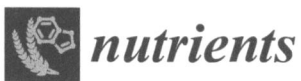

Article

Effectiveness of a Postpartum Breastfeeding Support Group Intervention in Promoting Exclusive Breastfeeding and Perceived Self-Efficacy: A Multicentre Randomized Clinical Trial

Isabel Rodríguez-Gallego [1,2], Isabel Corrales-Gutierrez [3,4,*], Diego Gomez-Baya [5,*] and Fatima Leon-Larios [6]

1. Foetal Medicine, Genetics and Reproduction Unit, Virgen del Rocío University Hospital, 41013 Seville, Spain; isroga@cruzroja.es
2. Red Cross Nursing University Centre, University of Seville, 41009 Seville, Spain
3. Surgery Department, Faculty of Medicine, University of Seville, 41009 Seville, Spain
4. Foetal Medicine Unit, Virgen Macarena University Hospital, 41009 Seville, Spain
5. Department of Social, Developmental and Educational Psychology, Universidad de Huelva, 21007 Huelva, Spain
6. Nursing Department, School of Nursing, Physiotherapy and Podiatry, University of Seville, 41009 Seville, Spain; fatimaleon@us.es
* Correspondence: icorrales@us.es (I.C.-G.); diego.gomez@dpee.uhu.es (D.G.-B.)

Abstract: There are numerous recognized benefits of breastfeeding; however, sociocultural, individual, and environmental factors influence its initiation and continuation, sometimes leading to breastfeeding rates that are lower than recommended by international guidelines. The aim of this study was to evaluate the effectiveness of a group intervention led by midwives supporting breastfeeding during the postpartum period in promoting exclusive breastfeeding, as well as to assess the impact of this intervention on perceived self-efficacy. This was a non-blind, multicentric, cluster-randomized controlled trial. Recruitment started October 2021, concluding May 2023. A total of 382 women from Andalusia (Spain) participated in the study. The results showed that at 4 months postpartum there was a higher prevalence of breastfeeding in the intervention group compared to formula feeding ($p = 0.01$), as well as a higher prevalence of exclusive breastfeeding ($p = 0.03$), and also at 6 months ($p = 0.01$). Perceived self-efficacy was similar in both groups for the first two months after delivery, which then remained stable until 4 months and decreased slightly at 6 months in both groups ($p = 0.99$). The intervention improved the average scores of perceived self-efficacy and indirectly caused higher rates of exclusive breastfeeding ($p = 0.005$). In conclusion, the midwife-led group intervention supporting breastfeeding proved to be effective at maintaining exclusive breastfeeding at 6 months postpartum and also at increasing perceived self-efficacy.

Keywords: breastfeeding; lactation; exclusive breastfeeding; self-efficacy; breastfeeding support groups; community health services; lactation support; midwifery; public health; randomized controlled trial

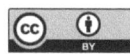

1. Introduction

The World Health Organization (WHO) advocates for breastfeeding as an unparalleled method of feeding that can provide all the nutrients a newborn needs for growth and immunological development in the first months of life. Breastfeeding provides half or more of a child's nutritional requirements during the second semester of life and up to a third during the second year [1]. Therefore, the current recommendation by the WHO, along with the United Nations Children's Fund, is that breast milk should be the exclusive food for newborns until the age of 6 months and that, until the age of 2 years, they should be fed a combination of breast milk and age-appropriate, nutritious foods [2].

There is increasing scientific evidence of the multiple benefits that breastfeeding brings the newborn, at physical, cognitive, and psychosocial levels [1–4], as well as the mother, by preventing pathologies related to physical and mental health [5–8]. In fact, there are numerous comprehensive reviews that summarize the benefits of breastfeeding and the mechanisms by which these are achieved by describing a series of increasingly well-understood complex pathways through which breast milk has evolved to optimize child survival. Even in recent epidemics, such as that caused by severe acute respiratory syndrome coronavirus, breastfeeding has been demonstrated to be superior to other types of infant feeding [9,10]. However, the global prevalence of breastfeeding indicates that, although the initiation of breastfeeding occurs in almost all countries, there is a progressive decrease in the number of mothers who continue breastfeeding over the first few months of a newborn's life [11–13].

In today's society, both social and cultural determinants, as well as support from health services, family and community support, social policies and work-life balance, and individual factors related to maternal and child health, influence the initiation and continuation of breastfeeding [14]. Specifically, the promotion and support of breastfeeding immediately after birth, skin-to-skin contact, avoidance of separating the newborn from the mother, and community support are prognostic factors for the success of breastfeeding [15,16].

Recent studies also indicate that group support interventions have a greater impact on breastfeeding rates than individual counselling. Prenatal advice has a positive effect, achieving better breastfeeding rates at 4–6 weeks postpartum, while the combination of prenatal and postnatal advice favours the prolongation of breastfeeding up to 6 months. Therefore, both prenatal and postnatal counselling and support are recommended to achieve better breastfeeding rates [17]. Furthermore, other studies [18–20] have shown that peer support has a greater effect on the initiation, maintenance, and duration of breastfeeding when led by professionals, reinforcing the idea of midwife-led group support interventions for breastfeeding mothers.

Various individual maternal factors, such as attitudes and expectations regarding breastfeeding and a lack of confidence in breastfeeding, can be modified through educational interventions during pregnancy and postpartum support. Maternal lack of confidence in breastfeeding is a point highlighted by mothers themselves when they discuss their experience and is an important predictor of premature cessation of breastfeeding [21]. Studies have shown that maternal self-efficacy in breastfeeding is a modifiable factor that can improve breastfeeding rates [22,23].

Numerous studies of environmental factors and, more specifically, work-life balance at the national and international levels [15,24–26] indicate that existing policies are insufficient, with the return to work being one of the main reasons for the early cessation of breastfeeding (before 6 months). Specifically, in Spain, maternity leave and leave for childcare generally last 16 weeks, which is less than the WHO's recommendation for exclusive breastfeeding [27].

The principal aim of this study was to evaluate the effectiveness of a midwife-led group intervention supporting breastfeeding during the postpartum period in promoting exclusive breastfeeding up to when newborns reached 6 months of age. The secondary objective was to assess the effect of this intervention on breastfeeding self-efficacy and its relationships with the duration and exclusivity of breastfeeding.

2. Materials and Methods

2.1. Study Setting

This was a multicentric cluster-randomized controlled trial with a control group and an intervention group and was not blinded. It was completed as described in our published protocol [28]. In addition, the trial was registered in the International Standard Registered Clinical/Social Study Number registry (Trial ID: ISRCTN17263529; date recorded: 17 June 2020).

2.2. Participants and Study Area

Eligible female participants were recruited in primary health centres in Andalusia, Spain. Andalusia is an autonomous community divided into eight provinces with a total of 8,472,407 inhabitants (data available in 2021) [29] and a birth rate of 7.72 per 1000 inhabitants (2021) [30]. By 1 July 2022, the number of women of reproductive age in Andalusia was 4,328,407 [31]. The study was conducted on the populations from the provinces of Seville, Cadiz, Huelva, Granada, and Jaen.

According to data provided by the National Statistical Institute of Spain, in 2021, there were a total of 65,650 births in Andalusia. Births in the provinces of Seville (15,655), Granada (7083), Huelva (4227), Jaen (4499), and Cadiz (8904) totalled 40,368, which represented 61.79% of the total births in the community [32].

2.3. Sample Design

The rate of exclusive breastfeeding at 6 months in Andalusia is 39% [33], which was estimated as the expected value in the control group. An estimated increase of 10%, as indicated by previous studies [14,34], in the rates of exclusive breastfeeding at 6 months was established. To achieve this difference between the two groups, a two-tailed hypothesis was posed, with a power of 80% and allowing for a type I error of 5%. The necessary sample size amounted to 371 women distributed between the two study groups.

2.4. Inclusion and Exclusion Criteria

Inclusion criteria:
1. Healthy women performing exclusive or partial breastfeeding 10 days after birth who attended antenatal lessons at the primary health centre.
2. Women over 18 years of age.
3. Women who accepted and signed the informed consent form.

Exclusion criteria:
1. Human immunodeficiency virus-positive.
2. Cancer.
3. Tuberculosis infection.
4. No intention to breastfeed.
5. Impossibility or contraindication to breastfeed due to medical conditions.
6. Premature and/or complicated labour or newborn in a neonatal intensive care unit during the first month of life.
7. Communication difficulties due to language barriers.

2.5. Randomization

Primary health centres were randomized into an intervention group or control group (usual care), considering whether any type of group breastfeeding support intervention was already being conducted there. The research technician assigned to the project, independent of the researchers who oversaw participant recruitment, performed this health centre allocation using a random sequence generated by the Oxford Minimization and Randomization system [35]. The technician assigned random unique identifiers to the health centres, differentiating between centres belonging to the control and intervention groups. Finally, out of a total of 23 primary health centres, 11 were included, 6 in the IG (2 centres in Seville, 1 centre in Huelva, 1 centre in Granada, 1 centre in Jaén, and 1 centre in Cádiz) and 5 in the CG (one centre per province). Each centre had a designated lead midwife responsible for recruiting participants and conducting the intervention, in the case of the intervention group.

After the randomization of centres for the recruitment of women into the intervention and control groups, each participant was assigned an identification code depending on the group to which she belonged.

2.6. Study Intervention

Women in the control group received the usual care regarding maternal education from the 28th week of pregnancy onward and postpartum visits, according to the Protocol for Care during Pregnancy, Childbirth, and Puerperium by the Andalusian Health and Social Welfare Council [36]. In the first 10 days after childbirth, they had an individual visit with the midwife, during which a breastfeeding session was observed using the WHO breastfeeding observation sheet [37], and concerns were resolved individually. Women also had the option of requesting on-demand individual postpartum consultations with the reference midwife of their health centre. All of this is included in standard care.

In addition, women in the intervention group received the usual prenatal and postpartum care, just like the control group. Subsequently, they participated in monthly 2 h face-to-face and/or virtual group sessions called breastfeeding support groups, for which the midwife acted as leader and moderator. These sessions had an educational component, through theoretical-practical presentations related to breastfeeding, based on the recommendations of the Baby-Friendly Hospital Initiative [38]. They also had a motivational component and a component based on the social or peer support established in the group. Thus, monthly, women were offered support by an organized and proactive professional. In addition to monthly meetings, participants had the option to interact with each other, with other breastfeeding women, and with the reference midwife via a Facebook™ and/or WhatsApp™ group established for this purpose. Thus, peer support was reinforced, and questions about the topic were resolved using information and communication technologies [39]. Likewise, participating women had the option of requesting on-demand individual consultations with the reference midwife, the same as women receiving usual care.

2.7. Instrument with Validity and Reliability

The study collected the following data: the participant's sociodemographic information (age, level of education, marital status, employment, ethnicity); obstetric outcomes (home labour and delivery, mode of delivery, gestation weeks); and neonatal outcomes (sex, weight, Apgar, neonatology admission, health problems). Incorrect or incomplete data were corrected via direct consultation with participants or were collected from their health medical records with their consent.

In relation to breastfeeding, outcomes were collected for previous experience in breastfeeding (multiparous women were asked about their experience with breastfeeding while raising previous children, as well as the reason for giving it up); the type of breastfeeding during the follow-up; and, in cases of interruption, the reason.

The types of breastfeeding were classified according to [15]:

- Exclusive breastfeeding: the newborn is fed only with breast milk, without using any other milk or food, from its birth up until the first 6 months of its corrected age.
- Partial breastfeeding: occasional administration of formula milk.
- Mixed breastfeeding: combination of breast and formula milk.
- Artificial breastfeeding: exclusively formula milk.

Breastfeeding self-efficacy was measured using a reduced version of the Breastfeeding Self-efficacy Scale-Short Form (BSES-SF), which was validated in Spanish by Oliver-Roig et al. [40]. This scale is a structured questionnaire that measures maternal confidence through 14 items grouped in only one dimension. The items are positively presented and preceded by the phrase 'I can always...'. Scoring is by a Likert-type scale from 1–5, where 1 indicates 'not sure at all' and 5 indicates 'very sure'. Higher scores indicate higher self-efficacy levels for breastfeeding. The reliability of the Spanish version of the BSES-SF, as measured with the Cronbach alpha coefficient, was 0.92.

2.8. Data Collection

Participant recruitment began in October 2021 and ended in May 2023. It was conducted by the midwives responsible for each health centre, who received prior training on the project and were also advised by a research technician midwife of the project who was not involved in the execution of the intervention.

The referring midwife of each health centre, in a consultation of week 35–37 to all women who met the established inclusion criteria, was informed of the nature and objectives of the study, as well as of the follow-ups to be carried out. In addition, at the postpartum visit, it was verified that the woman met the criteria for partial or exclusive breastfeeding at 10 days. Once the women agreed to participate, they signed the informed consent form in duplicate. Participants provided information through the web application project created for the study, which automatically sent them a reminder message and an email at the three assessment moments designed in the study.

The main control and outcome variables were collected before the start of the intervention (baseline) and at the 2-4- and 6-month follow-ups. The data relating to electronic follow-ups were coded and safeguarded by the research team. All data were stored in an electronic database accessible only to members of the research team.

2.9. Data Analysis

The analysis was conducted according to the intention-to-treat principle, regardless of whether participants adhered to the requirement to participate in the breastfeeding support group. The individual health centres were the randomization unit, and mother-infant dyads were the unit of analysis. All statistical tests and confidence intervals used a type I error rate set at alpha = 0.05 and were conducted using the SPSS v. 23 [41] statistical package (IBM).

First, an exploratory analysis of the different variables studied was performed. For the descriptive analysis of categorical variables, frequency distribution tables and percentages were generated. For continuous variables, means and standard deviations were calculated. Second, differences between the control and intervention groups in all descriptive study variables were analysed. The relationship between two categorical variables was analysed by developing contingency tables using Pearson's chi-square test. For continuous variables, to examine differences between two groups, the independent samples Student's t-test was conducted. To examine differences in continuous variables between three groups, ANOVA was used.

Third, the effectiveness analysis was conducted by comparing the proportion of women exclusively breastfeeding at 6 months in both groups using the McNemar test. Contingency tables were designed to examine the percentage of breastfeeding mothers based on whether or not they were in the intervention group. These tables were used to analyse the percentages before and after the intervention and after follow-up. To analyse changes in breastfeeding self-efficacy, a repeated measures ANOVA, controlling for the intervention group and the control group at the three evaluation time points of the study, was conducted. Additionally, the association between postpartum breastfeeding type and breastfeeding type after follow-up was examined using a chi-square test. Finally, the relationship between type of breastfeeding and employment status was examined using a chi-square test.

To examine the extent to which the use of breastfeeding after the intervention could be explained by the increase in breastfeeding self-efficacy, a partial mediation model was designed. In this model, based on regression analysis, the intervention acted as the independent variable (x), self-efficacy as the mediator (m), and breastfeeding as the dependent variable (y). The standardized coefficients of the model were analysed, as was the change in the total effect of the intervention on breastfeeding after including the mediating mechanism. These analyses were performed according to the method proposed by Hayes et al. [42] with the PROCESS macro v. 4.1 (2022) in SPSS v. 28.1 for Windows (IBM Corp. 2018, Armonk, NY, USA).

2.10. Ethical Considerations

Participation in the project was voluntary, as was the participation request. Verbal and written informed consent information was provided to every participant in the study.

The study was designed according to the Spanish regulation act No. 14/2007 of 3 July regarding biomedical research, and complied with the study suitability requirements and with the procedures regarding the study objectives. All patient-related data collected for this study were treated according to the Spanish Organic Law on Protection of Personal Data and Guarantee of Digital Rights (Spanish Organic Law 3/2018).

The study was approved by the Research Ethics Committees of the Virgen Macarena and Virgen del Rocío hospitals (Seville, Spain) on 24 February 2020 (Code 1936-N-19).

3. Results

3.1. Characteristics of the Sample

A total of 382 women participated in the study: 232 (60.5%) in the intervention group and 151 (39.5%) in the control group. Table 1 shows the main sociodemographic and obstetric characteristics of the participants. At the recruitment baseline, the average age of all participants was 33.41 (standard deviation (SD) = 4.66) years, with the majority being of Spanish nationality (93.45%), having a university education (64.39%), being employed (71.46%), and predominantly working less than 20 h per week (25.39%). In terms of obstetric characteristics, most births were of spontaneous onset (60.47%), had eutocic delivery (61.78%), and occurred on average at 39.45 (SD = 1.25) weeks of gestation. Approximately 51.04% of the newborns were male, with an average weight of 3262.58 g (SD = 463.76). Most participants (57.85%) had no previous breastfeeding experience. No statistically significant differences in any of these characteristics were observed between the groups, indicating a homogeneous sample (Table 1).

Table 1. Comparison of principal sociodemographic and obstetric characteristics of the groups.

Characteristic Baseline	Total (n = 382)	Group		χ^2	t	p-Value
		Intervention (n = 231)	Control (n = 151)			
Maternal age, years; mean ± SD	33.41 ± 4.66	33.50 ± 4.41	33.28 ± 5.03		−0.45	0.64
Nationality, n (%)				0.14		0.70
Spanish	357 (93.45)	215 (93.07)	142 (94.03)			
Other	25 (6.54)	16 (6.92)	9 (5.96)			
Education level, n (%)				0.81		0.84
Without	1 (0.26)	1 (0.4)	0 (0)			
Primary studies	11 (3.66)	9 (3.9)	5 (3.3)			
Secondary studies	121 (31.67)	74 (32)	47 (31.1)			
University studies	246 (64.39)	147 (63.6)	99 (65.6)			
Employment, n (%)				2.08		0.35
Employed	273 (71.46)	165 (71.4)	108 (71.5)			
Unemployed	109 (28.53)	66 (28.6)	43 (28.5)			
Work hours (per week), n (%)				34.46		0.44
<20	97 (25.39)	57 (34.5)	40 (37.0)			
20–30	75 (19.63)	44 (40.7)	31 (28.7)			
>20	57 (14.92)	33 (20)	24 (22.2)			
Gestation, weeks; mean ± SD	39.45 ± 1.25	39.45 ± 1.14	39.46 ± 1.38		0.13	0.89
Home labour and delivery (%)				0.13		0.71
Induced	151 (39.52)	61 (40.4)	90 (59.6)			
Spontaneous	231 (60.47)	89 (38.5)	142 (61.5)			
Mode of delivery, n (%)				2.88		0.41
Eutocic	236 (61.78)	140 (60.6)	96 (63.6)			
Dystocic	77 (20.15)	51 (22.1)	26 (17.2)			
SCS	17 (4.45)	12 (5.2)	5 (3.3)			
UCS	52 (13.61)	28 (12.1)	24 (15.9)			

Table 1. Cont.

Characteristic Baseline	Total (n = 382)	Group		χ²	t	p-Value
		Intervention (n = 231)	Control (n = 151)			
Infant sex, n (%)				0.16		0.68
Male	195 (51.04)	116 (50.2)	79 (52.3)			
Female	187 (48.95)	115 (49.8)	72 (47.7)			
Newborn weight, g; mean ± SD	3262.58 ± 463.76	3239.10 ± 483.92	3298.51 ± 430.19		1.22	0.22
Previous breastfeeding experience, n (%)				1.42		0.23
Yes	161 (42.14)	103 (44.6)	58 (38.4)			
No	221 (57.85)	128 (55.4)	93 (61.6)			

Note: χ^2, chi-square test; t, independent samples t-test; significant p-values < 0.05; SD, standard deviation; SCS, scheduled Caesarean section; UCS, urgent Caesarean section.

The dropout rate at the 4-month follow-up was similar in both groups (intervention group = 12.38% vs. control group = 17.8%; p = 0.81; Figure 1).

3.2. Effectiveness of the Intervention in Influencing the Type of Breastfeeding

From the start of breastfeeding to 6 months postpartum, higher rates of breastfeeding, specifically exclusive breastfeeding, were maintained over time in the intervention group than in the control group, and breastfeeding rates were considerably higher from 2 months postpartum onward.

At 2 months postpartum, 89.3% of women in the control group continued with breastfeeding of various types, compared to 93.5% of women in the intervention group (χ^2 (3) = 2.60, p = 0.44, Cramer's V = 0.10). However, at 4 months postpartum, when attendance at support groups had accumulated in the intervention group, a statistically significant difference in the prevalence of breastfeeding was observed between groups (intervention group = 88.9% vs. control group = 80.7%) compared to formula feeding, which was significantly higher in the control group (intervention group = 11.1% vs. control group = 19.3%; χ^2 (3) = 13.19, p < 0.01, Cramer's V = 0.24).

On the other hand, at 6 months postpartum, 95.2% of women continued breastfeeding, compared to 90.7% of participants in the control group. Especially different were the percentages of mixed breastfeeding at this time point between both groups (intervention group = 21.4% vs. control group = 31.3%; χ^2 (3) = 7.02, p = 0.07, Cramer's V = 0.17).

Table 2 shows the comparison of the type of breastfeeding between the intervention and control groups during the follow-up period up to 6 months postpartum.

3.3. Effectiveness of the Intervention in Promoting Exclusive Breastfeeding

At the start of the study, similar percentages of exclusive breastfeeding were observed in both groups, with slightly higher rates in women who received only routine care (intervention group = 77.9% vs. control group = 78.1%; χ^2 (1) = 0.002, p = 0.96, V = 0.002). However, after continued attendance of breastfeeding support groups by women in the intervention group, at 4 months postpartum, significant differences begin to be observed. A total of 69.4% of women in the intervention group were exclusively breastfeeding, compared to 51.4% in the control group (χ^2 (1) = 8.72, p = 0.03, V = 0.15). Similarly, at 6 months postpartum, 63.4% of women in the intervention group continued exclusive breastfeeding, compared to 47.9% of women in the control group (χ^2 (1) = 5.98, p = 0.01, V = 0.15).

Supplementary Table S1 shows changes in the type of breastfeeding from the start of the postpartum period to 2, 4, and 6 months later in both study groups.

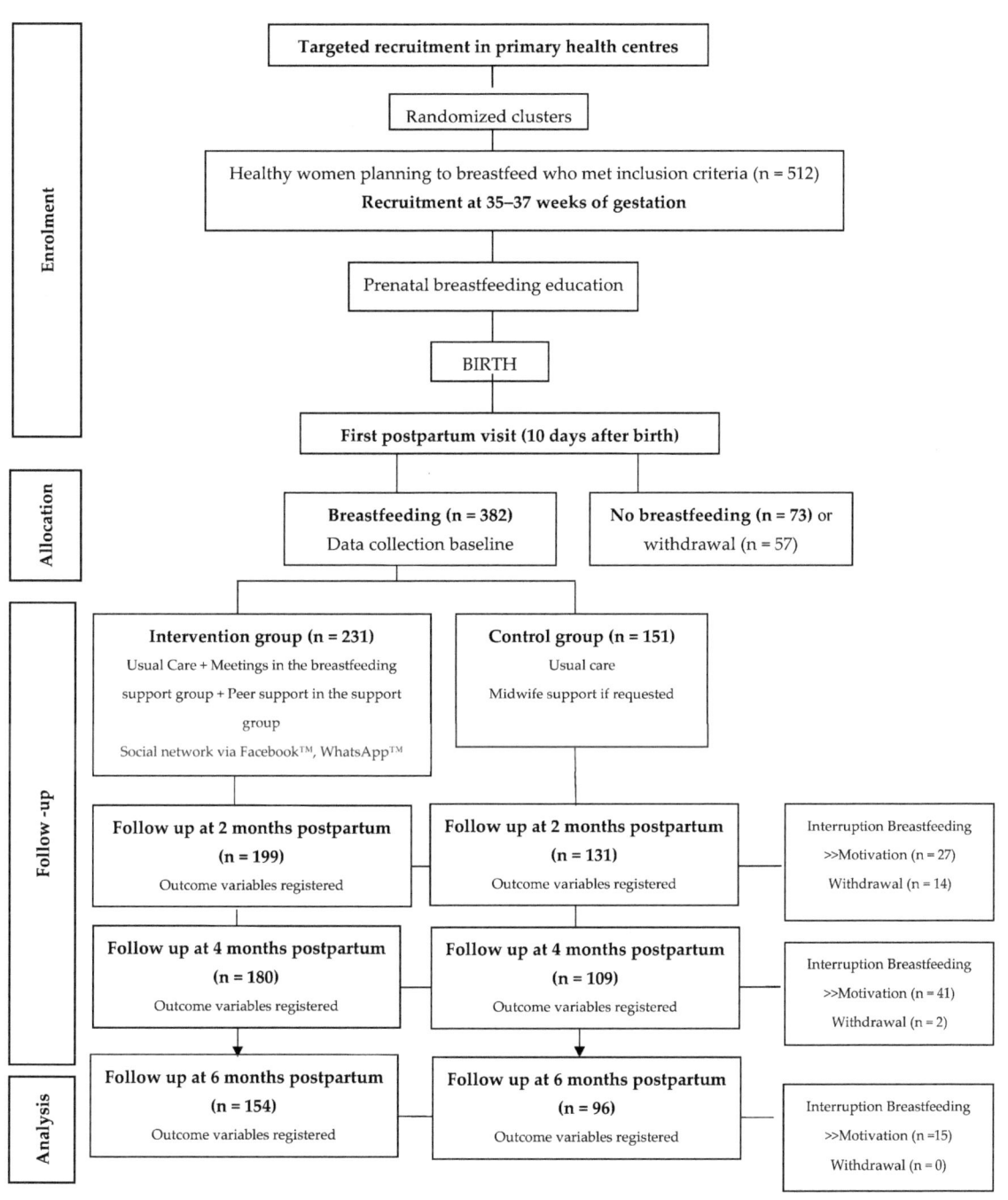

Figure 1. Participant selection flowchart.

Table 2. Comparison of type of breastfeeding between the intervention and control groups.

Type of Breastfeeding	Time Postpartum							
	T0 Group		T1 Group		T2 Group		T3 Group	
	IG n (%)	CG n (%)	IG n (%)	CG n (%)	IG n (%)	CG n (%)	IG n (%)	CG n (%)
Exclusive breastfeeding	180 (77.9)	118 (78.1)	144 (72.4)	85 (64.9)	125 (69.4)	56 (51.4)	98 (63.4)	46 (47.9)
z-value	−0.1	0.1	1.4	−1.4	3.1	−3.1	2.4	−2.4
Breastfeeding with occasional help	31 (13.4)	20 (13.2)	18 (9)	14 (10.7)	22 (11.7)	12 (11.0)	16 (10.4)	11 (11.5)
z-value	0.0	0.0	−0.5	0.5	0.2	−0.2	−0.3	0.3
Breastfeeding mixed	20 (8.7)	13 (8.6)	24 (12.1)	18 (13.7)	14 (7.8)	20 (18.3)	32 (21.4)	30 (31.3)
z-value	0.0	0.0	−0.4	0.4	−2.7	2.7	−1.7	1.7
Artificial breastfeeding	–	–	13 (6.5)	14 (10.7)	20 (11.1)	21 (19.3)	7 (4.5)	9 (9.4)
z-value			−1.3	1.3	−1.9	1.9	−1.5	1.5

Note: T0, postpartum; T1, 2 months postpartum; T2, 4 months postpartum; T3, 6 months postpartum IG, intervention group; CG, control group.

At two months postpartum, 86.5% of women who initiated exclusive breastfeeding continued with this type of feeding in the intervention group, compared to 72.8% of women in the control group (χ^2 (3) = 10.11, $p < 0.01$, V = 0.20). On the other hand, among women in the control group who exclusively breastfed at the beginning of the study, 57.5% continued exclusive breastfeeding at 4 months, while 11.5% continued with occasional help, 16.1% opted for mixed feeding, and 14.9% abandoned breastfeeding in favour of formula. However, in the intervention group, 78.5% of women who started with exclusive breastfeeding continued with this type of feeding until 4 months postpartum, and only 4.9% abandoned breastfeeding (χ^2 (3) = 16.8, $p < 0.01$, V = 0.26). At six months postpartum, a significant trend was observed towards a shift from occasional breastfeeding assistance to exclusive breastfeeding in the intervention group compared to the control (intervention group = 57.1% vs. control group = 8.3%; χ^2 (3) = 8.81, $p = 0.03$, V = 0.58).

3.4. Breastfeeding Self-Efficacy

At the start of the study, women in the intervention group had slightly higher average perceived breastfeeding self-efficacy scores than those in the control group (intervention group = 57.38 ± 10.70 vs. control group = 53.70 ± 12.83). From the start to 2 months postpartum, a slight increase in self-efficacy was observed (intervention group = 59.75 ± 9.64 vs. control group = 56.15 ± 11.01), after which scores remained similar until 4 months postpartum (intervention group = 59.96 ± 11.04 vs. control group = 55.87 ± 13.03). However, at 6 months postpartum, a decrease in perceived self-efficacy was observed in both groups, this being more pronounced in women who received usual care (intervention group = 52.85 ± 1.69 vs. control group = 47.44 ± 2.27). There were no statistically significant differences in breastfeeding self-efficacy between the two study groups (F (3) = 0.19, $p = 0.99$) (Figure 2).

Table 3 shows the results of the mediation analysis of the relationship between the intervention and exclusive breastfeeding at 4 months postpartum (where the highest ratio was observed) through the effects of breastfeeding self-efficacy. Figure 3 shows the standardized coefficients of the relationships included in the model. The results indicated that the effect of the intervention on exclusive breastfeeding at 4 months postpartum was fully mediated by the indirect effect of breastfeeding self-efficacy. The total effect of the intervention (before including the mediator) was $\beta = -0.32$ ($p = 0.002$), and it reduced to $\beta = -0.16$ ($p = 0.78$) after including the mediating variable of breastfeeding self-efficacy. Thus, the analysis revealed that the intervention improved average perceived self-efficacy scores, and, indirectly, this increase contributed to higher rates of exclusive breastfeeding, particularly at 4 months postpartum (F (2, 271) = 89.12, $p < 0.001$, $R^2 = 0.47$).

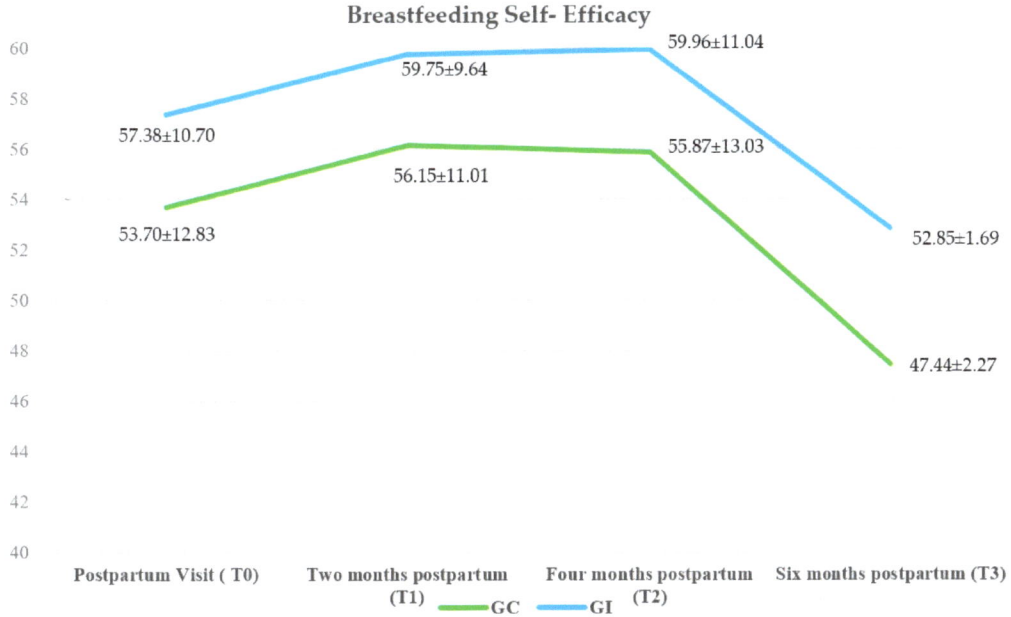

Figure 2. Changes in breastfeeding self-efficacy over time.

Table 3. Results of the partial mediation model.

		β	t	p	95% Confidence Interval Lower	Upper
Direct effect	Intervention → Exclusive breastfeeding T2	−0.16	−1.77	0.78	−0.34	−0.18
Total effect	Intervention → Exclusive breastfeeding T2	−0.32	−3.15	0.00	−0.53	−0.12
Effect on mediator	Intervention → Breastfeeding self-efficacy	0.35	2.77	0.005	0.10	0.60
Effect by mediator	Breastfeeding self-efficacy → Exclusive breastfeeding T2	−0.52	−12.55	<0.001	−0.60	−0.44

Note: T2, 4 months postpartum.

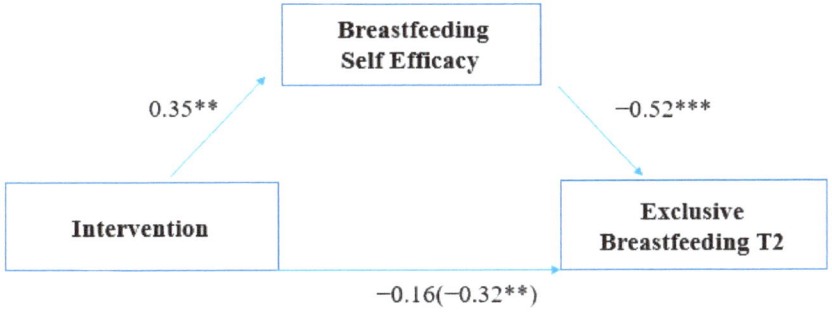

Figure 3. Mediational role of perceived breastfeeding self-efficacy on the relationship between intervention and exclusive breastfeeding at 4 months postpartum. Note: ** significant p-values < 0.01; *** significant p-values < 0.001.

3.5. Early Cessation of Breastfeeding

At 2 months postpartum, 13 participants (6.5%, $z = -1.6$) who attended the support groups prematurely abandoned breastfeeding, compared to 14 women (10.7%, $z = 1.6$) in the control group. The main reasons reported globally for this cessation were a feeling of low milk production (37.3%), weight loss in the newborn (33.3%), difficulty latching (22.2%), and difficulty with breastfeeding practices (7.40%) (χ^2 (1) = 2.50, $p = 0.11$, V = 0.08).

In contrast, at 4 months postpartum, the observed percentages of early breastfeeding cessation were nearly double in the control group ($n = 21$, 19.30%, $z = 1.9$) compared to the intervention group ($n = 20$, 11.1%, $z = -1.9$). At this time point, the main reasons for early cessation were returning to work (34.78%), difficulty latching (17.39%), weight loss in the newborn (15.21%), a feeling of low milk production (13.04%), mastitis (10.81%), and personal desire (8.69%) (χ^2 (1) = 8.49, $p = 0.04$, V = 0.17).

At 6 months postpartum, 7 women (4.5%; $z = -1.5$) in the intervention group chose to discontinue breastfeeding in favor of formula feeding, compared to 9 women (9.4%; $z = 1.5$) in the control group. The reasons for discontinuation were returning to work (43.75%), introduction of complementary feeding (43.75%), and personal desire (12.5) (χ^2 (1) = 2.30, $p = 0.12$, V = 0.96).

3.6. Employment and Breastfeeding

Participants in the intervention group who continued with their paid maternity leave at 4 months postpartum had higher percentages of exclusive breastfeeding (78.25%) than women in the same situation who received only standard care (50%). Additionally, women in the control group in the same employment situation more often stopped breastfeeding prematurely and had higher percentages of formula feeding (25%) than in the intervention group (10.3%) (χ^2 (3) = 11.66, $p = 0.09$, V = 0.29).

Similarly, among women who returned to work, a higher percentage of them continued with exclusive breastfeeding at 4 months postpartum in the intervention group (69.2%) than in the control group (44.4%). In women in the control group, a greater inclination towards formula feeding (22.2%) and, therefore, early cessation of breastfeeding, was observed (χ^2 (3) = 10.95, $p = 0.12$, V = 0.37; Table 4).

Table 4. Breastfeeding type by employment at 4 months postpartum.

Employment	Type of Breastfeeding								χ^2 (df)	p-Value	V
	Exclusive Breastfeeding (%) Group		Breastfeeding with Occasional Help (%) Group		Breastfeeding Mixed (%) Group		Artificial Breastfeeding (%) Group				
	IG n (%)	CG n (%)	IG n (%)	CG n (%)	IG n (%)	CG n (%)	IG n (%)	CG n (%)			
Paid maternity leave	58 (77.3)	28 (50.9)	4 (5.3)	6 (10.9)	5 (6.7)	8 (14.5)	8 (10.7)	13 (23.6)	9.90 (3)	0.01	0.28
z-value	3.1	−3.1	−1.2	1.2	−1.5	1.5	−2.0	2.0			
Active duty mothers	36 (69.2)	11 (52.4)	10 (19.2)	2 (9.5)	3 (5.8)	5 (23.8)	3 (5.8)	3 (14.3)	6.7 (3)	0.07	0.31
z-value	−0.1	−1.5	1.9	−0.9	−0.4	2.2	−1.4	1.2			
Unemployed	31 (62)	17 (56.7)	8 (16)	4 (13.3)	6 (12)	7 (23.3)	5 (10)	2 (6.7)	1.9 (3)	0.6	0.15
z-value	0.5	−0.5	0.3	−0.3	−1.3	1.3	0.5	−0.5			

Note: χ^2, chi-square test; df, degrees of freedom; V, Cramer's V; significant p-values < 0.05; IG, intervention group; CG, control group.

At 6 months postpartum, only 13.6% of women ($n = 34$) were still on paid maternity leave, compared to 57.2% ($n = 143$) of women who were employed. A notable difference was observed in the percentages of exclusive breastfeeding among employed women by study group (intervention group = 60% vs. control group = 45.1%), as well as for other types of breastfeeding (χ^2 (3) = 5.53, $p = 0.13$, V = 0.2; Table 5).

Table 5. Breastfeeding type by employment at 6 months postpartum.

Employment	Type of Breastfeeding								χ^2 (df)	p-Value	V
	Exclusive Breastfeeding (%) Group		Breastfeeding with Occasional Help (%) Group		Breastfeeding Mixed (%) Group		Artificial Breastfeeding (%) Group				
	IG n (%)	CG n (%)	IG n (%)	CG n (%)	IG n (%)	CG n (%)	IG n (%)	CG n (%)			
Paid maternity leave	17 (89.5)	10 (66.7)	--	3 (20)	2 (10.5)	2 (13.3)	--	--	4.40 (2)	0.11	0.36
z-value	1.6	−1.6	−2.0	2.0	−0.3	0.3	--	--			
Active duty mothers	56 (60.0)	23 (45.1)	11 (12)	5 (9.8)	21 (22.8)	17 (33.3)	4 (4.3)	6 (11.8)	5.55 (3)	0.13	0.2
z-value	1.8	−1.8	0.4	−0.4	−1.4	1.4	−1.7	1.7			
Unemployed	24 (60)	13 (44.8)	5 (12.5)	3 (10.3)	8 (20)	10 (34.5)	3 (7.5)	3 (10.3)	2.3 (3)	0.51	0.18
z-value	1.2	−1.2	0.3	−0.3	1.4	1.4	−0.4	0.4			

Note: χ^2, chi-square test; df, degrees of freedom; V, Cramer's V; significant p-values < 0.05; IG, intervention group; CG, control group.

4. Discussion

This multicentric cluster-randomized controlled trial aimed to analyse the impacts of a midwife-led group intervention that supported breastfeeding during the postpartum period and evaluate its effectiveness in promoting exclusive breastfeeding until newborns reached 6 months of age. Additionally, this study assessed the effect of this intervention on breastfeeding self-efficacy and its relationships with the duration and exclusivity of breastfeeding. This study provided evidence that additional support for routine breastfeeding care, in the form of a midwife-led group intervention with peer support, was an effective intervention that improved breastfeeding rates up to 6 months postpartum. Specifically, the designed intervention demonstrated that women who received additional support showed a relative increase of about 20% in exclusive breastfeeding rates at 4 months and a relative increase about 15% at 6 months postpartum. This key finding agrees with other studies that reported similar results [43,44]: exclusive breastfeeding increased in the intervention group when community-based interventions were conducted, including counselling or group support, immediate breastfeeding support during childbirth and postpartum, and breastfeeding management. The main increase in these rates was observed from 2 months postpartum onward, with the intervention becoming significantly effective at 4 months postpartum. This result was also observed in a study by Moudi et al. [45], which compared a routine care group with two experimental groups, one that received peer support and one that received support from healthcare providers.

In addition to the face-to-face support of the group, participants received online support through groups created on social networks that reinforced the main intervention, favoured peer support, and facilitated quick and safe access to information [46,47]. This strategy has been demonstrated by other studies [48–50] to be effective in maintaining exclusive breastfeeding rates when investigated as a single support component. However, in the present clinical trial, combined face-to-face and online support was provided, following the recommendations of recent meta-analyses [19,51] that have advocated for a multicomponent intervention involving a health professional as an effective strategy to improve global breastfeeding and exclusive breastfeeding. This recommended intervention involves theory taught face-to-face and subsequent online follow-up during the prenatal and postnatal periods.

With the rise of new technologies and the impact of the 2019 coronavirus disease pandemic on health services, social network support for breastfeeding, in addition to being effective, has become increasingly necessary, popular, and important for women [52]. This type of support is an indispensable resource, not only for providing information and solving breastfeeding-related problems, but also for emotional support [53]. Online support has also been shown to be effective in promoting attitudes related to breastfeeding [54], increasing the levels of breastfeeding self-efficacy of participating women [55,56], one of the main findings of the present study.

Additionally, this clinical trial confirmed that the effectiveness of support groups was enhanced by the effect of the intervention on perceived breastfeeding self-efficacy. The observed average scores were higher in all follow-up periods in the intervention group than for the women who received only routine support. Other studies [57–59] have reported similar findings for the intervention group and have also observed higher scores in mothers who breastfed exclusively than in those who did not. Franco-Antonio et al. [60] already observed, in their clinical trial on the effect of a brief motivational intervention conducted immediately postpartum, that higher breastfeeding self-efficacy scores predicted the durations of both exclusive and non-exclusive breastfeeding. This relationship between high self-efficacy and prolonged exclusive breastfeeding is partially explained by a study by Blyth et al. [61], in which the main finding was that mothers with higher self-efficacy were more likely to adapt and react more positively to breastfeeding difficulties and, therefore, were more likely to continue breastfeeding. Unlike other factors, breastfeeding self-efficacy is a potentially modifiable individual determinant that can improve breastfeeding rates, as reported by previous studies [59,62–65], when combined with interventions by health professionals [23,66,67]. Moreover, breastfeeding self-efficacy has been recognized as one of the factors positively associated with the establishment and duration of exclusive breastfeeding [68,69], even in premature newborns [70,71], and it has also been identified as a significant predictor of breastfeeding after future pregnancies [72]. These findings provide additional evidence that support aimed at improving breastfeeding rates also improves self-efficacy expectations and, therefore, the probability of successful exclusive breastfeeding.

In this study, which was conducted in the same country as the LACTEM [15] study in 2016, similar results were found on the subjective sensation of low milk production, which was one of the main reasons for the early cessation of breastfeeding. Additionally, other international studies [73] have shown this factor to be one of the most prevalent among those driving the cessation of breastfeeding. For example, Colin et al. [74] observed that this sensation, in addition to promoting the cessation of breastfeeding, generated substantial anxiety among mothers and that many of them experienced this anxiety for up to 6 months postpartum, inclusive. Another relevant factor promoting the cessation of breastfeeding is insufficient weight gain of the newborn, which emerged as an important maternal concern in a study by Odom et al. [75].

Previous national and international [76–78] studies have found a correlation between women's return to work and lower breastfeeding rates and, specifically, exclusive breastfeeding rates. The present study found similar results that, although not statistically significant, might have clinical relevance. However, women who attended the support groups showed higher breastfeeding rates at 6 months, as did participants in other studies who received additional support or resources, such as a favourable environment [79] or a support network [80].

There are some limitations of this study. First, there is a limitation in relation to the number of participants per research group, because the recruitment of women from the control group was more difficult because there was no hypothetical benefit related to the study and there was no blinding of the participants. For this reason, they declined to participate in the study in greater numbers. On the other hand, although a population may share the same nationality, it is crucial to recognize intra-cultural and health system differences that may influence the results of a study. Therefore, the importance of replicating studies in different contexts to validate and generalize the findings is emphasized, thus ensuring a more complete and accurate understating of the phenomena studied. Second, the success of the intervention may have been modulated by mothers' predispositions to participate in such groups and receive additional support. Additionally, adherence to group attendance may have been influenced by the degree of leadership shown by the midwife who guided and moderated the group, although all received prior training involving attitudes and knowledge. Third, the trial dropout rate by the 6-month follow-up was over 15%, although the sample size was adequate at the time of recruitment, the reasons for withdrawal were recorded, and the method of data collection was easy and accessible to women at any time and from any electronic device, without the need for travel. Fourth, data related to breastfeeding and self-efficacy were self-reported, which could introduce a memory or desirability bias. Finally, the 2019 coronavirus disease pandemic affected the follow-up of participants and ability to conduct the intervention in person, as instructions from the Ministry of Health changed due to variation in the incidence and prevalence of the disease.

In future research, a more personalized follow-up is suggested to prevent losses during the follow-up and the possibility of offering the control group a health intervention unrelated to breastfeeding could be considered to increase participation. On the other hand, it would also be interesting to explore the informal support received by the participants during the study, as well as whether there are differences between online and face-to-face groups, in order to offer results adjusted to the intervention modality. It would be advisable to monitor the long-term impact of the intervention, beyond the recommended period of exclusive breastfeeding. This way, results regarding the impact of the intervention on prolonged breastfeeding and the introduction of complementary feeding could be provided. The subjective results reported by the participants can be accompanied by objective observations made by midwives or detailed feeding diaries. Furthermore, assessing the satisfaction of women attending midwife-led support groups through focus groups would provide valuable insights.

5. Conclusions

Breastfeeding support groups, a group intervention led by midwives and aimed at supporting breastfeeding during the postpartum period, proved to be effective at maintaining exclusive breastfeeding up to 6 months postpartum. Additionally, the intervention improved perceived breastfeeding self-efficacy, which is a modifiable factor, so the effectiveness of this intervention was mediated by higher self-efficacy scores in women who attended the support groups.

One of the main factors for the early cessation of breastfeeding at 4 and 6 months postpartum, return to work, can be combated with additional face-to-face and online support in the form of support groups. However, additional measures are needed to attain the breastfeeding rates recommended by international organizations.

Once the effectiveness of this midwife-led group intervention is demonstrated, guidelines could be developed for professionals describing the implementation practices of this support resource. These findings should encourage a shift in the current breastfeeding support system towards an integrated network of support led by midwives to achieve improved maternal and child health.

Supplementary Materials: The following supporting information can be downloaded at: https://www.mdpi.com/article/10.3390/nu16070988/s1, Table S1. Breastfeeding type postpartum to 2, 4 and 6 months postpartum.

Author Contributions: Conceptualization and methodology: F.L.-L. & I.R.-G.; analysis of data: I.R.-G. & D.G.-B.; writing—original draft preparation, writing—review and editing: F.L.-L., I.R.-G., I.C.-G. & D.G.-B. All authors have read and agreed to the published version of the manuscript.

Funding: This is a project document that has received a public grant for its development in the call for Research, Development, and Innovation on Biomedicine and Health Sciences in Andalusia of the Health and Family Council (Consejería de Salud y Familias), Spain (Code PI-0008-2019).

Institutional Review Board Statement: The study was approved by the Research Ethics Committees of the Virgen Macarena and Virgen del Rocío Hospitals (Seville, Spain) on 24 February 2020 (Code 1936-N-19).

Informed Consent Statement: Informed consent was obtained from all subjects involved in the study.

Data Availability Statement: The data presented in this study are available on request from the corresponding author. The data are not publicly available due to confidentiality issues.

Acknowledgments: To all the mothers who have voluntarily and altruistically participated in this study. To the Health and Family Councial (Andalusia, Spain), for their support and funding for research in Biomedicine and Health Sciences.

Conflicts of Interest: The authors declare no conflict of interest. The funders had no role in the design of the study; in the collection, analyses, or interpretation of data; in the writing of the manuscript; or in the decision to publish the results.

References

1. Organización Mundial de la Salud. Lactancia Materna Exclusiva. Available online: https://www.who.int/news/item/15-01-2011-exclusive-breastfeeding-for-six-months-best-for-babies-everywhere (accessed on 25 July 2023).
2. Organización Mundial de la Salud, UNICEF. *Estrategia Mundial para la Alimentación del Lactante y el Niño Pequeño*; Organización Mundial de la Salud: Geneva, Switzerland, 2003. Available online: https://www.paho.org/es/documentos/estrategia-mundial-para-alimentacion-lactante-nino-pequeno-1 (accessed on 25 July 2023).
3. Alzate-Meza, M.C.; Arango, C.; Castaño-Castrillón, J.J.; Henao-Hurtado, A.M.; Lozano-Acosta, M.; Muñoz-Salazar, G.; Ocampo-Muñoz, N.A.; Rengifo-Calderón, S.V.; Tovar-Orozco, L.M.; Vallejo-Chávez, S.H. Lactancia materna como factor protector para enfermedades prevalentes en niños hasta de 5 años de edad en algunas instituciones educativas de Colombia 2009. Estudio de corte transversal. *Rev. Colomb. Obstet. Ginecol.* **2011**, *62*, 57–63. [CrossRef]
4. Woodward, L.J.; Liberty, K.A. Enciclopedia Sobre el Desarrollo de la Primera Infancia: Lactancia Materna y Desarrollo Psicosocial del Niño. 2017. Available online: https://www.enciclopedia-infantes.com/pdf/expert/lactancia-materna/segun-los-expertos/lactancia-materna-y-desarrollo-psicosocial-del-nino (accessed on 20 July 2023).
5. Chowdhury, R.; Sinha, B.; Sankar, M.J.; Taneja, S.; Bhandari, N.; Rollins, N.; Bahl, R.; Martines, J. Breastfeeding and maternal health outcomes: A systematic review and meta-analysis. *Acta Paediatr.* **2015**, *104*, 96–113. [CrossRef] [PubMed]
6. Tschiderer, L.; Seekircher, L.; Kunutsor, S.K.; Peters, S.A.E.; O'Keeffe, L.M.; Willeit, P. Breastfeeding Is Associated with a Reduced Maternal Cardiovascular Risk: Systematic Review and Meta-Analysis Involving Data from 8 Studies and 1 192 700 Parous Women. *J. Am. Heart Assoc.* **2022**, *11*, e022746. [CrossRef] [PubMed]
7. Aune, D.; Norat, T.; Romundstad, P.; Vatten, L.J. Breastfeeding and the maternal risk of type 2 diabetes: A systematic review and dose-response meta-analysis of cohort studies. *Nutr. Metab. Cardiovasc. Dis.* **2014**, *24*, 107–115. [CrossRef]
8. Dias, C.C.; Figueiredo, B. Breastfeeding and depression: systematic review of the literature. *J. Affect. Disord.* **2015**, *171*, 142–154. [CrossRef] [PubMed]
9. Prentice, A.M. Breastfeeding in the Modern World. *Ann. Nutr. Metab.* **2022**, *78*, 29–38. [CrossRef] [PubMed]
10. World Health Organization. *Clinical Management of COVID-19: Interim Guidance (27 May 2020)*; World Health Organization: Geneva, Switzerland, 2020.
11. Comité de Lactancia Materna; Asociación Española de Pediatría. Tasas de Inicio y Duración de Lactancia Materna en España y Otros Países. AEP, 2016. Available online: https://www.aeped.es/sites/default/files/documentos/201602-lactancia-materna-cifras.pdf (accessed on 25 July 2023).
12. From the First Hour of Life: Making the Case for Improved Infant and Young Child Feeding Everywhere. United Nations Children's Fund UNICEF, 2016. Available online: https://www.unicef.org/media/49801/file/From-the-first-hour-of-life-ENG.pdf (accessed on 25 July 2023).
13. Victora, C.G.; Bahl, R.; Barros, A.J.; França, G.V.; Horton, S.; Krasevec, J.; Murch, S.; Sankar, M.J.; Walker, N.; Rollins, N.C. Breastfeeding in the 21st century: Epidemiology, mechanisms, and lifelong effect. *Lancet* **2016**, *387*, 475–490. [CrossRef] [PubMed]
14. Rollins, N.C.; Bhandari, N.; Hajeebhoy, N.; Horton, S.; Lutter, C.K.; Martines, J.C.; Piwoz, E.G.; Richter, L.M.; Victora, C.G.; Lancet Breastfeeding Series Group. Why invest, and what it will take to improve breastfeeding practices? *Lancet* **2016**, *387*, 491–504. [CrossRef]
15. Cabedo, R.; Manresa, M.; Cambredó, M.V.; Montero, L.; Reyes, A.; Gol, R.; Falguera, G. Tipos de lactancia materna y factores que influyen en su abandono hasta los 6 meses. Estudio LACTEM. *Matronas Prof.* **2019**, *20*, 54–61.
16. Renfrew, M.J.; McCormick, F.M.; Wade, A.; Quinn, B.; Dowswell, T. Support for healthy breastfeeding mothers with healthy term babies. *Cochrane Database Syst. Rev.* **2012**, *5*, CD001141. [CrossRef]
17. Imdad, A.; Yakoob, M.Y.; Siddiqui, S.; Bhutta, Z.A. Screening and triage of intrauterine growth restriction (IUGR) in general population and high risk pregnancies: A systematic review with a focus on reduction of IUGR related stillbirths. *BMC Public Health* **2011**, *11*, S1. [CrossRef]
18. Srinivas, G.; Benson, M.; Worley, S.; Schulte, E. A clinic-based breastfeeding peer counselor intervention in an urban, low-income population: Interaction with breastfeeding attitude. *J. Hum. Lact.* **2015**, *31*, 120–128. [CrossRef] [PubMed]
19. Kim, S.; Park, S.; Oh, J.; Kim, J.; Ahn, S. Interventions promoting exclusive breastfeeding up to six months after birth: A systematic review and meta-analysis of randomized controlled trials. *Int. J. Nurs. Stud.* **2018**, *80*, 94–105. [CrossRef] [PubMed]
20. Zhu, J.; Chan, W.C.; Zhou, X.; Ye, B.; He, H.G. Predictors of breast feeding self-efficacy among Chinese mothers: A cross-sectional questionnaire survey. *Midwifery* **2014**, *30*, 705–711. [CrossRef] [PubMed]

21. Marco, T.D.; Martínez, D.; Muñoz, M.J.; Sayas, I.; Oliver-Roig, A.; Richart-Martínez, M. Valores de referencia españoles para la versión reducida de la Escala de Autoeficacia para la Lactancia Materna BSES-SF [Spanish reference values for the Breastfeeding Self-Efficacy Scale-Short Form BSES-SF]. *An. Sist. Sanit. Navar.* **2014**, *37*, 203–211. [CrossRef] [PubMed]
22. Mercan, Y.; Tari Selcuk, K. Association between postpartum depression level, social support level and breastfeeding attitude and breastfeeding self-efficacy in early postpartum women. *PLoS ONE* **2021**, *16*, e0249538. [CrossRef]
23. Brockway, M.; Benzies, K.; Hayden, K.A. Interventions to Improve Breastfeeding Self-Efficacy and Resultant Breastfeeding Rates: A Systematic Review and Meta-Analysis. *J. Hum. Lact.* **2017**, *33*, 486–499. [CrossRef] [PubMed]
24. Amer, S.; Kateeb, E. Mothers' Employment and Exclusive Breastfeeding Practices: A Brief Report from Jerusalem Governorate. *Int. J. Environ. Res. Public Health* **2023**, *20*, 2066. [CrossRef]
25. López de Aberasturi, A.; Santos, N.; Ramos, Y.; García, M.; Artola, C.; Arara, I. Prevalencia y determinantes de la lactancia materna: Estudio Zorrotzaurre [Prevalence and determinants of breastfeeding: The Zorrotzaurre study]. *Nutr. Hosp.* **2021**, *38*, 50–59. (In Spanish) [CrossRef]
26. Lechosa-Muñiz, C.; Paz-Zulueta, M.; Cayón-De Las Cuevas, J.; Llorca, J.; Cabero-Pérez, M.J. Declared Reasons for Cessation of Breastfeeding during the First Year of Life: An Analysis Based on a Cohort Study in Northern Spain. *Int. J. Environ. Res. Public Health* **2021**, *18*, 8414. [CrossRef]
27. Real Decreto-Ley 6/2019, de 1 de Marzo, de Medidas Urgentes para Garantía de la Igualdad de Trato y de Oportunidades Entre Mujeres y Hombres en el Empleo y la Ocupación. (Boletín Oficial del Estado, Número 57, de 7 de Marzo de 2019). Available online: https://www.boe.es/eli/es/rdl/2019/03/01/6/con (accessed on 25 July 2023).
28. Rodríguez-Gallego, I.; Leon-Larios, F.; Ruiz-Ferrón, C.; Lomas-Campos, M.D. Evaluation of the impact of breastfeeding support groups in primary health CENTRES in Andalusia, Spain: A study protocol for a cluster randomized controlled trial (GALMA project). *BMC Public Health* **2020**, *20*, 1129, Erratum in *BMC Public Health* **2020**, *20*, 1445. [CrossRef]
29. Instituto Nacional de Estadística. Oficina Estadística Española. Registro INE 2021. Available online: https://www.ine.es/jaxiT3/Datos.htm?t=2915 (accessed on 20 July 2023).
30. Instituto Nacional de Estadística. Oficina Estadística Española. Registro INE 2022. Available online: https://www.ine.es/jaxiT3/Datos.htm?t=1433#!tabs-tabla (accessed on 20 July 2023).
31. Instituto Nacional de Estadística (INE). Series Detalladas Desde 2002. Población Residente por Fecha, Sexo, Grupo de Edad y Nacionalidad (Agrupación de Países). Oficina Estadística Española. Registro INE 2023. Available online: https://www.ine.es/jaxiT3/Datos.htm?t=56942 (accessed on 20 July 2023).
32. Instituto Nacional de Estadística (INE). Movimiento Natural de la Población: Nacimientos. Fenómenos Demográficos por Comunidades y Ciudades Autónomas y Tipo de Fenómeno Demográfico. Oficina Estadística Española. Registro INE 2022. Available online: https://www.ine.es/jaxiT3/Datos.htm?t=6567 (accessed on 20 July 2023).
33. Ministerio de Sanidad. Encuesta Nacional de Salud de España 2017 (ENSE 2017). Determinantes de Salud. Tipo de Lactancia. Tabla 3.078. Según Sexo y Clase Social Basada en la Ocupación de la Persona de Referencia 2017. Available online: https://www.sanidad.gob.es/estadEstudios/estadisticas/encuestaNacional/encuestaNac2017/ENSE17_MOD3_REL.pdf (accessed on 20 July 2023).
34. Nabulsi, M.; Hamadeh, H.; Tamim, H.; Kabakian, T.; Charafeddine, L.; Yehya, N.; Sinno, D.; Sidani, S. A complex breastfeeding promotion and support intervention in a developing country: Study protocol for a randomized clinical trial. *BMC Public Health* **2014**, *14*, 36. [CrossRef] [PubMed]
35. Guillaumes, S.; O'Callaghan, C. Versión en español del software gratuito OxMaR para minimización y aleatorización de estudios clínicos. *Gac. Sanit.* **2019**, *33*, 395–397. [CrossRef] [PubMed]
36. Aceituno, L.; Maldonado, J.; Arribas, L.; Caño, A.; Corona, I.; Martín, J.E.; Mora, M.A.; Morales, L.; Ras, J.; Sánchez, T.; et al. *Embarazo, Parto y Puerperio. Proceso Asistencial Integrado*, 3rd ed.; Consejería De Igualdad, Salud y Políticas Sociales: Junta de Andalucía, Spain, 2014; pp. 24–46.
37. Organización Mundial de la Salud, UNICEF. *Consejería en Lactancia Materna: Curso de Capacitación*; WHO: Geneva, Switzerland, 1993.
38. World Health Organization, UNICEF. *Protecting, Promoting, and Supporting Breastfeeding in Facilities Providing Maternity and Newborn Services: The Revised Baby-Friendly Hospital Initiative 2018*; Implementation Guidance; WHO: Geneva, Switzerland, 2018.
39. Robinson, A.; Lauckner, C.; Davis, M.; Hall, J.; Anderson, A.K. Facebook support for breastfeeding mothers: A comparison to offline support and associations with breastfeeding outcomes. *Digit. Health* **2019**, *5*, 2055207619853397. [CrossRef]
40. Oliver-Roig, A.; d'Anglade-González, M.L.; García-García, B.; Silva-Tubio, J.R.; Richart-Martínez, M.; Dennis, C.L. The Spanish version of the Breastfeeding Self-Efficacy Scale-Short Form: Reliability and validity assessment. *Int. J. Nurs. Stud.* **2012**, *49*, 169–173. [CrossRef] [PubMed]
41. IBM Corp. *IBM SPSS Statistics for Windows*, version 23.0; IBM Corp.: Armonk, NY, USA, 2018.
42. Hayes, A.F. *Introduction to Mediation, Moderation, and Conditional Process Analysis: A Regression-Based Approach*; Guilford Publications: New York, NY, USA, 2013.
43. Jenkins, L.A.; Barnes, K.; Latter, A.; Edwards, R.A. Examining the Baby Café Model and Mothers' Breastfeeding Duration, Meeting of Goals, and Exclusivity. *Breastfeed. Med.* **2020**, *15*, 331–334. [CrossRef] [PubMed]
44. Schreck, P.K.; Solem, K.; Wright, T.; Schulte, C.; Ronnisch, K.J.; Szpunar, S. Both Prenatal and Postnatal Interventions Are Needed to Improve Breastfeeding Outcomes in a Low-Income Population. *Breastfeed. Med.* **2017**, *12*, 142–148. [CrossRef] [PubMed]

45. Moudi, S.; Tafazoli, M.; Boskabadi, H.; Ebrahimzadeh, S.; Salehiniya, H. Comparing the effect of breastfeeding promotion interventions on exclusive breastfeeding: An experimental study. *Biomed. Res. Ther.* **2016**, *3*, 910–927. [CrossRef]
46. Wagg, A.J.; Callanan, M.M.; Hassett, A. Online social support group use by breastfeeding mothers: A content analysis. *Heliyon* **2019**, *5*, e01245. [CrossRef]
47. Regan, S.; Brown, A. Experiences of online breastfeeding support: Support and reassurance versus judgement and misinformation. *Matern. Child Nutr.* **2019**, *15*, e12874. [CrossRef]
48. Cavalcanti, D.S.; Cabral, C.S.; de Toledo Vianna, R.P.; Osório, M.M. Online participatory intervention to promote and support exclusive breastfeeding: Randomized clinical trial. *Matern. Child Nutr.* **2019**, *15*, e12806. [CrossRef]
49. Wilson, J.C. Using Social Media for Breastfeeding Support. *Nurs. Women's Health* **2020**, *24*, 332–343. [CrossRef] [PubMed]
50. Blackmore, A.; Howell, B.; Romme, K.; Gao, Z.; Nguyen, H.; Allwood Newhook, L.A.; Twells, L. The Effectiveness of Virtual Lactation Support: A Systematic Review and Meta-Analysis. *J. Hum. Lact.* **2022**, *38*, 452–465. [CrossRef]
51. Wong, M.S.; Mou, H.; Chien, W.T. Effectiveness of educational and supportive intervention for primiparous women on breastfeeding related outcomes and breastfeeding self-efficacy: A systematic review and meta-analysis. *Int. J. Nurs. Stud.* **2021**, *117*, 103874. [CrossRef] [PubMed]
52. Rodríguez-Gallego, I.; Strivens-Vilchez, H.; Agea-Cano, I.; Marín-Sánchez, C.; Sevillano-Giraldo, M.D.; Gamundi-Fernández, C.; Berná-Guisado, C.; Leon-Larios, F. Breastfeeding experiences during the COVID-19 pandemic in Spain: A qualitative study. *Int. Breastfeed. J.* **2022**, *17*, 11. [CrossRef] [PubMed]
53. Clapton-Caputo, E.; Sweet, L.; Muller, A. A qualitative study of expectations and experiences of women using a social media support group when exclusively expressing breastmilk to feed their infant. *Women Birth* **2021**, *34*, 370–380. [CrossRef] [PubMed]
54. Skelton, K.R.; Evans, R.; LaChenaye, J.; Amsbary, J.; Wingate, M.; Talbott, L. Exploring Social Media Group Use among Breastfeeding Mothers: Qualitative Analysis. *JMIR Pediatr. Parent.* **2018**, *1*, e11344. [CrossRef]
55. Black, R.; McLaughlin, M.; Giles, M. Women's experience of social media breastfeeding support and its impact on extended breastfeeding success: A social cognitive perspective. *Br. J. Health Psychol.* **2020**, *25*, 754–771. [CrossRef]
56. Uzunçakmak, T.; Gökşin, İ.; Ayaz-Alkaya, S. The effect of social media-based support on breastfeeding self-efficacy: A randomised controlled trial. *Eur. J. Contracept. Reprod. Health Care* **2022**, *27*, 159–165. [CrossRef]
57. De Roza, J.G.; Fong, M.K.; Ang, B.L.; Sadon, R.B.; Koh, E.Y.L.; Teo, S.S.H. Exclusive breastfeeding, breastfeeding self-efficacy and perception of milk supply among mothers in Singapore: A longitudinal study. *Midwifery* **2019**, *79*, 102532. [CrossRef]
58. Wu, D.S.; Hu, J.; McCoy, T.P.; Efird, J.T. The effects of a breastfeeding self-efficacy intervention on short-term breastfeeding outcomes among primiparous mothers in Wuhan, China. *J. Adv. Nurs.* **2014**, *70*, 1867–1879. [CrossRef] [PubMed]
59. Chan, M.Y.; Ip, W.Y.; Choi, K.C. The effect of a self-efficacy-based educational programme on maternal breast feeding self-efficacy, breast feeding duration and exclusive breast feeding rates: A longitudinal study. *Midwifery* **2016**, *36*, 92–98. [CrossRef] [PubMed]
60. Franco-Antonio, C.; Calderón-García, J.F.; Santano-Mogena, E.; Rico-Martín, S.; Cordovilla-Guardia, S. Effectiveness of a brief motivational intervention to increase the breastfeeding duration in the first 6 months postpartum: Randomized controlled trial. *J. Adv. Nurs.* **2020**, *76*, 888–902. [CrossRef]
61. Blyth, R.; Creedy, D.K.; Dennis, C.L.; Moyle, W.; Pratt, J.; De Vries, S.M. Effect of maternal confidence on breastfeeding duration: An application of breastfeeding self-efficacy theory. *Birth* **2002**, *29*, 278–284. [CrossRef] [PubMed]
62. Awano, M.; Shimada, K. Development and evaluation of a self care program on breastfeeding in Japan: A quasi-experimental study. *Int. Breastfeed. J.* **2010**, *5*, 9. [CrossRef]
63. Ansari, S.; Abedi, P.; Hasanpoor, S.; Bani, S. The Effect of Interventional Program on Breastfeeding Self-Efficacy and Duration of Exclusive Breastfeeding in Pregnant Women in Ahvaz, Iran. *Int. Sch. Res. Not.* **2014**, *2014*, 510793. [CrossRef]
64. Shariat, M.; Abedinia, N.; Noorbala, A.A.; Zebardast, J.; Moradi, S.; Shahmohammadian, N.; Karimi, A.; Abbasi, M. Breastfeeding Self-Efficacy as a Predictor of Exclusive Breastfeeding: A Clinical Trial. *Iran. J. Neonatol.* **2018**, *9*, 26–34. [CrossRef]
65. Tseng, J.F.; Chen, S.R.; Au, H.K.; Chipojola, R.; Lee, G.T.; Lee, P.H.; Shyu, M.L.; Kuo, S.Y. Effectiveness of an integrated breastfeeding education program to improve self-efficacy and exclusive breastfeeding rate: A single-blind, randomised controlled study. *Int. J. Nurs. Stud.* **2020**, *111*, 103770. [CrossRef] [PubMed]
66. Chipojola, R.; Chiu, H.Y.; Huda, M.H.; Lin, Y.M.; Kuo, S.Y. Effectiveness of theory-based educational interventions on breastfeeding self-efficacy and exclusive breastfeeding: A systematic review and meta-analysis. *Int. J. Nurs. Stud.* **2020**, *109*, 103675. [CrossRef]
67. Franco-Antonio, C.; Santano-Mogena, E.; Sánchez-García, P.; Chimento-Díaz, S.; Cordovilla-Guardia, S. Effect of a brief motivational intervention in the immediate postpartum period on breastfeeding self-efficacy: Randomized controlled trial. *Res. Nurs. Health* **2021**, *44*, 295–307. [CrossRef]
68. Maleki-Saghooni, N.; Amel, M.; Moeindarbari, S.; Fatemeh, Z.K. Investigating the Breastfeeding Self-Efficacy and its Related Factors in Primiparous Breastfeeding Mothers. *Int. J. Pediatr.* **2017**, *5*, 6275–6283. [CrossRef]
69. Efrat, M.W. Breastfeeding Self-Efficacy and Level of Acculturation among Low-Income Pregnant Latinas. *Int. J. Child Health Nutr.* **2018**, *7*, 169–174. [CrossRef]
70. Brockway, M.; Benzies, K.M.; Carr, E.; Aziz, K. Breastfeeding self-efficacy and breastmilk feeding for moderate and late preterm infants in the Family Integrated Care trial: A mixed methods protocol. *Int. Breastfeed. J.* **2018**, *13*, 29. [CrossRef] [PubMed]
71. Brockway, M.; Benzies, K.M.; Carr, E.; Aziz, K. Does breastfeeding self-efficacy theory apply to mothers of moderate and late preterm infants? A qualitative exploration. *J. Clin. Nurs.* **2020**, *29*, 2872–2885. [CrossRef] [PubMed]

72. Bartle, N.C.; Harvey, K. Explaining infant feeding: The role of previous personal and vicarious experience on attitudes, subjective norms, self-efficacy, and breastfeeding outcomes. *Br. J. Health Psychol.* **2017**, *22*, 763–785. [CrossRef]
73. Morrison, A.H.; Gentry, R.; Anderson, J. Mothers' Reasons for Early Breastfeeding Cessation. *MCN Am. J. Matern. Child Nurs.* **2019**, *44*, 325–330. [CrossRef]
74. Colin, W.B.; Scott, J.A. Breastfeeding: Reasons for starting, reasons for stopping and problems along the way. *Breastfeed. Rev.* **2002**, *10*, 13–19. [PubMed]
75. Odom, E.C.; Li, R.; Scanlon, K.S.; Perrine, C.G.; Grummer-Strawn, L. Reasons for earlier than desired cessation of breastfeeding. *Pediatrics* **2013**, *131*, e726–e732. [CrossRef]
76. Ramiro, M.D.; Ortiz, H.; Arana, C.; Esparza, M.J.; Cortés, O.; Terol, M.; Ordovás, M. Prevalencia de la lactancia materna y factores asociados con el inicio y la duración de la lactancia materna exclusiva en la Comunidad de Madrid entre los participantes en el estudio ELOIN [Prevalence of breastfeeding and factors associated with the start and duration of exclusive breastfeeding in the Community of Madrid among participants in the ELOIN]. *An. Pediatr. (Engl. Ed.)* **2018**, *89*, 32–43. (In Spanish) [CrossRef]
77. Castetbon, K.; Boudet-Berquier, J.; Salanave, B. Combining breastfeeding and work: Findings from the Epifane population-based birth cohort. *BMC Pregnancy Childbirth* **2020**, *20*, 110. [CrossRef]
78. Santos, M.N.; Azeredo, C.M.; Rinaldi, A.E.M. Association Between Maternal Work and Exclusive Breastfeeding in Countries of Latin America and Caribbean. *Matern. Child Health J.* **2022**, *26*, 1496–1506. [CrossRef] [PubMed]
79. Tsai, S.Y. Shift-work and breastfeeding for women returning to work in a manufacturing workplace in Taiwan. *Int. Breastfeed. J.* **2022**, *17*, 27. [CrossRef] [PubMed]
80. Silva, I.A.; Silva, C.M.; Costa, E.M.; Ferreira, M.J.; Abuchaim, E.S.V. Continued breastfeeding and work: Scenario of maternal persistence and resilience. *Rev. Bras. Enferm.* **2023**, *76*, e20220191. [CrossRef] [PubMed]

Disclaimer/Publisher's Note: The statements, opinions and data contained in all publications are solely those of the individual author(s) and contributor(s) and not of MDPI and/or the editor(s). MDPI and/or the editor(s) disclaim responsibility for any injury to people or property resulting from any ideas, methods, instructions or products referred to in the content.

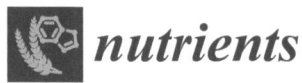

Article

Factors Associated with Exclusive Breastfeeding during Admission to a Baby-Friendly Hospital Initiative Hospital: A Cross-Sectional Study in Spain

Cristina Verea-Nuñez [1], Nuria Novoa-Maciñeiras [2], Ana Suarez-Casal [2] and Juan Manuel Vazquez-Lago [3,4,*]

[1] Resident Nurse in Pediatrics, Pediatric Service, University Hospital of Santiago de Compostela, Rua da Choupana s/n, 15705 Santiago de Compostela, Spain; cristina.verea.nunez@sergas.es
[2] Nurse Specialist in Pediatrics, Hospitalary Unit of Neonatology, University Hospital of Santiago de Compostela, Rua da Choupana s/n, 15705 Santiago de Compostela, Spain; nuria.novoa.macineiras@sergas.es (N.N.-M.); ana.suarez.casal@sergas.es (A.S.-C.)
[3] Preventive Medicine and Public Health Service, University Hospital of Santiago de Compostela, Rua da Choupana s/n, 15705 Santiago de Compostela, Spain
[4] UTAMI, Health Research Institute of Santiago de Compostela (IDIS), 15706 Santiago de Compostela, Spain
* Correspondence: juan.manuel.vazquez.lago@sergas.es

Abstract: Background: Breastfeeding is the optimal nourishment for infants and it is recommended that children commence breastfeeding within the first hour of birth and be exclusively breastfed for the initial 6 months of life. Our objective was to determine which factors related to mothers could influence the degree of exclusive breastfeeding during hospitalization, as well as to assess breastfeeding mothers' attitudes towards breastfeeding. Methods: A multicenter cross-sectional study was undertaken in the healthcare area of Santiago de Compostela, Spain. The necessary variables were collected using a specially designed ad hoc questionnaire. The researcher responsible for recruitment conducted the interviews with the participants. The reduced Iowa Infant Feeding Attitude Scale (IIFAS-s) was employed to gauge maternal attitudes toward feeding their baby. Results: In total, 64 women were studied. The overall score of IIFAS-s (mean ± standard deviation) was 36.95 ± 5.17. A positive attitude towards breastfeeding was therefore observed in our sample. No use of a pacifier by the newborn was associated with a positive attitude for breastfeeding. Having previous children (Ora = 6.40; IC95% 1.26–32.51) and previous experience with breastfeeding (Ora = 6.70; IC95% 1.31–34.27) increased the likelihood of exclusive breastfeeding during admission. Conclusions: In our study, exclusive breastfeeding during hospitalization is associated with having previous children and prior breastfeeding experience.

Keywords: breastfeeding; attitudes; baby-friendly hospital

1. Introduction

The World Health Organization (WHO) recognizes breastfeeding (BF) as the optimal nourishment for infants and recommends that children commence breastfeeding within the first hour of birth and be exclusively breastfed for the initial 6 months of life. Subsequently, they should begin consuming safe and suitable complementary foods while continuing breastfeeding for up to two years or beyond [1]. BF not only provides nutritional benefits but also confers psychological and emotional advantages to both the newborn (NB) and the mother [2–6]. Additionally, it contributes to the economic and social well-being of families by promoting better infant health outcomes [6–8].

According to the latest National Health Survey in Spain from 2017, breastfeeding was the most prevalent feeding method for babies during the first 6 weeks (73.9%), but it decreased to 63.9% by 3 months. By 6 months, 41.6% of babies were being fed with formula milk, thereby relegating breastfeeding to a secondary position (39%) [9]. This trend is associated with various sociodemographic, clinical, and psychological factors, including maternal insecurity and doubts during the breastfeeding process, as well as the absence of a supportive environment [10,11]. The sociolaboral and cultural shifts of recent decades have negatively impacted breastfeeding rates, with maternal return to work being a primary cause of breastfeeding cessation [10,12–14]. Insufficient maternal knowledge about breastfeeding is also a contributing factor to early breastfeeding discontinuation [13,14]. This may partly stem from the lack of or inadequate dissemination of information by health professionals, which in turn can lead to premature breastfeeding cessation [15–17]. Furthermore, nursing staff providing care to women in the early postpartum days may also have insufficient knowledge about breastfeeding [18].

Currently, healthcare services are beginning to establish breastfeeding support groups and programs [19,20]. The Initiative for the Humanization of Birth and Breastfeeding Care (BFHI) launched by the WHO and UNICEF aims to encourage hospitals, health services, and particularly maternity wards to adopt practices that protect, promote, and support exclusive breastfeeding from birth [21–23]. One of the standards for continuous improvement in these hospitals is that at least 75% of mothers should practice exclusive breastfeeding during hospitalization [24]. Our hospital has been part of the BFHI network since 2015, in Phase 2D since 2020. Hospitals in Phase 2D are required to conduct self-assessments to identify areas for improvement in factors that may influence exclusive breastfeeding [25]. Based on the aforementioned points, it could be expected that a BFHI hospital would have a high proportion of mothers who exclusively breastfeed during hospitalization and continue breastfeeding after discharge. If this is not the case, it is important to understand the factors that may influence these decisions. Our objectives were to determine the percentage of mothers who practiced exclusive BF during hospitalization and which factors related to mothers could influence the degree of exclusive breastfeeding during hospitalization, as well as to assess breastfeeding mothers' attitudes towards breastfeeding.

2. Materials and Methods

2.1. Study Design, Population, and Sample

The study was conducted from June 2023 to February 2024 in Galicia, a region in northwest Spain with a population of 2.7 million inhabitants, where breastfeeding abandonment stands at 58.8% within the first year of infant life [26]. To address the study objectives, a multicenter cross-sectional study was undertaken in the healthcare area of Santiago de Compostela, covering a population of 450,000. In 2023, there were 1948 births in this healthcare area.

The sample size was calculated prior to starting the study. Based on the number of births in our healthcare area in 2023, the percentage of exclusive breastfeeding at discharge was estimated at 87.5% [27]. Using a binomial distribution, a sample of at least 62 women was needed, with a 10% absolute error and a 95% confidence level. Once the sample size was determined, primary healthcare centers (PHCs) were randomly selected. From a list of 74 PHCs, 5 were randomly chosen: 2 urban (Concepción Arenal PHC and Vite PHC) and 3 rural (Boqueixón PHC, O Pino PHC, and Touro PHC). Women meeting the selection criteria were invited to participate during routine check-ups through purposive sampling.

2.2. Sample Selection and Procedure

To achieve the study objectives, women aged 18 or older, mothers of infants under 12 months who had chosen breastfeeding or started but switched to formula feeding before 6 months, and who gave birth at the clinical hospital of Santiago de Compostela, were randomly selected from the participating PHCs. Participation was offered during contact with the pediatric nurse. Mothers of children older than 12 months or those opting for formula feeding were excluded.

Data were collected using a specific data collection notebook comprising sections on the sociodemographic variables of women, variables related to children, and variables related to breastfeeding, including type of breastfeeding during admission and discharge, support and information on breastfeeding during admission and follow-up in the HC, and family support for breastfeeding.

Additionally, the Reduced Iowa Infant Feeding Attitude Scale (IIFAS-s) was employed to gauge maternal attitudes toward feeding their baby, validated for the Spanish population [28,29].

IIFAS-s scale consists of 9 items, each rated from 1 (completely disagree) to 5 (completely agree) on a Likert scale. It has a unidimensional structure with adequate reliability and validity results [27,28]. This scale also serves as a predictive indicator of the choice of feeding method (breastfeeding, formula, or mixed) and breastfeeding duration. It assesses maternal attitudes towards infant feeding pre- and postpartum, identifying women at risk of not initiating breastfeeding. Item scores were grouped into three categories: disagree/positive towards formula feeding (Scores 1 and 2), neutral (Score 3), and agree/positive towards breastfeeding (Scores 4 and 5). Based on the average score, values below 18 classify the sample as "positive attitude towards formula feeding"; values between 18 and 36 as "neutral attitude"; and values above 36 as "positive attitude towards breastfeeding".

The IIFAS-s questionnaire was used because it is a valid and reliable tool for measuring mothers' attitudes towards breastfeeding. This allows us to estimate, based on the scores of this questionnaire, the effect that a positive attitude towards breastfeeding has on maintaining exclusive breastfeeding during hospitalization. The IIFAS-s was administered either on paper or online via a QR code, voluntarily and anonymously, through the nurse or midwife.

2.3. Ethical and Legal Considerations

The study was approved by the Territorial Committee of Ethics in Research of Santiago-Lugo (registration code: 2023/199), ensuring informed consent from participants.

2.4. Variables and Statistical Analysis

Sociodemographic variables (mother's age, child's age, educational level, economic status, type of delivery, social and family support, return to work) and hospitalization-related variables (previous breastfeeding experience, skin-to-skin contact, child's admission, information received about breastfeeding, type of breastfeeding during admission) were collected.

Qualitative variables were presented as numbers and percentages, and quantitative variables as the mean and standard deviation or median and interquartile range.

Bivariate analyses explored the relationship between maternal characteristics or hospitalization-related variables and those measured through the IIFAS-s. Logistic regression models calculated crude and adjusted odds ratios (ORs), with confounding variables included based on significance in the bivariate analysis ($p < 0.1$). All analyses adhered to a 95% confidence level and significance at $p < 0.05$.

3. Results

3.1. Sample Description

A total of 64 women were studied, with a participation rate of 100%. All women offered participation in the study accepted. The mean age of the mothers was 36.6 ± 4.1 years, with 45 (70.3%) being ≥ 35 years old. The mean age of the children was 6.3 ± 3.6 months.

Nine (14.1%) newborns were admitted to the hospital's neonatology unit at the time of birth. Further characteristics of the participating women can be seen in Table 1.

Regarding the assistance received from professionals during their hospitalization, 41 (64.1%) women considered it good, while 23 (35.9%) considered it improvable. Regarding the information received during hospitalization about breastfeeding, 36 women (56.3%) considered it good, while 28 (43.7%) considered it improvable.

Table 1. Characteristics of women (*n* = 64).

Variable	n	%
Age		
<35 years	19	20.7
≥35 years	45	70.3
Type of population		
Urban	45	70.3
Rural	19	29.7
Family income		
<18.000 €/año	12	18.8
≥18.000 €/año	52	81.3
Type of childbirth		
Cesarean	15	23.4
Vaginal	49	76.6
Previous children		
Yes	27	42.2
No	37	57.8
Use of pacifier by newborn		
Yes	26	40.6
No	38	59.4
Previous experience in breastfeeding		
Yes	27	42.2
No	37	57.8
Skin-to-skin contact in first 30 min		
Yes	52	81.3
No	12	18.8
Exclusive breastfeeding during hospital admission		
Yes	47	73.4
No	17	26.6
Exclusive breastfeeding at hospital discharge		
Yes	54	84.4
No	10	15.6

In total, 30 (46.9%) of the women had received information about breastfeeding at their PHC from the pediatric nurse, 20 (31.3%) considered they did not need it, and 14 (21.9%) did not receive any information at their PHC. Regarding the level of satisfaction received, 5 (7.8%) women declared not being satisfied at all, 4 (6.3%) declared being somewhat satisfied, 6 (9.4%) fairly satisfied, and 15 (23.4%) very satisfied.

Despite receiving information about breastfeeding in the hospital and PHC, 31 (48.4%) had contacted breastfeeding support groups/counseling, and 58 (90.6%) declared having good family support for breastfeeding.

A high percentage of women did not receive assistance from healthcare professionals regarding breastfeeding during hospitalization. It was also observed that the women who did receive assistance and information about breastfeeding during hospitalization or in their PHC found that the information could be improved. These results may explain why around half of the sample (48.4%) had contacted breastfeeding support groups/counseling.

3.2. Attitudes towards Breastfeeding

Table 2 shows women's attitudes towards breastfeeding through the IIFAS-s. The overall score (mean ± standard deviation) of the test was 36.95 ± 5.17. Items 5 and 6 had the lowest and highest scores, respectively. In our sample, we did not observe any women who fell into the negative attitude towards breastfeeding category. Twenty-one (32.8%) women exhibited a neutral attitude, and forty-three (67.2%) showed a positive attitude towards breastfeeding.

Table 2. Women's attitudes towards breastfeeding (IIFAS-s).

Ítem. Variable (a)	M	SD	Agreement (%)	Neutral (%)	Disagreement (%)
1. Formula feeding is more convenient than breastfeeding (b)	4.63	0.84	92.2	4.7	3.1
2. Breastfeeding strengthens the bond between mother and child	4.63	0.84	92.2	4.7	3.1
3. Formula feeding is the best option if the mother intends to work outside the home (b)	3.8	1.04	64.1	23.4	12.5
4. Mothers who do not breastfeed miss out on one of the best experiences of motherhood	3.53	1.19	50	34.4	15.6
5. Breastfed babies are healthier than formula-fed babies	3.44	1.27	50	29.7	20.3
6. Breast milk is the ideal food for the baby	4.78	0.58	95.3	3.1	1.6
7. Breast milk is more easily digested than formula milk	4.31	0.94	75	23.4	1.6
8. Formula milk is as healthy for the baby as breast milk (b)	3.7	1.11	57.8	28.1	14.1
9. Breastfeeding your baby is more convenient than not doing so	4.14	1.14	76.6	15.6	7.8
Total	36.95	5.17	72.6	18.6	8.8

(a) Participants ($n = 64$) were asked if they agreed with each statement on a 5-point Likert scale ranging from 1 (strongly disagree) to 5 (strongly agree). These scores were then grouped into the following three categories: disagree/positive towards formula feeding (Scores 1 and 2), neutral (Score 3), and agree/positive towards breastfeeding (Scores 4 and 5). (b) These items were reversed when calculating the score. M: mean. SD: standard deviation.

It was observed that the mean score for each item is above three, indicating that the studied sample has a positive attitude towards breastfeeding, with Items 3, 4, 5, and 8 being closest to neutrality. Additionally, 72.57% of the women scored the IIFAS-s items with values of four or five, demonstrating a positive attitude towards breastfeeding, compared to 8.85% of the women who scored the items with values of one or two, indicating a positive attitude towards formula feeding (Table 2).

Women whose newborns do not use pacifiers show higher scores on the IIFAS-s, indicating a more favorable attitude towards breastfeeding (see Table 3). Conversely, no differences are observed between women's demographic variables and the mean scores of the IIFAS-s.

Table 3. Differences in attitudes towards breastfeeding by demographic factor, as determined by scores on the IIFAS-s scale. Higher IIFAS-s scores reflect more positive attitudes towards breastfeeding.

Factor (a)	Category	Mean Score (SD)	p
Mother's age	<35 years	35.32 (6.05)	0.145
	≥35 years	37.64 (4.66)	

Table 3. *Cont.*

Factor (a)	Category	Mean Score (SD)	p
Type of population	Rural	36.58 (6.24)	0.741
	Urban	37.11 (4.72)	
Family incomes	<18,000 €/year	37.08 (5.73)	0.924
	≥18,000 €/year	36.92 (5.10)	
Type of childbirth	Cesarean	37.13 (4.44)	0.879
	Vaginal	36.90 (5.42)	
Previous children	Yes	37.30 (4.58)	0.537
	No	36.48 (5.94)	
Use of pacifier by the newborn	Yes	35.35 (5.61)	0.039 *
	No	38.05 (4.61)	
Previous breastfeeding experience	Yes	36.67 (6.01)	0.708
	No	37.16 (4.54)	
Skin-to-skin contact during the first 30 min	Yes	36.92 (5.34)	0.924
	No	37.08 (4.56)	
Admission of the newborn to neonatology	Yes	37.22 (4.94)	0.868
	No	36.91 (5.25)	
Exclusive breastfeeding at hospital discharge	Yes	37.31 (5.14)	0.196
	No	35.00 (5.14)	
Perception of proper assistance from healthcare professional during admission	Yes	36.34 (5.26)	0.209
	No	38.04 (4.94)	
Perception of proper information about breastfeeding from healthcare professional during admission	Yes	35.86 (5.21)	0.055
	No	38.36 (4.86)	
Contact with breastfeeding support groups	Yes	37.84 (5.34)	0.186
	No	36.12 (4.94)	
Family support for breastfeeding	Yes	36.91 (4.99)	0.852
	No	37.33 (7.29)	

(a) n = 64. SD: Standard deviation. * $p < 0.05$ test *t*-Student.

3.3. Factors Influencing Exclusive Breastfeeding during Hospitalization

The following table (Table 4) shows factors associated with the woman or certain hospitalization characteristics that may influence the implementation of exclusive breastfeeding during hospitalization. It can be observed that having previous children, prior experience with breastfeeding, and the newborn not being admitted to the neonatology unit increase the likelihood of exclusive breastfeeding during admission.

Table 4. Factors influencing exclusive breastfeeding during hospitalization. n = 64.

	Exclusive Breastfeeding during Hospital Admission			
Factor	YES n (%)	NO n (%)	ORc (IC 95%)	ORa (IC 95%)
Mother's age ≥ 35 years	36 (76.6)	9 (52.9)	2.91 (0.91–9.35)	1.89 (0.50–7.06)
Urban population	31 (66.0)	14 (82.4)	2.41 (0.60–9.62)	3.21 (0.55–18.82)
Incomes ≥ 18.000 €/year	39 (83.0)	13 (76.5)	1.50 (0.39–5.81)	2.08 (0.43–10.10)
Vaginal childbirth	36 (76.6)	13 (76.5)	1.01 (0.27–3.73)	1.34 (0.28–6.41)

Table 4. Cont.

	Exclusive Breastfeeding during Hospital Admission			
Factor	YES n (%)	NO n (%)	ORc (IC 95%)	ORa (IC 95%)
≥1 previous children	25 (53v2)	2 (11.8)	8.52 (1.75–41.49)	6.40 (1.26–32.51)
Previous breastfeeding experience	25 (53.2)	2 (11.8)	8.52 (1.75–41.49)	6.70 (1.31–34.27)
Skin-to-skin contact during the first 30 min	40 (85.1)	12 (70.6)	2.38 (0.64–8.88)	1.18 (0.22–6.19)
No admission of the newborn to neonatology	43 (91.5)	12 (70.6)	4.48 (1.04–19.33)	3.41 (0.68–17.02)
Use of pacifier by the newborn	20 (42.6)	6 (35.3)	1.36 (0.43–4.29)	1.71 (0.45–6.50)
Perception of proper assistance from healthcare professional during admission	31 (66.0)	10 (58.8)	1.36 (0.43–4.24)	1.67 (0.45–6.20)
Perception of proper information about breastfeeding from healthcare professional during admission	29 (61.7)	7 (41.2)	2.30 (0.74–7.13)	1.92 (0.54–6.86)
Contact with breastfeeding support groups	24 (51.1)	7 (41.2)	1.49 (0.48–4.58)	1.59 (0.46–5.57)
Family support for breastfeeding	43 (91.5)	15 (88.2)	1.43 (0.24–8.64)	1.04 (0.14–7.87)

ORc: Crude odds ratio. ORa: Adjusted odds ratio. Adjusted for the following variables: mother's age, information regarding breastfeeding during hospitalization, performing skin-to-skin contact in the first 30 min.

When adjusting the odds ratio (OR) associated with these variables for possible confounding variables, having previous children and prior experience with breastfeeding remain associated with exclusive breastfeeding during hospitalization. Among the most important findings, it is worth highlighting that having previous children increases the probability of exclusive breastfeeding during hospitalization by 6.4 times. Additionally, prior breastfeeding experience increases this probability by 6.7 times.

4. Discussion

To our knowledge, this is the first study to evaluate factors associated with exclusive breastfeeding, especially during hospital admission. Our results show that factors such as having previous children or prior experience with breastfeeding increase the likelihood of exclusive breastfeeding during subsequent births. Studies have linked multiparity with a positive association with breastfeeding duration [29]. Additionally, other studies have confirmed that previous breastfeeding experiences, unsuccessful attempts at breastfeeding, and the inability to breastfeed the first child have been associated with lower breastfeeding initiation rates in subsequent children [30–32].

The results of our study show a percentage of women exclusively breastfeeding during admission of 73.4%, with 75% being the sentinel indicator for the rate of exclusive breastfeeding at discharge for BFHI accreditation [33]. This study identified that the number of women breastfeeding exclusively post-discharge increased by seven respondents (10% more), possibly explained by the role of the primary care pediatric nurse or the mother's contact with breastfeeding support groups. In our sample, we observed that a high percentage of mothers contacted breastfeeding support groups. Despite giving birth in a BFHI hospital, 35.9% of the women did not receive assistance or information about breastfeeding from the healthcare professionals who cared for them during their stay. Among those who did receive assistance, a high percentage considered it could be improved. A similar situation occurred at the primary healthcare level. This could be explained by the need to improve training activities for healthcare professionals. Evidence demonstrates that interventions to support breastfeeding in primary care have a positive effect on breastfeeding rates, duration, or exclusive maintenance [34]. A systematic review by Balogun et al. asserts that the rate of breastfeeding initiation improves among women who receive breastfeeding education and support led by healthcare professionals compared to those who receive standard care [35].

Skin-to-skin contact, performed by 81.3% of participants, appears to be beneficial for breastfeeding in the short and long term, as shown in a systematic review that observed improvements in both breastfeeding status and duration [32]. Regarding factors influencing exclusive breastfeeding during hospitalization, we observed that if the child is not admitted to the neonatal unit, there is an increased probability of establishing exclusive breastfeeding during admission, as well as having previous experience with exclusive breastfeeding. This is consistent with studies demonstrating that rooming-in mother/child in neonatal units increases the probability of successful exclusive breastfeeding [36–38]. Two areas have been identified where specific interventions could be focused on the healthcare staff who care for women during their hospital stay. By concentrating training interventions on promoting skin-to-skin contact within the first 30 min, as well as equipping hospitals with more humanized and open neonatal units that encourage activities like the kangaroo mother care technique and skin-to-skin contact, the likelihood that mothers will choose exclusive breastfeeding during their stay would increase. Additionally, the duration of breastfeeding is likely to extend once they are discharged from the hospital. There is evidence that addressing the two identified areas would achieve these goals [39,40].

The total score of the IIFAS-s scale in our study does not differ from the available evidence, where it can be observed that women present positive attitudes towards exclusive breastfeeding, especially during pregnancy and hospital admission [41,42]. In this study, we did not observe any women who fell into the negative attitude towards breastfeeding category and 67.2% showed a positive attitude towards breastfeeding. This result is much higher than those found in previous studies [43,44]. It should be taken into account when interpreting these results that the women who participated did so after their hospital stay, while they were being followed up by pediatric nurses at their PHCs. This may be influenced by the fact that the women received advice at that time from their pediatric nurse and breastfeeding support groups. Regarding the results extracted from the IIFAS-s scale, it can be observed that mothers' attitudes towards breastfeeding through the IIFAS-s scale do not show statistically significant differences by demographic factor. Concerning pacifier use, this was systematically questioned since numerous studies demonstrate that pacifier use is related to a lower rate of exclusive breastfeeding, although some demonstrate the opposite [20]. Our data reflect that women whose newborns do not use pacifiers show higher scores on the IIFAS-s, indicating a more favorable attitude towards breastfeeding. Additionally, it is noteworthy that only 50% of the surveyed mothers reported that breast-fed babies are healthier than formula-fed babies, when no literature has been found to demonstrate otherwise.

As a strength of this study, we would like to highlight the survey as a cost-effective and efficient tool for obtaining data: its accessibility, ease of use, and availability in both paper and QR code formats have allowed us to reach the target population in a short period. Additionally, the IIFAS-s scale is considered a good predictor of attitudes towards initiating exclusive breastfeeding, although not as a predictor of maintaining exclusive breastfeeding during hospital admission [28]. By using these two methods in this study, we consider that we used the appropriate tool to obtain a representative picture of the attitudes and characteristics of our group.

Another strength of this study is that it allows us to identify areas for improvement or gaps to target and focus interventions on, both for mothers and healthcare professionals, as well as the healthcare system. This is consistent with similar studies [45].

Regarding the study's limitations, it is worth mentioning the inherent limitations of a cross-sectional design, although our results serve to generate hypotheses on the topic of the work. On the other hand, the achieved sample size may not be sufficient to provide high power to our results. It would be necessary to carry out studies with prospective designs to corroborate our results.

5. Conclusions

In our study, exclusive breastfeeding during hospitalization is associated with having previous children and prior breastfeeding experience. It also appears to be linked to the likelihood of the newborn not being admitted to neonatal units. This association is influenced by the mother's age, breastfeeding information provided during hospitalization, and skin-to-skin contact within the first 30 min. Exclusive breastfeeding during hospitalization could be improved by increasing healthcare staff training and encouraging their involvement in achieving goals according to the BFHI criteria. Future research with prospective designs is needed to measure the effect of multifaceted interventions focused on our findings, in order to estimate the association with exclusive breastfeeding during hospitalization and its duration after discharge.

Author Contributions: Conceptualization, C.V.-N. and N.N.-M.; methodology, C.V.-N. and N.N.-M.; validation, J.M.V.-L.; formal analysis, J.M.V.-L.; investigation, C.V.-N. and A.S.-C.; resources, C.V.-N., A.S.-C. and N.N.-M.; data curation, J.M.V.-L.; writing—original draft preparation, C.V.-N. and J.M.V.-L.; writing—review and editing, C.V.-N. and J.M.V.-L.; visualization, N.N.-M. and A.S.-C.; supervision, N.N.-M.; project administration, C.V.-N. and N.N.-M. All authors have read and agreed to the published version of the manuscript.

Funding: This research received no external funding.

Institutional Review Board Statement: This study was conducted in accordance with the Declaration of Helsinki, and approved by the Ethics Committee of Santiago-Lugo, protocol code 2023/199 and date of approval 07/28/2023.

Informed Consent Statement: Informed consent was obtained from all subjects involved in the study.

Data Availability Statement: Data availability is under petition.

Conflicts of Interest: The authors declare no conflicts of interest.

References

1. WHO. Breastfeeding [Internet]. Available online: https://www.who.int/health-topics/breastfeeding#tab=tab_1 (accessed on 3 January 2024).
2. Bachrach, V.R.; Schwarz, E.; Bachrach, L.R. Breastfeeding and the risk of hospitalization for respiratory disease in infancy: A metaanalysis. *Arch. Pediatr. Adolesc. Med.* **2003**, *157*, 237–243. [CrossRef]
3. De Kroon, M.L.; Renders, C.M.; Buskermolen, M.P.; Van Wouwe, J.P.; van Buuren, S.; Hirasing, R.A. The Terneuzen Birth Cohort. Longer exclusive breastfeeding duration is associated with leaner body mass and a healthier diet in young adulthood. *BMC Pediatr.* **2011**, *11*, 33. [CrossRef] [PubMed]
4. Wallby, T.; Lagerberg, D.; Magnusson, M. Relationship Between Breastfeeding and Early Childhood Obesity: Results of a Prospective Longitudinal Study from Birth to 4 Years. *Breastfeed Med.* **2017**, *22*, 48–53. [CrossRef] [PubMed]
5. Harder, T.; Bergmann, R.; Kallischnigg, G.; Plagemann, A. Duration of Breastfeeding and Risk of Overweight: A Meta-Analysis. *Am. J. Epidemiol.* **2005**, *162*, 397–403. [CrossRef] [PubMed]
6. Krol, K.M.; Grossmann, T. Psychological effects of breastfeeding on children and mothers. *Bundesgesundheitsblatt Gesundheitsforschung Gesundheitsschutz* **2018**, *61*, 977–985. [CrossRef] [PubMed]
7. Quesada, J.A.; Méndez, I.; Martín-Gil, R. The economic benefits of increasing breastfeeding rates in Spain. *Int. Breastfeed J.* **2020**, *15*, 34. [CrossRef] [PubMed]
8. National Institute of Statistics [Internet]. Health Determinants (Overweight, Fruit and Vegetable Consumption, Type of Breastfeeding, Physical Activity, Care in the Family Environment). Available online: https://www.ine.es/ss/Satellite?c=INESeccion_C&p=1254735110672&pagename=ProductosYServicios/PYSLayout&cid=1259926457058&L=1 (accessed on 8 February 2024).

9. Maleki-Saghooni, N.; Amel Barez, M.; Karimi, F.Z. Investigation of the relationship between social support and breastfeeding self-efficacy in primiparous breastfeeding mothers. *J. Matern. -Fetal Neonatal Med.* **2020**, *33*, 3097–3102. [CrossRef] [PubMed]
10. Santacruz-Salas, E.; Segura-Fragoso, A.; Cobo-Cuenca, A.I.; Carmona-Torres, J.M.; Pozuelo-Carrascosa, D.P.; Laredo-Aguilera, J.A. Factors associated with the abandonment of exclusive breastfeeding before three months. *Children* **2020**, *7*, 298. [CrossRef]
11. Cortés-Rúa, L.; Díaz-Grávalos, G.J. Early interruption of breastfeeding. A qualitative study. *Enfermería Clínica* **2019**, *29*, 207–215. [CrossRef]
12. Ramiro González, M.D.; Ortiz Marrón, H.; Arana Cañedo-Argüelles, C.; Esparza Olcina, M.J.; Cortés Rico, O.; Terol Claramonte, M. Prevalence of breastfeeding and factors associated with the start and duration of exclusive breastfeeding in the Community of Madrid among participants in the ELOIN. *An. De Pediatría* **2018**, *89*, 32–43. [CrossRef]
13. Wu, Q.; Tang, N.; Wacharasin, C. Factors influencing exclusive breastfeeding for 6 months postpartum: A systematic review. *Int. J. Nurs. Knowl.* **2022**, *33*, 290–303. [CrossRef]
14. Hernández, M.I.N.; Riesco, M.L. Exclusive breastfeeding abandonment in adolescent mothers: A cohort study within health primary services. *Rev. Lat.-Am. De Enferm.* **2022**, *30*, e3786. [CrossRef] [PubMed]
15. Beake, S.; Pellowe, C.; Dykes, F.; Schmied, V.; Bick, D. A systematic review of structured compared with non-structured breastfeeding programmes to support the initiation and duration of exclusive and any breastfeeding in acute and primary health care settings. *Matern. Child Nutr.* **2012**, *8*, 141–161. [CrossRef] [PubMed]
16. Robert, E.; Michaud-Létourneau, I.; Dramaix-Wilmet, M.; Swennen, B.; Devlieger, R. A comparison of exclusive breastfeeding in Belgian maternity facilities with and without Baby-friendly Hospital status. *Matern. Child Nutr.* **2019**, *15*, e12845. [CrossRef]
17. Pérez-Escamilla, R.; Martinez, J.L.; Segura-Pérez, S. Impact of the Baby-friendly Hospital Initiative on breastfeeding and child health outcomes: A systematic review. *Matern. Child Nutr.* **2016**, *12*, 402–417. [CrossRef] [PubMed]
18. Gavine, A.; MacGillivray, S.; Renfrew, M.J.; Siebelt, L.; Haggi, H.; McFadden, A. Education and training of healthcare staff in the knowledge, attitudes and skills needed to work effectively with breastfeeding women: A systematic review. *Int. Breastfeed J.* **2017**, *12*, 6. [CrossRef] [PubMed]
19. Dykes, F. The education of health practitioners supporting breastfeeding women: Time for critical reflection. *Matern. Child Nutr.* **2006**, *2*, 204–216. [CrossRef]
20. Martín-Ramos, S.; Domínguez-Aurrecoeche, B.; García Vera, C.; Lorente García Mauriño, A.M.; Sánchez Almeida, E.; Solís-Sánchez, G. Breastfeeding in Spain and the factors related to its establishment and maintenance: LAyDI Study (PAPenRed). *Aten. Primaria* **2024**, *56*, 102772. [CrossRef]
21. UNICEF/WHO. BFHI Spain [Internet]. Ihan.es. Available online: https://www.ihan.es/ (accessed on 8 February 2024).
22. UNICEF/WHO. BFHI Spain. Grupos de Apoyo [Internet]. Ihan.es. Available online: https://www.ihan.es/grupos-apoyo/ (accessed on 2 February 2024).
23. García García, N.; Fernández Gutiérrez, P. Conocimientos y actitudes de las madres ante la lactancia materna en un hospital IHAN. *Metas De Enfermería* **2018**, *21*, 50–58. [CrossRef]
24. UNICEF/WHO. BFHI Spain [Internet]. Global Criteria. 2021. Available online: https://www.ihan.es/wp-content/uploads/2023/12/Criterios-Globales_IHAN-Espan83a-2021.pdf (accessed on 22 February 2024).
25. Work Group BFHI Hospitals [Internet]. Guía Para La Solicitud Del Certificado de Fase 2D-Maternidad. UNICEF/OMS. BFHI Spain. 2021. Available online: https://www.ihan.es/wp-content/uploads/2023/12/02.-Gui81a_F2D_Hospitales-2021.pdf (accessed on 22 February 2024).
26. Candal-Pedreira, C.; Pérez-Ríos, M.; Pérez-Franco, D.; Vila-Farinas, A.; Santiago-Pérez, M.I.; Rey-Brandariz, J.; Mourino, N.; Ruano-Ravina, A. Abandono de la lactancia materna en Galicia: ¿cuándo se produce y por qué? *Galicia Clin.* **2023**, *84*, 7–12. [CrossRef]
27. Tomás-Almarcha, R.; Oliver-Roig, A.; Richart-Martinez, M. Reliability and Validity of the Reduced Spanish Version of the Iowa Infant Feeding Attitude Scale. *J. Obstet. Gynecol. Neonatal Nurs.* **2016**, *45*, e26–e40. [CrossRef]
28. Duque de Rodriguez, G.; Laredo, S.; Soriano, J.M. Cuestionarios validados en español para la investigación en lactancia materna: Una revisión sistemática. *Nutr. Clín. Diet. Hosp.* **2022**, *42*, 43–57. [CrossRef]
29. Cohen, S.S.; Alexander, D.D.; Krebs, N.F.; Young, B.E.; Cabana, M.D.; Erdmann, P.; Hays, N.P.; Bezold, C.P.; Levin-Sparenberg, E.; Turini, M.; et al. Factors associated with breastfeeding initiation and continuation: A meta-analysis. *J. Pediatr.* **2018**, *203*, 190–196.e21. [CrossRef] [PubMed]
30. Hobbs, A.J.; Mannion, C.A.; McDonald, S.W.; Brockway, M.; Tough, S.C. The impact of caesarean section on breastfeeding initiation, duration and difficulties in the first four months postpartum. *BMC Pregnancy Childbirth* **2016**, *16*, 90. [CrossRef]
31. Sutherland, T.; Pierce, C.B.; Blomquist, J.L.; Handa, V.L. Breastfeeding practices among first-time mothers and across multiple pregnancies. *Matern. Child Health J.* **2012**, *16*, 1665–1671. [CrossRef] [PubMed]
32. Rius, J.M.; Ortuño, J.; Rivas, C.; Maravall, M.; Calzado, M.A.; López, A.; Aguar, M.; Vento, M. Factors associated with early weaning in a Spanish region. *An. De Pediatr.* **2014**, *80*, 6–15. [CrossRef] [PubMed]
33. UNICEF/WHO [Internet]. Innocenti Declaration On the Protection, Promotion and Support of Breastfeeding. 1 August, 1990 Florence, Italy. Available online: https://waba.org.my/v3/wp-content/uploads/2019/04/1990-Innocenti-Declaration.pdf (accessed on 22 February 2024).

34. Pallás Alonso, C.R.; Soriano Faura, J.; Colomer Revuelta, J.; Cortés Rico, O.; Olcina, M.J.; Galbe Sánchez-Ventura, J.; Iborra, A.G.; Aguado, J.G.; Moína, M.M.; Diego, Á.R.; et al. Support for breastfeeding in Primary Care. *Pediatr. De Aten. Primaria* **2019**, *21*, 191–201. Available online: https://scielo.isciii.es/pdf/pap/v21n82/1139-7632-pap-21-82-191.pdf (accessed on 24 February 2024).
35. Balogun, O.O.; O'Sullivan, E.J.; McFadden, A.; Ota, E.; Gavine, A.; Garner, C.D.; Renfrew, M.J.; MacGillivray, S. Interventions for promoting the initiation of breastfeeding. *Cochrane Database Syst. Rev.* **2016**, *2016*. [CrossRef] [PubMed]
36. Tolppola, O.; Renko, M.; Sankilampi, U.; Kiviranta, P.; Hintikka, L.; Kuitunen, I. Pacifier use and breastfeeding in term and preterm newborns-a systematic review and meta-analysis. *Eur. J. Pediatr.* **2022**, *181*, 3421–3428. [CrossRef]
37. Miñones Suarez, L.; Fernández Morales, M.; García Pérez, L.; Huguet Gorriz, A.; Fernández Romasanta, A.; Aldaz Calvo, M.; Ramillete Bandrés, S. Ingreso neonatal en alojamiento conjunto: Efecto sobre la lactancia materna durante los 6 primeros meses de vida. *Rev. De Lact. Matern.* **2024**, *2*, e30790. [CrossRef]
38. Ragusa, R.; Marranzano, M.; La Rosa, V.L.; Giorgianni, G.; Commodari, E.; Quattrocchi, R.; Cacciola, S.; Guardabasso, V. Factors Influencing Uptake of Breastfeeding: The Role of Early Promotion in the Maternity Hospital. *Int. J. Environ. Res. Public Health* **2021**, *18*, 4783. [CrossRef] [PubMed]
39. Song, J.T.; Kinshella, M.W.; Kawaza, K.; Goldfarb, D.M. Neonatal Intensive Care Unit Interventions to Improve Breastfeeding Rates at Discharge Among Preterm and Low Birth Weight Infants: A Systematic Review and Meta-Analysis. *Breastfeed Med.* **2023**, *18*, 97–106. [CrossRef] [PubMed]
40. Renfrew, M.J.; Dyson, L.; McCormick, F.; Misso, K.; Stenhouse, E.; King, S.E.; Williams, A.F. Breastfeeding promotion for infants in neonatal units: A systematic review. *Child Care Health Dev.* **2010**, *36*, 165–178. [CrossRef]
41. Bednarek, A.; Bodys-Cupak, I.; Serwin, A.; Cipora, E. Mothers' Attitudes Towards Breastfeeding in Terms of Health Safety and Professional Lactation Education: A National Survey of Women. *J. Multidiscip. Healthc.* **2023**, *16*, 3273–3286. [CrossRef]
42. Cole, J.; Bhatt, A.; Chapple, A.G.; Buzhardt, S.; Sutton, E.F. Attitudes and barriers to breastfeeding among women at high-risk for not breastfeeding: A prospective observational study. *BMC Pregnancy Childbirth* **2024**, *24*, 81. [CrossRef] [PubMed]
43. Alkhaldi, S.M.; Al-Kuran, O.; AlAdwan, M.M.; Dabbah, T.A.; Dalky, H.F.; Badran, E. Determinants of breastfeeding attitudes of mothers in Jordan: A cross-sectional study. *PLoS ONE* **2023**, *18*, e0285436. [CrossRef] [PubMed]
44. Han, F.L.; Ho, Y.J.; McGrath, J.M. The influence of breastfeeding attitudes on breastfeeding behavior of postpartum women and their spouses. *Heliyon* **2023**, *9*, e13987. [CrossRef]
45. Al-Thubaity, D.D.; Alshahrani, M.A.; Elgzar, W.T.; Ibrahim, H.A. Determinants of High Breastfeeding Self-Efficacy among Nursing Mothers in Najran, Saudi Arabia. *Nutrients* **2023**, *15*, 1919. [CrossRef]

Disclaimer/Publisher's Note: The statements, opinions and data contained in all publications are solely those of the individual author(s) and contributor(s) and not of MDPI and/or the editor(s). MDPI and/or the editor(s) disclaim responsibility for any injury to people or property resulting from any ideas, methods, instructions or products referred to in the content.

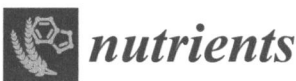

Article

Effect of Holder Pasteurization, Mode of Delivery, and Infant's Gender on Fatty Acid Composition of Donor Breast Milk

Réka Anna Vass [1,2,3,*], Miaomiao Zhang [4], Livia Simon Sarkadi [4], Márta Üveges [5], Judit Tormási [6], Eszter L. Benes [6], Tibor Ertl [1,2] and Sandor G. Vari [7]

[1] Department of Obstetrics and Gynecology, Medical School University of Pécs, 7624 Pécs, Hungary; ertl.tibor@pte.hu
[2] National Laboratory on Human Reproduction, University of Pécs, 7624 Pécs, Hungary
[3] Obstetrics and Gynecology, Magyar Imre Hospital, 8400 Ajka, Hungary
[4] Department of Nutrition, Faculty of Food Science and Technology, Hungarian University of Agriculture and Life Sciences, 1118 Budapest, Hungary; zhang.miaomiao@phd.uni-mate.hu (M.Z.); simonne.sarkadi.livia@uni-mate.hu (L.S.S.)
[5] Division of Chemical, Noise, Vibration, and Lighting Technology Laboratories, Department of Methodology and Public Health Laboratories, National Center for Public Health and Pharmacy, 1096 Budapest, Hungary; uveges.marta@uni-mate.hu
[6] Department of Food Chemistry and Analysis, Faculty of Food Science and Technology, Hungarian University of Agriculture and Life Sciences, 1118 Budapest, Hungary; tormasi.judit@uni-mate.hu (J.T.); benes.eszter.luca@uni-mate.hu (E.L.B.)
[7] International Research and Innovation in Medicine Program, Cedars-Sinai Medical Center, Los Angeles, CA 90048, USA; sandor.vari@cshs.org
* Correspondence: rekaanna.vass@gmail.com; Tel.: +36-302532000

Abstract: Breast milk (BM) plays a crucial role in providing essential fatty acids (FA) and energy for the growing infant. When the mother's own BM is not available, nutritional recommendations suggest donor milk (DM) in clinical and home practices. BM was collected from a variety of donor mothers in different lactation stages. Holder pasteurization (HoP) eliminates potential contaminants to ensure safety. FA content of BM samples from the Breast Milk Collection Center of Pécs, Hungary, were analyzed before and after HoP. HoP decreases the level of C6:0, C8:0, C14:1n-5c, C18:1n-9c, C18:3n-6c, C18:3n-3c, and C20:4n-6c in BM, while C14:0, C16:0, C18:1n-9t, C22:0, C22:1n-9c, C24:0, C24:1n-9c, and C22:6n-3c were found in elevated concentration after HoP. We did not detect time-dependent concentration changes in FAs in the first year of lactation. BM produced for girl infants contains higher C20:2n-6c levels. In the BM of mothers who delivered via cesarean section, C12:0, C15:0, C16:0, C17:0, C18:0, C18:1n-9t, C22:1n-9c levels were higher, while C18:2n-6c, C22:0, C24:0, and C22:6n-3c concentrations were lower compared to mothers who gave birth spontaneously. FAs in BM are constant during the first year of lactation. Although HoP modifies the concentration of different FAs, pasteurized DM provides essential FAs to the developing infant. Current data providing information about the FA profile of BM gives origination to supplementation guidelines.

Keywords: capric acid; lauric acid; myristic acid; palmitic acid; stearic acid; linoleic acid; oleic acid; donor milk

1. Introduction

Human milk is a remarkable and complex fluid that has evolved over time to meet the nutritional and developmental needs of infants [1,2]. Fatty acids are crucial components of human milk and play a vital role in the growth and well-being of the child [3,4]; on average, breast milk is composed of about 3–5% fat [5]. However, it is important to note that individual variations are common. Human milk contains a variety of fatty acids that are crucial for the growth and development of infants. These fatty acids are essential in developing the nervous system, brain, and overall health [6,7]. The composition of fatty acids in human milk can vary depending on factors such as the mother's diet [8,9], and breast milk (BM) is a concentrated source of calories, essential fatty acids, and fat-soluble vitamins. FAs synthesized de novo in the mammary gland, such as caprylic acid (8:0), capric acid (10:0), lauric acid (12:0), and myristic acid (14:0), are known as medium-chain saturated fatty acids (MCFAs) [10]. It was found that the content of MCFAs increased from colostrum to transitional and mature milk, irrespective of the region or gestational age of mothers [11,12]. The two main types of FAs found in human milk are saturated and unsaturated FAs [13].

Saturated fatty acids (SFAs): These fatty acids have no double bonds between carbon atoms. Examples include lauric acid, myristic acid, and palmitic acid. Palmitic acid is one of human milk's most abundant saturated fatty acids [14].

Two subtypes of unsaturated fatty acids (UFAs) are distinguished: monounsaturated fatty acids (MUFAs) and polyunsaturated fatty acids (PUFAs) [14].

MUFAs are FAs that have one double bond between carbon atoms. Oleic acid is human milk's primary monounsaturated fatty acid [15]. MUFAs have been associated with various health benefits, particularly cardiovascular health. They help improve blood lipid profiles by reducing levels of low-density lipoprotein (LDL) cholesterol while maintaining or increasing levels of high-density lipoprotein (HDL) cholesterol [16].

PUFAs have two or more double bonds between carbon atoms. The two main types of polyunsaturated fatty acids in human milk are omega-3 (e.g., docosahexaenoic acid and alpha-linolenic acid) and omega-6 (e.g., linoleic acid (LA) and arachidonic acid) [8,11]. Omega-3 fatty acids are alfa-linolenic acid (ALA), arachidonic acid (ARA), eicosatrienoic acid (ETE), eicosapentaenoic acid (EPA), and docosahexaenoic acid (DHA). DHA is a major structural component of the brain and is crucial for neurodevelopment and function. EPA and DHA have been shown to have cardiovascular benefits through triglyceride level reduction, lowering blood pressure, having anti-inflammatory effects, and impacting immune responses [17]. DHA is present in high concentrations in the retina, and adequate intake is associated with a reduced risk of age-related macular degeneration (AMD) and other disorders [18]. The placenta is crucial in nutrient transport from the mother to the fetus. Fatty acids, including essential ones like LA and ALA, are transferred across the placenta to support fetal development. In the case of preterm birth, this transfer is disrupted, therefore the only postnatal source is the BM of FAs for the developing infant [3,4,19].

Based on the number of carbon atoms in the alkyl chain length, fatty acids can be classified into short-chain (2–4 carbon atoms), medium-chain (6–10 carbon atoms), and long-chain fatty acids (12–26 carbon atoms) [20,21]. Medium-chain (saturated) fatty acids (MCFA) include caproic (6:0), caprylic (8:0), and capric (10:0) acids. Long-chain (saturated) fatty acids (LCFA) include linoleic acid (C18:2n-6; LA), alfa-linolenic acid (C18:3n-3; ALA), arachidonic acid (C20:4n-6; ARA), docosahexaenoic acid (C22:6n-3; DHA), eicosapentaenoic acid (C20:5n-3; EPA), behenic (22:0), lignoceric (24:0) acid [3,22].

Human breast milk also contains LCPUFAs, which play a role in the immune system. Breastfeeding protects against childhood infections [23] and may protect against childhood allergies and asthma [24], and part of this protection seems likely to be due to optimized immune development in breastfed infants. They control and participate in pain signaling pathways, inflammation, thrombosis, and vasoconstriction [25,26]. Fatty acids play a crucial role in intrauterine development, contributing to the formation and growth of various tissues and organs in the developing fetus. The availability of essential fatty acids during pregnancy is critical to developing the nervous and immune systems and other physiological processes [3,4]. Fatty acids are structural components of cell membranes, influencing membrane fluidity and stability [25]. This is particularly important during rapid cell division and differentiation in the developing fetus [3,4]. A cohort study suggests that higher mean daily serum levels of DHA during the early postnatal period are associated with less severe retinopathy of prematurity (ROP), but only in infants with elevated arachidonic acid values [27].

For infants who rely on pasteurized donor milk for various reasons, including prematurity or medical conditions or their own mother's milk is not available, pasteurized donor milk ensures safety and nutritional support [28]. Holder pasteurization (HoP) is knowingly influencing the composition of BM [29–33], although when the mother's own milk is not available this is the recommended feeding form [34]. The present work is focused on providing information about the general FA composition of BM and DM, to optimize nutritional supplementation of newborns.

2. Materials and Methods

2.1. Donor Milk Samples

After the approval of the Regional and Local Research Ethics Committee of the University of Pécs, Pécs, Hungary (PTE KK 7072-2018). Waivers for participant consent were obtained. To determine the effect of HoP on breast milk composition, 56 registered donor mothers were recruited from the Breast Milk Collection Center of the Unified Health Institution at Pécs, Hungary. Freshly pumped BM was collected according to the center's protocol. We have chosen donations on 10 random occasions. Samples were taken individually and immediately stored at −80 °C, then the donated BM samples were pooled, and Holder pasteurized (30 min at 62.5 °C) at the Unified Health Institution (Pécs, Hungary) (Figure 1). Three samples were taken from the holder pasteurized donor milk pool and stored at −80 °C until further analysis, similar to our previous works [30–33]. Then, 3–4 mL aliquots were taken with a sterile pipette and placed into microtubes (Eppendorf, Hamburg, Germany). After labeling sample containers, they were immediately placed in a freezer at —20 °C. Samples were processed at the Department of Food Chemistry and Analysis (Budapest, Hungary).

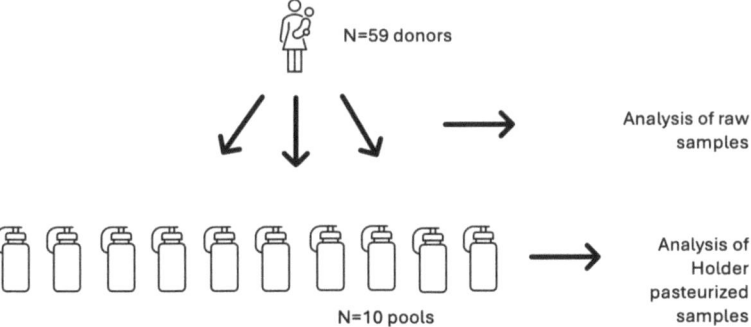

Figure 1. Schematic figure of sample collection and analysis.

2.2. Gas Chromatographic Analysis of Samples

Gas chromatographic analysis was performed to detect FAs in BM samples. The study of BM samples was conducted based on a reference ISO method [35]. The reference method was slightly modified regarding sample preparation. The frozen BM samples were thawed to room temperature and vortexed effectively to gain homogeneity, and then 0.5 g of each BM sample was transferred into conical centrifuge tubes. Following the ISO method 2.5 mL of tert-butyl methyl ether was added to the samples. During sample transesterification reactions, the reaction times were noted. First, 2.5 mL of 5% (w/v) methanolic sodium hydroxide solution was added to the tube and mixed for 10 s using a LABINCO L46 Power Mixer (Breda, The Netherlands). After a specific time (180 s), the tube was opened, and 1 mL isooctane was added to the mixture; 30 s later, the reaction was stopped when a 5 mL neutralization mixture was added. The neutralization was performed with a 10% (w/v) disodium hydrogen citrate and 15% (w/v) sodium chloride aqueous solution. Samples were centrifuged by Hettich Mikro 22R Centrifuge (Hetting Zentrifugen, Tuttlingen, Germany) for 5 min at 1750 rpm (g = 375) to obtain two different phases. The upper layer was transferred into a gas chromatography vial for GC analysis.

The resulting volatile fatty acid methyl ester compounds (FAMEs) were analyzed by an Agilent 6890 GC-FID system (GC ChemStation B.04.002 [98] (2001–2009 Agilent Technologies Inc.) Palo Alto, CA, USA), which was equipped with an autosampler (Agilent 7683), for the separation of FAMEs Phenomenex Zebron ZB-FAME (Phenomenex, Torrance, CA, USA) (60 m, 0.25 mm, 0.20 µm with cyanopropyl stationary phase) column was applied. The flow of the mobile phase (hydrogen gas) was set to 1.2 mL min^{-1}. The inlet and detector temperatures were set to 250 °C and 260 °C, respectively. A 1 µL amount was injected with sample supernatants while a 50:1 split ratio was used. The gradient temperature program was as follows: 100 °C of starting oven temperature was held for 3 min, then the column was heated applying 20 °C min^{-1} rate to 166 °C (held for 5 min), then 1 °C min^{-1} gradient was used to reach 180 °C, the final temperature (240 °C) was held for 3 min that was achieved with a temperature gradient of 10 °C min^{-1}. Mass Hunter software (MSD Chemstation F.01.03.2357 (1989–2015 Agilent Technologies Inc.) Palo Alto, CA, USA) was used to control GC-FID system. Chromatographic separation was carried out in 40 min per sample [36].

The investigated compounds were identified by a FAME (fatty acid methyl ester) standard mixture solution (Supelco 37 Component FAME Mix—Supleco Analytical chromatography division of Sigma Aldrich, Burlington, MA, USA) based on retention times. Results (fatty acid composition of the investigated human milk samples) were expressed as a percentage of the peak area of total fatty acid content measured in the sample.

2.3. Data Analysis

The Kolmogorov–Smirnov test results were considered to test the data's normality. Multivariate data analysis was performed using principal component analysis (PCA). A support vector machine (SVM) was used to classify the datasets. SPSS Statistics 23 (IBM, New York, NY, USA) software was used to evaluate. Differences between groups were tested by Kruskal–Wallis test. Results were considered statistically significant in case p SPSS Statistics 23 (IBM, New York, NY, USA) software was used to evaluate. The Kruskal–Wallis test was performed to compare the different groups since the distribution of fatty acids did not follow the normal distribution in the analyzed samples. Subgroups were analyzed according to the mode of delivery, the infant's gender, and different time points during lactation—1–3 vs. 3–6 vs. 6–12 months. Data were expressed as mean ± SD. Principal component analysis (PCA) was performed for data visualization and pattern recognition. The Hotelling's T2 and F-residual values were used for outlier detection. Random sevenfold cross-validation was used to verify the model. A support vector machine (SVM) was performed to classify the data based on the fatty acid profile of the pasteurized and non-pasteurized samples. The classification was run on the scores of the samples after PCA. Linear, quadratic, and cubic kernel functions were used for the modeling. Random eleven-fold cross-validation was used to verify the model performance.

3. Results

3.1. Maternal Data

Donor mothers were generally 30.53 ± 5.44 years old at the time of donation. Their body mass index (BMI) was 24.45 ± 3.38. Infants were born between 38th and 42nd weeks of gestation, on average 39.06 ± 2.71 weeks. Of the recruited mothers, 57.6% gave birth vaginally, while in 42.4% of the cases, a cesarian section was performed. Boy infants were born in 40.6%, and girls in 59.4% of deliveries. Primiparous mothers donated 35.5% of the BM samples, while 64.5% were from multiparous mothers. None of the volunteers had chronic diseases, and every one of them took a kind of vitamin supplementation during breastfeeding. BM samples were collected in the Breast Milk Collection Center on 10 different occasions, and the pool sizes were variable from 4 to 9 samples.

3.2. Fatty Acids in Breast Milk

The main fatty acids of BM produced for term infants are lauric, myristic, palmitic, stearic, cis-9-octadecenoic, and methyl linoleate acids. The other 24 FAs are presented in 6.36%. The general FA composition of the analyzed raw BM samples is shown in Table 1. Of the tested fatty acids, the samples did not contain the following: C15:1n-5c; C21:0; and C20:3n-3c (Table 1).

Table 1. Fatty acid composition of the analyzed breast milk samples (% of total fatty acid profile in mean ± STD).

Fatty Acids	Common Name	Value (%)	Fatty Acids	Common Name	Value (%)
C6:0	Caproic acid	0.01 ± 0.01	C18:2n-6t	Linolelaidic acid	<0.01
C8:0	Caprylic acid	0.06 ± 0.03	C18:2n-6c	Linoleic acid (LA)	15.13 ± 5.02
C10:0	Capric acid	0.98 ± 0.20	C18:3n-6c	γ-Linolenic acid (GLA)	0.10 ± 0.06
C11:0	Undecanoic acid	<0.01	C18:3n-3c	α-Linolenic acid (ALA)	0.54 ± 0.18
C12:0	Lauric acid	5.46 ± 1.92	C20:0	Arachidic acid	0.18 ± 0.08
C13:0	Tridecylic acid	0.03 ± 0.02	C20:1n-9c	Eicosenoic acid	0.40 ± 0.11
C14:0	Myristic acid	7.02 ± 1.99	C20:2n-6c	Eicosadienoic acid	0.30 ± 0.09
C14:1n-5c	Myristoleic acid	0.14 ± 0.06	C20:3n-6c	Eicosatrienoic acid (ETE)	0.35 ± 0.08
C15:0	Pentadecylic acid	0.31 ± 0.15	C20:4n-6c	Arachidonic acid (ARA)	0.40 ± 0.08
C16:0	Palmitic acid	26.01 ± 4.38	C22:0	Behenic acid	0.01 ± 0.03
C16:1n-7c	Palmitoleic acid	1.90 ± 0.44	C22:1n-9c	Erucic acid	0.02 ± 0.03
C17:1n-7c	Heptadecenoic acid	0.12 ± 0.10	C20:5n-3c	Eicosapentaenoic acid (EPA)	<0.01
C17:0	Margaric acid	0.27 ± 0.09	C22:2n-6c	Docosadienoic acid	0.01 ± 0.02
C18:0	Stearic acid	7.73 ± 1.87	C24:0	Lignoceric acid	0.02 ± 0.05
C18:1n-9t	Elaidic acid	0.12 ± 0.27	C24:1n-9c	Nervonic acid	0.02 ± 0.08
C18:1n-9c	Oleic acid	32.29 ± 4.06	C22:6n-3c	Docosahexaenoic acid (DHA)	0.07 ± 0.16

3.3. Effect of Holder Pasteurization on Breast Milk Samples

Holder pasteurization changed the amount of 14 fatty acids in BM (Table 2). The concentration of caproic acid (C6:0), caprylic acid (C8:0), capric acid (C10:0), myristoleic acid (C14:1n-5c), oleic acid (C18:1n-9c), γ-linolenic acid (C18:3n-6c), α-linolenic acid (C18:3n-3c), and ARA (C20:4n-6c) decreased after HoP. In the case of myristic acid (C14:0), palmitic acid (C16:0), elaidic acid (C18:1n-9t), lignoceric acid (C24:0), nervonic acid (C24:1n-9c), and DHA (C22:6n-3c) increased concentrations were detected after HoP (Table 2).

Table 2. Effect of Holder pasteurization on breast milk (% of total fatty acid profile in mean ± STD).

Fatty Acid	Raw	S	Pasteurized	Fatty Acid	Raw	S	Pasteurized
C6:0	0.07 ± 0.03	*	0.01 ± 0.00	C18:2n-6t	<0.01		<0.01
C8:0	0.19 ± 0.04	*	0.06 ± 0.02	C18:2n-6c	17.10 ± 2.47		15.21 ± 1.63
C10:0	1.26 ± 0.14	*	1.00 ± 0.07	C18:3n-6c	0.15 ± 0.03	*	0.10 ± 0.03
C11:0	<0.01		<0.01	C18:3n-3c	0.65 ± 0.12	*	0.54 ± 0.07
C12:0	5.88 ± 0.83		5.55 ± 0.65	C20:0	0.19 ± 0.02		0.18 ± 0.02
C13:0	<0.01		0.03 ± 0.01	C20:1n-9c	0.38 ± 0.05		0.39 ± 0.06
C14:0	6.05 ± 0.89	*	7.03 ± 0.68	C20:2n-6c	0.31 ± 0.05		0.30 ± 0.05
C14:1n-5c	0.16 ± 0.02	*	0.14 ± 0.02	C20:3n-6c	0.39 ± 0.07		0.36 ± 0.05
C15:0	0.25 ± 0.04		0.29 ± 0.06	C20:4n-6c	0.51 ± 0.06	*	0.40 ± 0.05
C16:0	22.98 ± 2.06	*	26.10 ± 1.16	C22:0	<0.01		0.014 ± 0.015
C16:1n-7c	1.94 ± 0.18		1.90 ± 0.18	C22:1n-9c	<0.01		0.02 ± 0.02
C17:0	0.24 ± 0.02		0.27 ± 0.03	C20:5n-3c	<0.01		<0.01
C17:1n-7c	0.08 ± 0.09		0.11 ± 0.03	C22:2n-6c	<0.01		<0.01
C18:0	6.98 ± 0.75		7.71 ± 0.61	C24:0	0.01 ± 0.03	*	0.02 ± 0.03
C18:1n-9t	0.01 ± 0.03	*	0.11 ± 0.13	C24:1n-9c	0.02 ± 0.05	*	0.03 ± 0.05
C18:1n-9c	34.16 ± 3.59	*	32.05 ± 2.46	C22:6n-3c	0.02 ± 0.07	*	0.07 ± 0.09

S = significance * $p < 0.05$.

3.4. Analysis of Different Co-Variants

The examined FAs showed no changes during the first 12 months of lactation. In BM produced for girl infants, C20:2n-6c presented in significantly higher concentration. When analyzing FAs based on maternal postpartum BMI, we did not find significant differences, although the donors were mainly in between the average weight BMI range. In BM samples of mothers who delivered via C-section, lower lauric acid (C12:0), pentadecylic acid (C15:0), palmitic acid (C16:0), margaric acid (C17:0), stearic acid (C18:0), elaidic acid (C18:1n-9t), and eicosenoic acid (C22:1n-9c) concentrations were determined compared to samples of mothers who delivered vaginally. Levels of linoleic acid (C18:2n-6c), behenic acid (C22:0), lignoceric acid (C24:0), and docosahexaenoic acid (C22:6n-3c) were significantly lower in the BM of mothers after spontaneous delivery (Table 3).

Table 3. Fatty acid content of BM in case of mothers who delivered spontaneously or via C-section (% of total fatty acid profile in mean ± STD).

Fatty Acid	Spontaneously	S	C-Section	Fatty Acid	Spontaneously	S	C-Section
C6:0	0.01 ± 0.01		0.01 ± 0.01	C18:2n-6t	<0.01		<0.01
C8:0	0.06 ± 0.03		0.06 ± 0.03	C18:2n-6c	14.59 ± 4.84	*	15.25 ± 4.74
C10:0	1.01 ± 0.19		0.95 ± 0.21	C18:3n-6c	0.08 ± 0.06		0.11 ± 0.06
C11:0	<0.01		<0.01	C18:3n-3c	0.53 ± 0.16		0.54 ± 0.20
C12:0	5.60 ± 1.90	*	5.19 ± 1.98	C20:0	0.17 ± 0.10		0.20 ± 0.06
C13:0	0.03 ± 0.02		0.03 ± 0.02	C20:1n-9c	0.40 ± 0.11		0.40 ± 0.11
C14:0	7.19 ± 1.80		6.83 ± 2.22	C20:2n-6c	0.29 ± 0.11		0.30 ± 0.08
C14:1n-5c	0.14 ± 0.06		0.14 ± 0.06	C20:3n-6c	0.34 ± 0.08		0.36 ± 0.08
C15:0	0.31 ± 0.16	*	0.29 ± 0.14	C20:4n-6c	0.38 ± 0.07		0.42 ± 0.08
C16:0	26.57 ± 4.53	*	26.19 ± 4.37	C22:0	0.01 ± 0.03	*	0.02 ± 0.03
C16:1n-7c	1.88 ± 0.37		1.92 ± 0.51	C22:1n-9c	0.02 ± 0.03	*	0.02 ± 0.04
C17:0	0.29 ± 0.09	*	0.26 ± 0.08	C20:5n-3c	0.01 ± 0.03		<0.01
C17:1n-7c	0.10 ± 0.10		0.14 ± 0.09	C22:2n-6c	<0.01		0.01 ± 0.02
C18:0	8.15 ± 1.96	*	7.45 ± 1.57	C24:0	0.02 ± 0.06	*	0.03 ± 0.07
C18:1n-9t	0.14 ± 0.31	*	0.11 ± 0.22	C24:1n-9c	0.03 ± 0.10		0.03 ± 0.11
C18:1n-9c	31.58 ± 4.33		32.66 ± 4.03	C22:6n-3c	0.07 ± 0.17	*	0.09 ± 0.18

S = significance * $p < 0.05$.

3.5. Results of Principal Component Analysis (PCA)

3.5.1. Fatty Acid Profile of BM Samples

Based on the results of PCA, the first three principal components (PC) described the variance of the dataset at 98% (PC1: 60%; PC2: 28%; PC3: 10%). No outliers were found based on the values of Hotelling T2 and F-residuals. The position of the samples for the first two PCs was mainly influenced by C16:0, C17:0, C18:0, C18:1n-9c, and C18:2n-6c fatty acids. In addition, the amount of C12:0, C15:0, and C20:3n-6c fatty acids present in the samples also had a significant effect. However, according to the results obtained for the first two PCs, the samples did not separate according to the groups tested (Figure 2).

3.5.2. Influence of Infant's Gender

However, when the third PC was considered, there was a separation between the samples based on the sex of the infant. For the second and third PCs, the differences between the samples are visible. For PC2, the amount of C18:1n-9c fatty acid, while for PC3, the amount of C14:0, C12:0, and C10:0 fatty acids had a substantial effect on the position of the samples and thus on the separation. The location in the negative range for PC2 was explained by a higher amount of C18:2n-6c fatty acid, while for the samples in the positive range, it was due to C17:0. BM produced for girl infants contained higher C20:2n-6c level. The latter effect was much smaller according to the correlation loading (Figure 3).

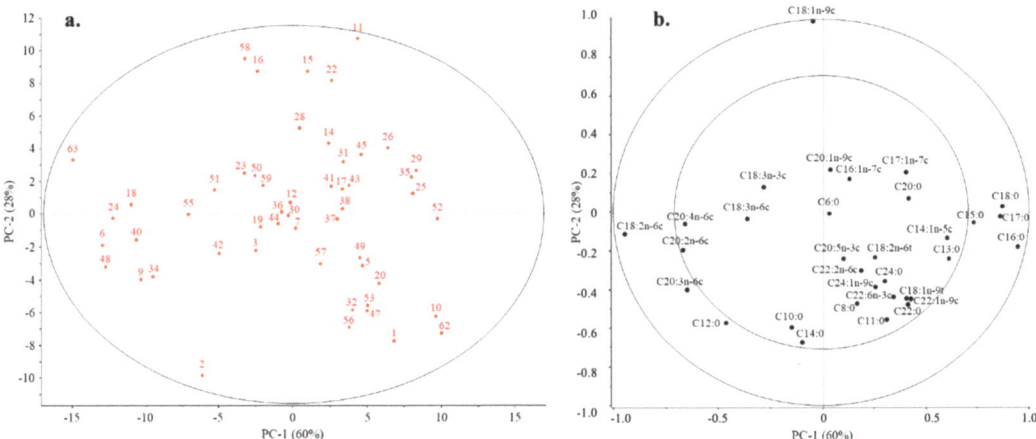

Figure 2. PCA scores (**a**) and correlation loadings (**b**) obtained for all of the investigated BM samples based on their fatty acid profile.

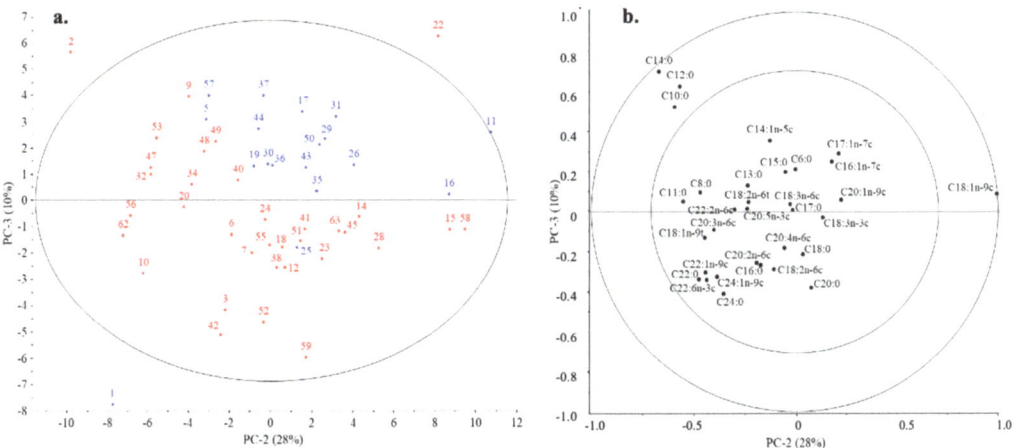

Figure 3. Influence of infant's gender on the separation (PC2–PC3) of BM samples according to the fatty acid profile. On scores plot (**a**) the samples were marked with colors according to the sex of the infant: girl—red; boy—blue. Fatty acids influence the position of the samples presented on the correlation loadings plot (**b**).

3.5.3. Effect of Holder Pasteurization

PCA was also performed on the fatty acid profiles of the pasteurized and untreated samples, the results of which are summarized in Figure 4. The first two PCs explain 93% of the variance in the data. The results clearly showed that pasteurization had a relevant effect on the fatty acid profile of the samples. This suggests that the samples, except for p10, are well separated along PC1 and PC2. Both principal components have a significant effect on the position of the samples. The pasteurized samples, except sample p1, were in the negative region of PC1, which was mainly associated with a higher percentage of C18:1n-9c fatty acid. The importance of this can be supported by the significant difference ($p < 0.05$) found for the Kruskal–Wallis test. The position in the positive region of PC1 was mainly explained by a higher proportion of C16:0 fatty acid, which was more prevalent for untreated samples (Figure 4). A classification method was also run to evaluate the effect of pasteurization. The best results were obtained with cubic support vector machines, resulting in the complete separation of samples. The accuracy of the model was 100% (Figure 4).

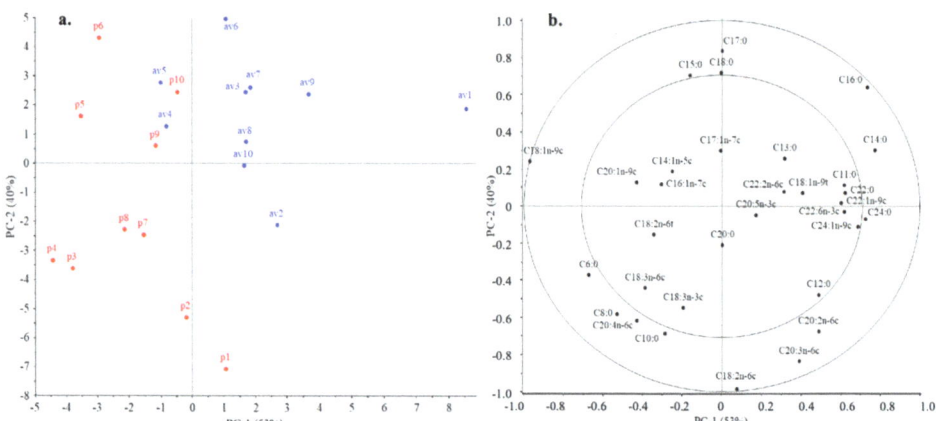

Figure 4. Separation of Holder pasteurized pooled BM samples (indicated with red color) and raw BM samples (indicated with blue color) based on the fatty acid profiles can be seen on scores plot (**a**). Correlation loadings (**b**) present fatty acids and their effect on the position of the scores.

3.5.4. Mode of Delivery

When the samples are labeled according to the mode of delivery in the PCA plot (Figure 5), they are separated based on the fatty acid profiles. In the case of PC1, this is most affected by the amount of each saturated and unsaturated fatty acid. Mothers who deliver by cesarean section have higher levels of C18:2n-6c fatty acids in their breast milk than mothers who deliver vaginally. In addition, the amounts of C20:4n-6c and C20:2n-6c fatty acids were also found to be higher. For PC2, the position of the samples is most dominated by C20:3n-6c, C12:0, and C18:1n-9c fatty acids. Samples with higher amounts of these fatty acids are in the negative region of PC1. In contrast, samples in the positive range of PC1 have a higher percentage of C16:0, C17:0, C18:0, and C15:0 fatty acids (Figure 5).

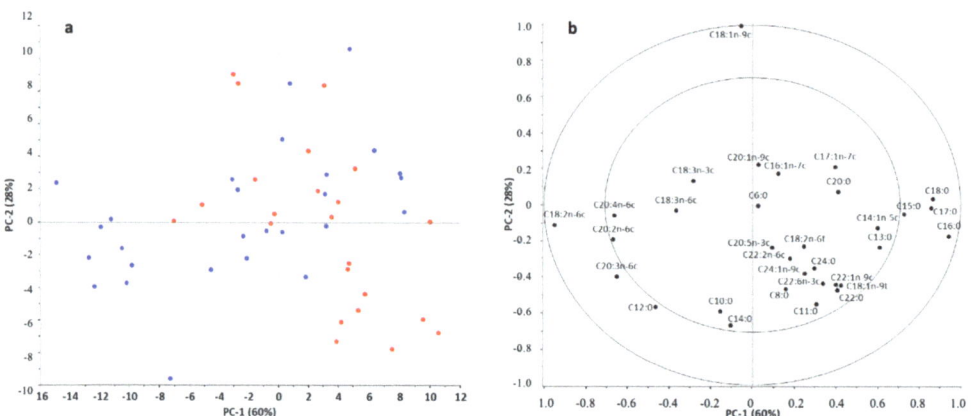

Figure 5. Effect of mode of delivery on the PCA (scores (**a**) and correlation loadings (**b**) of PC1-PC-2) results based on the fatty acids measured in breast milk samples. BMs provided by mothers with cesarean sections are labeled with blue dots, while samples provided by mothers with spontaneous delivery are colored with red dots.

4. Discussion

Fatty acids are a major infant energy source, providing a dense and easily digestible form of calories. They are essential for the development of the nervous system, including the brain, and contribute to the overall growth and development of the infant [4,5]. For instance, some mothers may have milk with a higher fat content, while others may have milk with a lower fat content. The fat content is influenced by several factors, including the mother's diet, the feeding duration, and the lactation stage. FA absorption through the gastrointestinal system is known; some FAs are synthesized by the mammary gland from carbohydrates [37].

In this study, we provide information about the general FA composition of BM and DM. The main FAs in BM are lauric, myristic, palmitic, stearic, cis-9-octadecenoic, and methyl linoleate acids. The other 24 examined FAs are present in only 6.36% [13]. This rate remains unaltered after HoP treatment.

Fatty acids in human milk also contribute to the immunological protection of the infant. Some fatty acids, such as lauric acid, have antimicrobial properties that help protect the infant from infections [38]. Breast milk provides a diverse array of fatty acids that support the development and function of the immune system [6,39]. DHA, an omega-3 fatty acid, is essential for developing the central nervous system, especially the brain. It is a major component of neuronal cell membranes and is critical for cognitive function and visual acuity. Breast milk is a significant source of DHA for infants. DHA is also crucial for developing the retina and overall visual system. Adequate levels of DHA are associated with improved visual and cognitive outcomes in infants [40–43]. Oleic acid is a monounsaturated omega-9 fatty acid, one of nature's most common fatty acids. It is classified as a non-essential fatty acid because the human body can synthesize it, but it is also obtained through diet [44]. Oleic acid has a variety of biological functions, has an anti-inflammatory effect, and is a significant component of human milk [45,46].

Fatty acids are structural components of cell membranes. They contribute to membrane fluidity and stability, influencing cell function and signaling. This is particularly relevant in rapidly growing tissues during postnatal development [7,19]. LCPUFAs serve as a dense and easily metabolizable energy source for infants. This is essential for supporting rapid growth and providing energy demands during the early stages of life. FAs are precursors to various signaling molecules, including hormones. They play a role in hormonal regulation, essential for developing endocrine organs and overall hormonal balance [47].

Essential fatty acids, including omega-3 and omega-6 fatty acids, have multifunctional effects in preventing some diseases, such as cardiovascular, myocardial, and bowel diseases, and play a role in bone health [48]. They are involved in forming and maintaining bone tissue and can influence the balance of bone-forming and bone-resorbing cells [49]. Lauric acid has antimicrobial properties that contribute to the infant's immune defense [50].

Breastfeeding and the unique composition of human milk have been associated with numerous long-term health benefits for infants, including a reduced risk of certain infections, allergies, and chronic diseases later in life [51–53]. Maternal diet influences the composition of BM [43,54] and the fetal outcome of the pregnancy [42]. In our study, the recruited mothers, based on questionnaires, followed no special diets, and all of them reportedly took vitamin supplementation.

HoP is chosen as it strikes a balance between ensuring the safety of DM and preserving as many of its nutritional components as possible. In everyday practice, no precaution is taken to prevent oxidation during pasteurization, resulting in fluctuation of FA composition of DM. Lepri et al. reported an 83% increase in FFA content after heat treatment [55]. Another study detected that after HoP, the proportion of MCFAs was increased [56]. Present result showed that HoP decreased the level of caproic (C6:0), caprylic (C8:0), cis-9-tetradecenoic (C14:1n-5c), oleic (C18:1n-9c), C18:3n-6c, alfa-linoleic (C18:3n-3c), and eicosatetraenoic (C20:4n-6c) acids in BM, while myristic (C14:0), palmitic acid (C16:0), C18:1n-9t, behenic (C22:0), C22:1n-9c, lignoceric (C24:0), C24:1n-9c, and C22:6n-3c were found in elevated concentration after HoP. Similarly to our results, in a review that analyzed over 55 publications, the authors concluded that the most abundant FAs (palmitic, linoleic, and oleic acid) remained stable over time [57]. The changes detected by our research group maintained that increase-free FAs are known to be more absorbable in the gastrointestinal system.

BM-derived components play essential roles in early life immune development. Still, exposure to antigens (e.g., from microbes and foods) and an adequate immune response are critical in shaping the infant's gut microbiota and MCFAs, mainly 10:0, 12:0, and 14:0. These FAs stabilize the bacterial flora in the child's digestive tract [58].

LCPUFAs in BM [43] have been identified to impact the development of the visual and cognitive systems of the infant [52]. After birth, preterm infants become dependent on external sources of LCPUFAs. Although studies indicated the potential positive effects of LCPUFA supplementation on neurodevelopment and vision, recent large, randomized trials revealed concerns about the possible increase in risk [59]. A recent meta-analysis concluded that supplementation with DHA alone increased necrotizing enterocolitis (NEC), but when ARA and DHA supplementation were combined, it increased NEC incidence [59]. LCPUFA supplementation modulated the inflammatory process in the pathophysiology of NEC [59]. Also, results indicate that enteral DHA supplementation reduced NEC incidence among preterm infants due to their immunoregulatory effect [59–61].

Infants who had received LCPUFAs had a lower risk of wheezing/asthma, wheezing/asthma plus atopic dermatitis, any allergy, and upper respiratory tract infection. Infants receiving LCPUFAs were less likely to develop bronchitis or bronchiolitis at 5, 7, and 9 months [38,41,62]. Also, there were fewer allergic illnesses and skin allergic illnesses in the first year compared to infants in the control group, and these outcomes remained lower at the age of 4 years. LCPUFAs reduced wheeze/asthma in infants of allergic mothers [38]. Infants with higher plasma DHA or higher plasma EPA and docosapentaenoic acid and DHA at age 6 months were less likely to develop recurrent wheezing by age 12 months [63]. In a later follow-up study, when the children were five, there was no difference between groups for any clinical outcome related to lung function or allergy [64]. A birth cohort study in Iceland identified that 2.5-year-old children who had received n-3 LCPUFA supplements in infancy were less likely to have been diagnosed with food sensitization [65,66]. n-3 LCPUFAs also decreased the severity of allergies [65]. Early n-3 and n-6 LCPUFA supply may moderate the impact of hypoxia and oxidative damage, thus affecting the recovery from injury, later organ development, and neurodevelopmental outcomes [67]. The European Food Safety Authority recommends supplementation with DHA [68].

Results indicated that the mode of delivery impacts the composition of BM FAs. In our study, similarly to previous findings [69], the BM of mothers who delivered spontaneously contained significantly higher n-3 PUFA, stearic, and palmitoleic acid levels, which are knowingly anti-inflammatory components. Similar to other results, in our work, the BM of mothers undergoing C-sections had elevated DHA BM levels [69]. Our results showed that inflammatory FA content and n-6/n-3 ratio were higher in the BM of mothers who delivered via C-section.

Previous studies reported significant sex-based differences in the FA composition of BM; fat content produced for boy infants was significantly higher than for girl infants [70]. A higher ratio of ARA/DHA in female infants may reduce the risk of food sensitization and atopic dermatitis [71]. We found that BM produced for female infants contains higher eicosadienoic acid levels. Low temperature treatments, like Holder pasteurization, create oxidative environments, resulting in modest changes in FA concentration [72].

Our results give information about the fatty acid profile of BM, supporting the aims of supplementation among preterm infants. Although HoP resulted in changes in the detected proportion of FAs in BM, due to the statistically significant but infinitesimal modification, pasteurized DM provides an alternative to own mother's milk during postnatal adaptation. Pooled DM is a safe way to merge BM from different lactation sessions and to evenly distribute nutrients. Different treatment technologies are applied to ensure the microbiological safety of DM, like high-temperature, short-time (HTST), or ultra-violet processing. Previous works investigating these techniques had no significant effect on the

FA composition of BM [73,74]. Serum hormone levels in preterm infants, e.g., leptin, predict early childhood developmental assessment scores [75]. Studies proving the ability of fatty acids to improve cognitive functions among adults are known. However, the possible predictive effects of fatty acids are still unknown despite their multifunctional effect on neurodevelopment [76,77]. Fatty acid supplementation for preterm infants is a common practice in neonatal care to support their growth and development [78], and it is especially relevant because these infants are born before they have had the chance to accumulate sufficient fat stores in utero.

5. Conclusions

The adaptability of human milk to the child's specific needs is a fascinating aspect of breastfeeding and highlights the evolutionary importance of this unique source of nourishment. The FA profile of human milk is a critical aspect of its nutritional and immunological properties, contributing to the overall health and well-being of the breastfed infant. Based on our results, the fatty acid composition of BM differs based on the gender of the infants, the course of delivery, the maternal age, and BMI. While the decrease in fatty acids is a concern, the reduction in nutritional components, including PUFAs, needs to be balanced against the primary goal of pasteurization, which is to destroy harmful microorganisms while minimizing the impact on milk quality. Holder pasteurization has been widely used because it effectively reduces microbial contamination while, as our measurements strengthen previous results, minimizing the impact on the overall composition of breast milk. Data from the present study provides detailed information about the FA profile of BM; therefore, it may contribute to protocols for FA supplementation of premature or formula-fed infants. Fatty acid supplementation is one component of the comprehensive care approach, which provides optimal nutrition with the supplementation of fatty acids and supports development and growth.

Author Contributions: Conceptualization, R.A.V., L.S.S., T.E. and S.G.V.; methodology, R.A.V., M.Ü., E.L.B., M.Z., L.S.S., J.T., T.E. and S.G.V.; formal analysis, R.A.V., M.Ü., E.L.B., J.T. and M.Z.; investigation, R.A.V., M.Ü., J.T. and E.L.B.; data curation, R.A.V., M.Ü. and E.L.B.; writing—original draft preparation, R.A.V., M.Ü. and E.L.B.; writing—review and editing, R.A.V., M.Ü., E.L.B., M.Z., J.T., L.S.S., T.E. and S.G.V.; project administration, R.A.V.; funding acquisition, S.G.V. All authors have read and agreed to the published version of the manuscript.

Funding: This research was funded by the Association for Regional Cooperation of Health, Science and Technology (RECOOP HST Association) and Cedars-Sinai Medical Center—RECOOP Research Centers (CRRCs) by the RECOOP Grant No. 16: 2019-2022.

Institutional Review Board Statement: The study was conducted according to the guidelines of the Declaration of Helsinki and approved by the Regional and Local Research Ethics Committee of the University of Pécs, Pécs, Hungary (PTE KK 7072-2018, approval date: 15 June 2018).

Informed Consent Statement: Informed consent was obtained from all subjects involved in the study.

Data Availability Statement: The data is not publicly available due to ethical reasons, on request it is available from the corresponding author.

Conflicts of Interest: The authors declare no conflicts of interest.

References

1. Kumari, P.; Raval, A.; Rana, P.; Mahto, S.K. Regenerative potential of human breast milk: A natural reservoir of nutrients, bioactive components and stem cells. *Stem Cell Rev. Rep.* **2023**, *19*, 1307–1327. [CrossRef]
2. Nuzzi, G.; Trambusti, I.; DI Cicco, M.E.; Peroni, D.G. Breast milk: More than just nutrition! *Minerva Pediatr.* **2021**, *73*, 111–114. [CrossRef] [PubMed]
3. Koletzko, B.; Rodriguez-Palmero, M. Polyunsaturated fatty acids in human milk and their role in early infant development. *J. Mammary Gland. Biol. Neoplasia.* **1999**, *4*, 269–284. [CrossRef] [PubMed]
4. Mitguard, S.; Doucette, O.; Miklavcic, J. Human milk polyunsaturated fatty acids are related to neurodevelopmental, anthropometric, and allergic outcomes in early life: A systematic review. *J. Dev. Orig. Health Dis.* **2023**, *14*, 763–772. [CrossRef] [PubMed]

5. Ballard, O.; Morrow, A.L. Human milk composition: Nutrients and bioactive factors. *Pediatr. Clin. N. Am.* **2013**, *60*, 49–74. [CrossRef] [PubMed]
6. Ramiro-Cortijo, D.; Singh, P.; Liu, Y.; Medina-Morales, E.; Yakah, W.; Freedman, S.D.; Martin, C.R. Breast milk lipids and fatty acids in regulating neonatal intestinal development and protecting against intestinal injury. *Nutrients* **2020**, *12*, 534. [CrossRef] [PubMed]
7. Basak, S.; Mallick, R.; Duttaroy, A.K. Maternal docosahexaenoic acid status during pregnancy and its impact on infant neurodevelopment. *Nutrients* **2020**, *12*, 3615. [CrossRef] [PubMed]
8. Simon Sarkadi, L.; Zhang, M.; Muránszky, G.; Vass, R.A.; Matsyura, O.; Benes, E.; Vari, S.G. Fatty acid composition of milk from mothers with normal weight, obesity, or gestational diabetes. *Life* **2022**, *12*, 1093. [CrossRef] [PubMed]
9. Argov-Argaman, N.; Mandel, D.; Lubetzky, R.; Hausman Kedem, M.; Cohen, B.C.; Berkovitz, Z.; Reifen, R. Human milk fatty acids composition is affected by maternal age. *J. Matern. Fetal Neonatal Med.* **2017**, *30*, 34–37. [CrossRef] [PubMed]
10. Boersma, E.R.; Offringa, P.J.; Muskiet, F.A.; Chase, W.M.; Simmons, I.J. Vitamin E, lipid fractions, and fatty acid composition of colostrum, transitional milk, and mature milk: An international comparative study. *Am. J. Clin. Nutr.* **1991**, *53*, 1197–1204. [CrossRef] [PubMed]
11. Bitman, J.; Wood, L.; Hamosh, M.; Hamosh, P.; Mehta, N.R. Comparison of the lipid composition of breast milk from mothers of term and preterm infants. *Am. J. Clin. Nutr.* **1983**, *38*, 300–312. [CrossRef] [PubMed]
12. Giuffrida, F.; Cruz-Hernandez, C.; Bertschy, E.; Fontannaz, P.; Masserey Elmelegy, I.; Tavazzi, I.; Marmet, C.; Sanchez-Bridge, B.; Thakkar, S.K.; De Castro, C.A.; et al. Temporal changes of human breast milk lipids of chinese mothers. *Nutrients* **2016**, *8*, 715. [CrossRef] [PubMed]
13. Bokor, S.; Koletzko, B.; Decsi, T. Systematic review of fatty acid composition of human milk from mothers of preterm compared to full-term infants. *Ann. Nutr. Metab.* **2007**, *51*, 550–556. [CrossRef] [PubMed]
14. Ahmed, T.B.; Eggesbø, M.; Criswell, R.; Uhl, O.; Demmelmair, H.; Koletzko, B. Total fatty acid and polar lipid species composition of human milk. *Nutrients* **2021**, *14*, 158. [CrossRef] [PubMed]
15. Catassi, G.; Aloi, M.; Giorgio, V.; Gasbarrini, A.; Cammarota, G.; Ianiro, G. The role of diet and nutritional interventions for the Infant Gut Microbiome. *Nutrients* **2024**, *16*, 400. [CrossRef] [PubMed]
16. Cao, X.; Xia, J.; Zhou, Y.; Wang, Y.; Xia, H.; Wang, S.; Liao, W.; Sun, G. The effect of MUFA-rich food on lipid profile: A meta-analysis of randomized and controlled-feeding trials. *Foods* **2022**, *11*, 1982. [CrossRef] [PubMed]
17. von Schacky, C.; Harris, W.S. Cardiovascular benefits of omega-3 fatty acids. *Cardiovasc. Res.* **2007**, *73*, 310–315. [CrossRef] [PubMed]
18. Skowronska-Krawczyk, D.; Chao, D.L. Long-chain polyunsaturated fatty acids and age-related macular degeneration. *Adv. Exp. Med. Biol.* **2019**, *1185*, 39–43. [PubMed]
19. Innis, S.M. Fatty acids and early human development. *Early Hum. Dev.* **2007**, *83*, 761–766. [CrossRef] [PubMed]
20. Shete, H.; Patravale, V. Long chain lipid based tamoxifen NLC. Part I: Preformulation studies, formulation development and physicochemical characterization. *Int. J. Pharm.* **2013**, *454*, 573–583. [CrossRef] [PubMed]
21. Tvrzicka, E.; Kremmyda, L.S.; Stankova, B.; Zak, A. Fatty acids as biocompounds: Their role in human metabolism, health and disease—A review. Part 1: Classification, dietary sources and biological functions. *Biomed. Pap. Med. Fac. Palacky Univ. Olomouc* **2011**, *155*, 117–130. [CrossRef] [PubMed]
22. Sinanoglou, V.J.; Cavouras, D.; Boutsikou, T.; Briana, D.D.; Lantzouraki, D.Z.; Paliatsiou, S.; Volaki, P.; Bratakos, S.; Malamitsi-Puchner, A.; Zoumpoulakis, P. Factors affecting human colostrum fatty acid profile: A case study. *PLoS ONE* **2017**, *12*, e0175817. [CrossRef] [PubMed]
23. Sankar, M.J.; Sinha, B.; Chowdhury, R.; Bhandari, N.; Taneja, S.; Martines, J.; Bahl, R. Optimal breastfeeding practices and infant and child mortality: A systematic review and meta-analysis. *Acta Paediatr.* **2015**, *104*, 3–13. [CrossRef] [PubMed]
24. Oddy, W.H. Breastfeeding, childhood asthma, and allergic disease. *Ann. Nutr. Metab.* **2017**, *70* (Suppl. S2), 26–36. [CrossRef] [PubMed]
25. Kotlyarov, S.; Kotlyarova, A. Involvement of fatty acids and their metabolites in the development of inflammation in atherosclerosis. *Int. J. Mol. Sci.* **2022**, *23*, 1308. [CrossRef] [PubMed]
26. Mallick, R.; Duttaroy, A.K. Modulation of endothelium function by fatty acids. *Mol. Cell Biochem.* **2022**, *477*, 15–38. [CrossRef]
27. Hellström, A.; Pivodic, A.; Gränse, L.; Lundgren, P.; Sjöbom, U.; Nilsson, A.K.; Söderling, H.; Hård, A.L.; Smith, L.E.H.; Löfqvist, C.A. Association of docosahexaenoic acid and arachidonic acid serum levels with retinopathy of prematurity in preterm infants. *JAMA Netw. Open* **2021**, *4*, e2128771. [CrossRef] [PubMed]
28. Vass, R.A.; Kiss, G.; Bell, E.F.; Roghair, R.D.; Miseta, A.; Bódis, J.; Funke, S.; Ertl, T. Breast milk for term and preterm infants-own mother's milk or donor milk? *Nutrients* **2021**, *13*, 424. [CrossRef]
29. Vass, R.A.; Mikó, É.; Gál, C.; Kőszegi, T.; Vass, C.I.; Bokor, S.; Molnár, D.; Funke, S.; Kovács, K.; Bódis, J.; et al. The effect of Holder pasteurization and different variants on breast milk antioxidants. *Antioxidants* **2023**, *12*, 1857. [CrossRef] [PubMed]
30. Vass, R.A.; Bell, E.F.; Colaizy, T.T.; Schmelzel, M.L.; Johnson, K.J.; Walker, J.R.; Ertl, T.; Roghair, R.D. Hormone levels in preterm and donor human milk before and after Holder pasteurization. *Pediatr. Res.* **2020**, *88*, 612–617. [CrossRef]
31. Vass, R.A.; Roghair, R.D.; Bell, E.F.; Colaizy, T.T.; Schmelzel, M.L.; Johnson, K.J.; Walker, J.R.; Ertl, T. Pituitary glycoprotein hormones in human milk before and after pasteurization or refrigeration. *Nutrients* **2020**, *12*, 687. [CrossRef] [PubMed]

32. Vass, R.A.; Kiss, G.; Bell, E.F.; Miseta, A.; Bódis, J.; Funke, S.; Bokor, S.; Molnár, D.; Kósa, B.; Kiss, A.A.; et al. Thyroxine and thyroid-stimulating hormone in own mother's milk, donor milk, and infant formula. *Life* **2022**, *12*, 584. [CrossRef] [PubMed]
33. Vass, R.A.; Bell, E.F.; Roghair, R.D.; Kiss, G.; Funke, S.; Bokor, S.; Molnár, D.; Miseta, A.; Bódis, J.; Kovács, K.; et al. Insulin, testosterone, and albumin in term and preterm breast milk, donor milk, and infant formula. *Nutrients* **2023**, *15*, 1476. [CrossRef]
34. Committee on Nutrition; Section on Breastfeeding; Committee on Fetus and Newborn. Donor human milk for the high-risk infant: Preparation, safety, and usage options in the United States. *Pediatrics* **2017**, *139*, e20163440. [CrossRef] [PubMed]
35. ISO 16958:2015; Milk, Milk Products, Infant Formula and Adult Nutritionals, Determination of Fatty Acids Composition, Capillary Gas Chromatographic Method. ISO: Geneva, Switzerland, 2015.
36. Tormási, J.; Abrankó, L. Assessment of fatty acid-specific lipolysis by in vitro digestion and GC-FID. *Nutrients* **2021**, *13*, 3889. [CrossRef] [PubMed]
37. Annison, E.; Linzell, J.; Fazakerley, S.; Nichols, B. The oxidation and utilization of palmitate, stearate, oleate and acetate by the mammary gland of the fed goat in relation to their overall metabolism, and the role of plasma phospholipids and neutral lipids in milk-fat synthesis. *Biochem. J.* **1967**, *102*, 637–647. [CrossRef] [PubMed]
38. Foiles, A.M.; Kerling, E.H.; Wick, J.A.; Scalabrin, D.M.F.; Colombo, J.; Carlson, S.E. Formula with long-chain polyunsaturated fatty acids reduces incidence of allergy in early childhood. *Pediatr. Allergy Immunol.* **2016**, *27*, 156–161. [CrossRef] [PubMed]
39. Field, C.J. The immunological components of human milk and their effect on immune development in infants. *J. Nutr.* **2005**, *135*, 1–4. [CrossRef] [PubMed]
40. Marc, I.; Boutin, A.; Pronovost, E.; Perez Herrera, N.M.; Guillot, M.; Bergeron, F.; Moore, L.; Sullivan, T.R.; Lavoie, P.M.; Makrides, M. Association between enteral supplementation with high-dose Docosahexaenoic Acid and risk of bronchopulmonary dysplasia in preterm infants: A systematic review and meta-analysis. *JAMA Netw Open.* **2023**, *6*, e233934. [CrossRef]
41. Pastor, N.; Soler, B.; Mitmesser, S.H.; Ferguson, P.; Lifschitz, C. Infants fed docosahexaenoic acid- and arachidonic acid-supplemented formula have decreased incidence of bronchiolitis/bronchitis the first year of life. *Clin. Pediatr.* **2006**, *45*, 850–855. [CrossRef] [PubMed]
42. Krauss-Etschmann, S.; Shadid, R.; Campoy, C.; Hoster, E.; Demmelmair, H.; Jiménez, M.; Gil, A.; Rivero, M.; Veszprémi, B.; Decsi, T.; et al. Effects of fish-oil and folate supplementation of pregnant women on maternal and fetal plasma concentrations of docosahexaenoic acid and eicosapentaenoic acid: A European randomized multicenter trial. *Am. J. Clin. Nutr.* **2007**, *85*, 1392–1400. [CrossRef] [PubMed]
43. Brenna, J.T.; Varamini, B.; Jensen, R.G.; Diersen-Schade, D.A.; Boettcher, J.A.; Arterburn, L.M. Docosahexaenoic and arachidonic acid concentrations in human breast milk worldwide. *Am. J. Clin. Nutr.* **2007**, *85*, 1457–1464. [CrossRef] [PubMed]
44. Igarashi, M.; Iwasa, K.; Hayakawa, T.; Tsuduki, T.; Kimura, I.; Maruyama, K.; Yoshikawa, K. Dietary oleic acid contributes to the regulation of food intake through the synthesis of intestinal oleoylethanolamide. *Front. Endocrinol.* **2023**, *13*, 1056116. [CrossRef] [PubMed]
45. Carrillo, C.; Cavia Mdel, M.; Alonso-Torre, S. Role of oleic acid in immune system; mechanism of action; a review. *Nutr. Hosp.* **2012**, *27*, 978–990. [PubMed]
46. Santa-María, C.; López-Enríquez, S.; Montserrat-de la Paz, S.; Geniz, I.; Reyes-Quiroz, M.E.; Moreno, M.; Palomares, F.; Sobrino, F.; Alba, G. Update on anti-inflammatory molecular mechanisms induced by oleic acid. *Nutrients* **2023**, *15*, 224. [CrossRef] [PubMed]
47. Miles, E.A.; Childs, C.E.; Calder, P.C. Long-Chain Polyunsaturated Fatty Acids (LCPUFAs) and the developing immune system: A narrative review. *Nutrients* **2021**, *13*, 247. [CrossRef] [PubMed]
48. Dou, Y.; Wang, Y.; Chen, Z.; Yu, X.; Ma, D. Effect of n-3 polyunsaturated fatty acid on bone health: A systematic review and meta-analysis of randomized controlled trials. *Food Sci. Nutr.* **2021**, *10*, 145–154. [CrossRef] [PubMed]
49. Khalesi, N.; Bordbar, A.; Khosravi, N.; Kabirian, M.; Karimi, A. The efficacy of omega-3 supplement on prevention of retinopathy of prematurity in premature infants: A randomized double-blinded controlled trial. *Curr. Pharm. Des.* **2018**, *24*, 1845–1848. [CrossRef] [PubMed]
50. Matsue, M.; Mori, Y.; Nagase, S.; Sugiyama, Y.; Hirano, R.; Ogai, K.; Ogura, K.; Kurihara, S.; Okamoto, S. Measuring the antimicrobial activity of lauric acid against various bacteria in human gut microbiota using a new method. *Cell Transplant.* **2019**, *28*, 1528–1541. [CrossRef] [PubMed]
51. Zhang, M.; Simon Sarkadi, L.; Üveges, M.; Tormási, J.; Benes, E.; Vass, R.A.; Vari, S.G. Gas chromatographic determination of fatty acid composition in breast milk of mothers with different health conditions. *Acta Alimentaria.* **2022**, *51*, 625–635. [CrossRef]
52. Demmelmair, H.; Koletzko, B. Importance of fatty acids in the perinatal period. *World Rev. Nutr. Diet.* **2015**, *112*, 31–47. [PubMed]
53. Embleton, N.D.; Jennifer Moltu, S.; Lapillonne, A.; van den Akker, C.H.P.; Carnielli, V.; Fusch, C.; Gerasimidis, K.; van Goudoever, J.B.; Haiden, N.; Iacobelli, S.; et al. Enteral nutrition in preterm infants (2022): A position paper from the ESPGHAN Committee on nutrition and invited experts. *J. Pediatr. Gastroenterol. Nutr.* **2023**, *76*, 248–268. [CrossRef] [PubMed]
54. Keikha, M.; Shayan-Moghadam, R.; Bahreynian, M.; Kelishadi, R. Nutritional supplements and mother's milk composition: A systematic review of interventional studies. *Int. Breastfeed. J.* **2021**, *16*, 1. [CrossRef] [PubMed]
55. Lepri, L.; Del Bubba, M.; Maggini, R.; Donzelli, G.P.; Galvan, P. Effect of pasteurization and storage on some components of pooled human milk. *J. Chromatogr. B Biomed. Sci. Appl.* **1997**, *704*, 1–10. [CrossRef]
56. Ewaschuk, J.B.; Unger, S.; O'Connor, D.L.; Stone, D.; Harvey, S.; Clandinin, M.T.; Field, C.J. Effect of pasteurization on selected immune components of donated human breast milk. *J. Perinatol.* **2011**, *31*, 593–598. [CrossRef] [PubMed]

57. Floris, L.M.; Stahl, B.; Abrahamse-Berkeveld, M.; Teller, I.C. Human milk fatty acid profile across lactational stages after term and preterm delivery: A pooled data analysis. *Prostaglandins Leukot. Essent. Fatty Acids* **2020**, *156*, 102023. [CrossRef] [PubMed]
58. Marounek, M.; Skrivanova, E.; Rada, V. Susceptibility of Escherichia coli to C2–C18 fatty acids. *Folia Microbiol.* **2003**, *48*, 731–735. [CrossRef] [PubMed]
59. Alshaikh, B.N.; Reyes Loredo, A.; Yusuf, K.; Maarouf, A.; Fenton, T.R.; Momin, S. Enteral long-chain polyunsaturated fatty acids and necrotizing enterocolitis: A systematic review and meta-analysis. *Am. J. Clin. Nutr.* **2023**, *117*, 918–929. [CrossRef] [PubMed]
60. Alshaikh, B.N.; Reyes Loredo, A.; Knauff, M.; Momin, S.; Moossavi, S. The role of dietary fats in the development and prevention of necrotizing enterocolitis. *Nutrients* **2021**, *14*, 145. [CrossRef] [PubMed]
61. Abou El Fadl, D.K.; Ahmed, M.A.; Aly, Y.A.; Darweesh, E.A.G.; Sabri, N.A. Impact of Docosahexaenoic acid supplementation on proinflammatory cytokines release and the development of Necrotizing enterocolitis in preterm Neonates: A randomized controlled study. *Saudi Pharm. J.* **2021**, *29*, 1314–1322. [CrossRef] [PubMed]
62. Lapillonne, A.; Pastor, N.; Zhuang, W.; Scalabrin, D.M.F. Infants fed formula with added long chain polyunsaturated fatty acids have reduced incidence of respiratory illnesses and diarrhea during the first year of life. *BMC Prediatr.* **2014**, *14*, 168. [CrossRef] [PubMed]
63. D'Vaz, N.; Meldrum, S.J.; Dunstan, J.A.; Martino, D.; McCarthy, S.; Metcalfe, J.; Tulic, M.K.; Mori, T.A.; Prescott, S.A. Postnatal fish oil supplementation in high-risk infants to prevent allergy: Randomized controlled trial. *Pediatrics* **2012**, *130*, 674–682. [CrossRef] [PubMed]
64. Marks, G.B.; Mihrshahi, S.; Kemp, A.S.; Tovey, E.R.; Webb, K.; Almqvist, C.; Ampon, R.D.; Crisafulli, D.; Belousova, E.G.; Mellis, C.M.; et al. Prevention of asthma during the first 5 years of life: A randomized controlled trial. *J. Allergy Clin. Immunol.* **2006**, *118*, 53–61. [CrossRef] [PubMed]
65. Clausen, M.; Jonasson, K.; Keil, T.; Beyer, K.; Sigurdardottir, S.T. Fish oil in infancy protects against food allergy in Iceland—Results from a birth cohort study. *Allergy* **2018**, *73*, 1305–1312. [CrossRef] [PubMed]
66. Almqvist, C.; Garden, F.; Xuan, W.; Mihrshahi, S.; Leeder, S.R.; Oddy, W.; Webb, K.; Marks, G.B.; CAPS team. Omega-3 and omega-6 fatty acid exposure from early life does not affect atopy and asthma at age 5 years. *J. Allergy Clin. Immunol.* **2007**, *119*, 1438–1444. [CrossRef] [PubMed]
67. Uauy, R.; Mena, P. Long-chain polyunsaturated fatty acids supplementation in preterm infants. *Curr. Opin. Pediatr.* **2015**, *27*, 165–171. [CrossRef] [PubMed]
68. Crawford, M.A.; Wang, Y.; Forsyth, S.; Brenna, J.T. The European Food Safety Authority recommendation for polyunsaturated fatty acid composition of infant formula overrules breast milk, puts infants at risk, and should be revised. *Prostaglandins Leukot. Essent. Fatty Acids.* **2015**, *102–103*, 1–3. [CrossRef]
69. Samuel, T.M.; Thielecke, F.; Lavalle, L.; Chen, C.; Fogel, P.; Giuffrida, F.; Dubascoux, S.; Martínez-Costa, C.; Haaland, K.; Marchini, G.; et al. Mode of neonatal delivery influences the nutrient composition of human milk: Results from a multicenter European cohort of lactating women. *Front. Nutr.* **2022**, *9*, 834394. [CrossRef] [PubMed]
70. Khelouf, N.; Haoud, K.; Meziani, S.; Fizir, M.; Ghomari, F.N.; Khaled, M.B.; Kadi, N. Effect of infant's gender and lactation period on biochemical and energy breast milk composition of lactating mothers from Algeria. *J. Food Compos. Anal.* **2023**, *115*, 104889. [CrossRef]
71. Miliku, K.; Richelle, J.; Becker, A.B.; Simons, E.; Moraes, T.J.; Stuart, T.E.; Mandhane, P.J.; Sears, M.R.; Subbarao, P.; Field, C.J.; et al. Sex-specific associations of human milk long-chain polyunsaturated fatty acids and infant allergic conditions. *Pediatr. Allergy Immunol.* **2021**, *32*, 1173–1182. [CrossRef] [PubMed]
72. Rodríguez-Alcalá, L.M.; Alonso, L.; Fontecha, J. Stability of fatty acid composition after thermal, high pressure, and microwave processing of cow milk as affected by polyunsaturated fatty acid concentration. *J. Dairy. Sci.* **2014**, *97*, 7307–7315. [CrossRef] [PubMed]
73. Christen, L.; Lai, C.T.; Hartmann, B.; Hartmann, P.E.; Geddes, D.T. Ultraviolet-C irradiation: A novel pasteurization method for donor human milk. *PLoS ONE* **2013**, *8*, e68120. [CrossRef] [PubMed]
74. Wesolowska, A.; Sinkiewicz-Darol, E.; Barbarska, O.; Bernatowicz-Lojko, U.; Borszewska-Kornacka, M.K.; van Goudoever, J.B. Innovative Techniques of Processing Human Milk to Preserve Key Components. *Nutrients* **2019**, *11*, 1169. [CrossRef] [PubMed]
75. Roghair, R.D.; Colaizy, T.T.; Steinbrekera, B.; Vass, R.A.; Hsu, E.; Dagle, D.; Chatmethakul, T. Neonatal leptin levels predict the early childhood developmental assessment scores of preterm infants. *Nutrients* **2023**, *15*, 1967. [CrossRef] [PubMed]
76. Marriott, B.P.; Turner, T.H.; Hibbeln, J.R.; Newman, J.C.; Pregulman, M.; Malek, A.M.; Malcolm, R.J.; Burbelo, G.A.; Wismann, J.W. Impact of fatty acid supplementation on cognitive performance among United States (US) military officers: The ranger resilience and improved performance on phospholipid-bound Omega-3's (RRIPP-3) Study. *Nutrients* **2021**, *13*, 1854. [CrossRef] [PubMed]

77. Wei, B.Z.; Li, L.; Dong, C.W.; Tan, C.C.; Alzheimer's Disease Neuroimaging Initiative; Xu, W. The relationship of Omega-3 fatty acids with dementia and cognitive decline: Evidence from prospective cohort studies of supplementation, dietary intake, and blood markers. *Am. J. Clin. Nutr.* **2023**, *117*, 1096–1109. [CrossRef] [PubMed]
78. Embleton, N.D.; van den Akker, C.H.P. Protein intakes to optimize outcomes for preterm infants. *Semin. Perinatol.* **2019**, *43*, 151154. [CrossRef] [PubMed]

Disclaimer/Publisher's Note: The statements, opinions and data contained in all publications are solely those of the individual author(s) and contributor(s) and not of MDPI and/or the editor(s). MDPI and/or the editor(s) disclaim responsibility for any injury to people or property resulting from any ideas, methods, instructions or products referred to in the content.

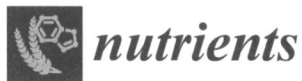

Article

Presepsin in Human Milk Is Delivery Mode and Gender Dependent

Ebe D'Adamo [1], Chiara Peila [2], Mariachiara Strozzi [3], Roberta Barolo [2], Antonio Maconi [4], Arianna Nanni [1], Valentina Botondi [1], Alessandra Coscia [2], Enrico Bertino [2], Francesca Gazzolo [5], Ali Saber Abdelhameed [6], Mariangela Conte [1], Simonetta Picone [7], Marianna D'Andrea [1], Mauro Lizzi [1], Maria Teresa Quarta [1] and Diego Gazzolo [1,*]

1. Neonatal Intensive Care Unit, "G. D'Annunzio" University, 66100 Chieti, Italy; ebe.dadamo@yahoo.com (E.D.); arianna.nanni.98@gmail.com (A.N.); valentina.botondi91@gmail.com (V.B.); conte.mariangela@virgilio.it (M.C.); mary.dandrea1988@libero.it (M.D.); mauro.lizzi.med@gmail.com (M.L.)
2. Neonatology Unit, Department of Public Health and Pediatrics, University of Turin, 10124 Torino, Italy; chiara.peila@unito.it (C.P.); roberta.barolo@unito.it (R.B.); alessandra.coscia@unito.it (A.C.); enrico.bertino@unito.it (E.B.)
3. Department of Pediatrics and Neonatology, Cardinal Massaia Hospital, 14100 Asti, Italy; chiara.strozzi@libero.it
4. Department of Maternal, Fetal and Neonatal Medicine, ASO SS Antonio, Biagio and C. Arrigo, 15121 Alessandria, Italy; amaconi@ospedale.al.it
5. Department of Medical and Surgical Sciences, Magna Graecia University, 88100 Catanzaro, Italy; francesca.gazzolo@libero.it
6. Department of Pharmaceutical Chemistry, College of Pharmacy, King Saud University, Riyadh 11451, Saudi Arabia; asaber@ksu.edu.sa
7. Neonatal Intensive Care Unit, Policlinico Casilino, 00169 Rome, Italy; simpico@libero.it
* Correspondence: dgazzolo@hotmail.com; Tel.: +39-0871358219

Abstract: Breast milk (BM) is a unique food due to its nutritional composition and anti-inflammatory characteristics. Evidence has emerged on the role of Presepsin (PSEP) as a reliable marker of early sepsis diagnosis. In the present study, we aimed to investigate the measurability of PSEP in BM according to different maturation stages (colostrum, C; transition, Tr; and mature milks, Mt) and corrected for delivery mode and gender. We conducted a multicenter prospective case–control study in women who had delivered 22 term (T) and 22 preterm (PT) infants. A total of 44 human milk samples were collected and stored at -80 °C. BM PSEP (pg/mL) levels were measured by using a rapid chemiluminescent enzyme immunoassay. PSEP was detected in all samples analyzed. Higher ($p < 0.05$) BM PSEP concentrations were observed in the PT compared to the T infants. According to the grade of maturation, higher ($p < 0.05$) levels of PSEP in C compared to Tr and Mt milks were observed in the whole study population. The BM subtypes' degrees of maturation were delivery mode and gender dependent. We found that PSEP at high concentrations supports its antimicrobial action both in PT and T infants. These results open the door to further studies investigating the role of PSEP.

Keywords: presepsin; breastmilk; newborn; nutrition; preterm; sCD14

1. Introduction

There is general consensus that breast milk (BM), due to its unique properties, constitutes the ideal product for the feeding of newborns [1–3]. The data in the literature support the notion that exclusive breastfeeding for the first 4–6 months of life is advised to ensure healthy growth and primary prevention against potential infectious pathogens at a stage when the neonatal immune system is completing its development [4,5]. BM is a specific–dynamic biofluid since its maturation is time-dependent and varies according to maternal diet and diseases [6]. Health benefits associated with breastfeeding lie in the combined action of the nutritional and bioactive components of BM [7–14], among which the glycoprotein CD14 aids neonatal gut function and development, modulates immune function, and regulates inflammation [15,16]. Membrane CD14 (mCD14) is a multifunctional glycoprotein expressed on the surface of various cells including monocytes, macrophages and neutrophils. Indeed, CD14 is a recognition receptor for Gram-negative and Gram-positive bacteria and lipopolysaccharides [17]. Notably, the soluble cluster of differentiation CD14 sub-type (sCD14), also called Presepsin (PSEP), has recently been put forward as a promising biomarker of sepsis [18]. Increased PSEP levels have been found in response to existing infections in adults, in children, and in infants [19,20]. In the perinatal period, the properties of PSEP, as reliable early diagnostic indicators of sepsis, can regard: (i) the fact that acute and chronic hypoxia insults do not constitute confounding factors as to its reliability in sepsis diagnosis [21]; (ii) its measurability in different biological fluids including urine and saliva [22], under several pathological conditions such as early neonatal sepsis, perinatal asphyxia, and fetal chronic hypoxia [23]; and (iii) its thermostability at room temperature and after thawing [24]. While PSEP has been established as a marker for sepsis in various biological fluids, its role and variability in breast milk across different stages of lactation and its impact on neonatal health remain unexplored.

Therefore, in the present study we aimed to investigate whether, in a cohort of preterm and term infants fed with BM, PSEP (i) was measurable in BM, (ii) varied according to different maturation stages (colostrum, transition, and mature milks), and (iii) was gestational age and gender dependent.

2. Materials and Methods

2.1. Study Population

Between March 2022 and December 2023, we conducted a multicenter prospective case–control study in 55 women who delivered term (T; n = 22) and preterm (PT; n = 22) infants at our third level referral centers for neonatal intensive care (NICU). The local ethics committees (Presap.ASO.Neonat.19.02/23.05.19) approved the study and informed and signed consent was obtained from all parents of the subjects before inclusion in the study. For sample size calculation, we used changes in PSEP as the main parameter [25]. As no basic data are available for PSEP levels in BM, we assumed an increase of 0.5 standard deviation (SD) in PSEP to be clinically significant. Considering an $\alpha = 0.05$ and using a two-sided test, we estimated a power of 0.95, recruiting 18 PT and T infants fed with BM. To allow for dropouts and withdrawn consent, we added 4 cases. Therefore, the study population consisted of n = 22 PT and T mothers from whom milk (colostrum, C; transition, Tr; mature, Mt) samples, defined according to Playford et al. [25], were collected from birth up to 30 days of age (Figure 1).

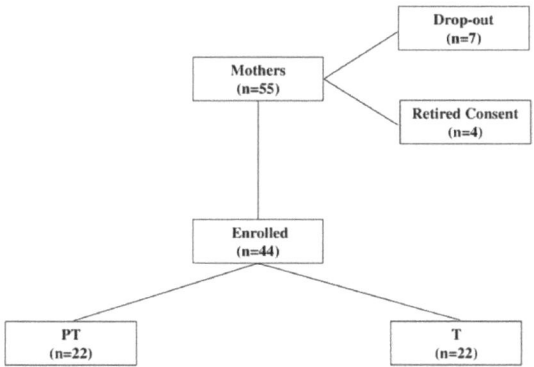

Figure 1. Flow chart describing patients' recruitment. Abbreviations: PT, preterm; T, Term.

Gestational age (GA) was determined using clinical data and a first trimester ultrasound scan. Appropriate growth was defined by the presence of ultrasonographic signs in accordance with current guidelines, and by a post-natal confirmation of a birthweight (BW) ranging between the 10th and 90th percentiles according to our population standards, after adjusting for the mother's height, weight, parity, and the sex of the newborn [26].

At birth, healthy newborns were defined in agreement with the criteria of the American Academy of Pediatrics [27]: no maternal illness, no signs of fetal distress, a pH greater than 7.2 in cord or venous blood, and Apgar scores greater than 7 at 1 and 5 min.

Exclusion criteria were infants with any malformations, chromosomal abnormalities, cardiac or hemolytic disease, chorioamnionitis, maternal systemic infection/inflammation, maternal fever, premature rupture of membranes, early and late onset sepsis, mastitis, and other diseases of the breast.

2.2. Perinatal Outcomes

The following main perinatal and neonatal outcomes were recorded in the studied groups: maternal age; gestational diabetes mellitus (GDM); pregnancy induced hypertension (PIH) and intrauterine growth retardation (IUGR) incidences; GA; BW; delivery mode (vaginal delivery, VD; cesarean section, CS); gender (Male, M; Female, F); and Apgar scores at 1st and 5th min.

2.3. Standard Monitoring Procedures

Laboratory parameters (venous blood pH; partial venous pressure of carbon monoxide, pCO_2; partial venous pressure of oxygen, pO_2; base excess, BE; red blood cell count RBC; hemoglobin blood concentrations, Hb; hematocrit rate, Ht; glucose and ions) were recorded in all infants on admission to NICU.

2.4. BM Collection

Fresh Milk samples were collected into sterile, disposable, high-density polyethylene sealed bottles. Milk was collected with standard extraction methods by means of an electric breast pump (Medela Symphony, Baar, Switzerland). According to current guidelines, in order to collect full pumping samples, the extraction session was stopped 2 min after the outflow of the last drops of milk. From the total amount of milk of each mother, a sample of 5 mL of milk was collected and then stored at $-80\ °C$ until analysis.

2.5. P-SEP Measurements

PSEP milk levels were measured quantitatively (pg/mL) in 5 mL of BM. The detection was performed using a chemiluminescent enzyme immunoassay with the point-of-care automated analyzer PATHFAST-TM (Gepa Diagnostics, Milan, Italy) according to the manufacturer's instructions. The assay detection limit was 200 pg/mL, the coefficient of variability intra-assay was $\leq 5.0\%$, and the coefficient of variability inter-assay was $\leq 10\%$.

The PATHFAST-TM analyzer was chosen for its high sensitivity and specificity for PSEP detection. Each 5 mL milk sample was determined to be optimal for ensuring consistent and reliable results based on preliminary trials.

2.6. Statistical Analysis

The demographic characteristics of maternal and neonatal outcomes were reported as mean $\pm$ SD. PSEP concentrations were expressed as median and interquartile ranges. Statistical analysis was performed by using a two-tailed paired t-test and a Mann–Whitney two-sided U-test when data did not follow a Gaussian distribution. A comparison between the groups was performed by using an ANOVA one-way test. Linear regression analysis was performed for correlations between PSEP levels in different milks and perinatal outcomes. Statistical analysis was performed using Sigma Stat 3.5 (GmBH, Mannheim, Germany). A $p < 0.05$ was considered significant.

3. Results

Perinatal characteristics and the main neonatal outcomes are reported in Table 1.

Table 1. Characteristics of milk donors and perinatal parameters recorded in preterm (PT) and term (T) infants admitted into the study.

Parameters	PT (n = 22)	T (n = 22)	p
Perinatal characteristics			
Maternal age (yrs)	34 ± 5	33.9 ± 4	NS
GDM (n/tot)	5/22	1/22	<0.05
PIH (n/tot)	7/22	0/22	<0.05
IUGR	4/22	1/22	<0.05
Neonatal characteristics			
GA (wks)	33 ± 3.8	39 ± 4	<0.05
BW (g)	1950 ± 650	3100 ± 510	<0.05
CS (n/tot)	13/22	9/22	<0.05
VD (n/tot)	9/22	13/22	<0.05
Gender (M/F)	10/12	9/13	NS
Apgar 1'	8 ± 1	9 ± 0.9	NS
Apgar 5'	9 ± 1	9 ± 1	NS
Monitoring parameters			
pH > 7.20 (n/total)	22/22	22/22	NS
pCO_2 (mmHg)	42 ± 3	41.6 ± 2.8	NS
pO_2 (mmHg)	42.9 ± 1.2	43.1 ± 1.1	NS
BE	−1.1 ± 0.6	−1 ± 0.7	NS
RBC count (10^{12}/L)	4.4 ± 0.3	4.3 ± 0.2	NS
Hb (g/L)	14.5 ± 3	13.8 ± 2.9	NS
Ht (%)	41 ± 0.07	41.5 ± 0.08	NS
Plasma glucose (mmol/L)	5.1 ± 0.2	5.2 ± 0.4	NS
Na^+ (mmol/L)	138.5 ± 0.9	139 ± 1	NS
Ca^{++} (mmol/L)	1.12 ± 0.02	1.13 ± 0.03	NS
K^+ (mmol/L)	3.8 ± 0.25	3.9 ± 0.2	NS

Abbreviations: PT, preterm; T, term; yrs, years; GDM, gestational diabetes mellitus; n, number; tot, total; PIH, pregnancy induced hypertension; IUGR, intrauterine growth retardation; GA, gestational age; wks, weeks; BW, birthweight; g, grams; CS, cesarean section; VD vaginal delivery; M, male; F, female; pCO_2, partial carbon dioxide venous pressure; pO_2, partial oxygen venous pressure; BE, base excess; RBC, red blood cell count; Hb, hemoglobin blood concentrations; Ht, hematocrit rate; Na+, sodium; Ca++, calcium; K+, potassium.

All enrolled mothers were Caucasian. Higher ($p < 0.05$, for all) incidences of GDM (6%), PIH (32%), and IUGR (18%) occurred in the PT group. As expected, GA and BW were lower ($p < 0.05$, for both) in the PT than in the T group. Moreover, the incidences of CS and VD ($p < 0.05$, for both) were higher and lower in the PT group, respectively. No differences ($p > 0.05$, for all) in maternal age, Apgar score at 1'–5' min, or gender were observed between the studied groups.

Laboratory parameters recorded at admission to our NICUs are reported in Table 2. No significant differences ($p > 0.05$, for all) were observed between groups for blood, pH, pCO_2, pO_2, BE, RBC, Hb, Ht, blood glucose, or ion levels.

Table 2. Presepsin levels in preterm (PT) and term (T) infants corrected for delivery mode and gender. Values are expressed in median and interquartile ranges. $p < 0.05$: [a] PSEP C vs. Tr and Mt; [b] PSEP C vs. Tr; [c] PSEP Tr vs. Mt; [d] PSEP C vs. Mt; * PT C, Tr and Mt vs. TC, Tr and Mt; ** PT C and Tr vs. T C and Tr; [&] M Mt vs. F Mt.

Presepsin (pg(mL)	PT (n = 22)			T (n = 22)	
	Median	25°	75°	Median	25°
Delivery Mode					
C VD	15.906 [d]**	11.326	19.789	5.843 [b]*	4.545
Tr VD	9.185	2.356	16.014	3.836	2.741
Mt VD	6.458	5.501	7.502	6.334	2.125
C CS	16.718 [a]	10.976	19.934	5.609 [cd]	4.260
Tr CS	11.303 [c]	9.228	19841	5.032	3.932
Mt CS	7.392	6.804	11938	1.738	1.637
Gender					
C M	16.447 [a]*	11.314	19.471	6.596	5.051
Tr M	11.303	8.668	19.841	3.932	3.862
Mt M	9.800 [&]	7.155	12.134	4.532	2.879
C F	16.888 [a]**	10.638	19.879	5.609	3.877
Tr F	10.458	6.502	11.766	3.836	2.127
Mt F	6.804	6.555	7.391	6.334	1.681

Abbreviations: PT, preterm; T, term; C, colostrum; Tr, transition; Mt, mature; VD, vaginal delivery; CS, cesarean section; M, male; F, female.

All infants admitted into the study were discharged in good clinical condition and no overt damage to any organs was detectable.

3.1. PSEP BM Levels in Total Population

PSEP was detectable in all BM samples collected. When milk samples were corrected for the grade of maturation in the whole study population, the level of PSEP in C was higher ($p < 0.001$, for both) than in the Tr and Mt fluids. No significant differences ($p > 0.05$) were observed in PSEP between the Tr and Mt fluids (Figure 2).

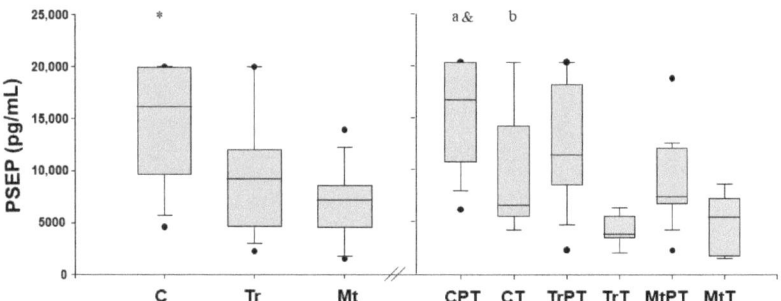

Figure 2. Presepsin (PSEP) milk levels (pg/mL) measured in colostrum (C), transition (Tr) and mature (Mt) milk fluids in the preterm (PT) and term (T) groups. Values are expressed in median and interquartile ranges. $p < 0.05$; * PSEP C vs. Tr vs. Mt; a PT PSEP C vs. Tr vs. Mt; b T PSEP C vs. Tr; & PT PSEP C, Tr, Mt vs. T PSEP C, Tr, Mt.

3.2. PSEP BM Levels in PT and T Infants

The PSEP BM levels in the PT and T infants are reported in Figure 2. In the PT infants, the PSEP levels in the C fluid were significantly higher ($p < 0.001$) than those in the Tr and Mt, whilst no differences ($p > 0.05$) were detectable between the Tr and Mt fluids.

In T infants, the PSEP levels in the C fluid were significantly higher ($p < 0.05$) than those in Tr, whilst no differences ($p > 0.05$, for both) were detectable between C and Mt or between Tr and Mt.

Higher ($p < 0.001$) PSEP levels were observed in the PT compared to the T infants when comparing the total amount of the protein. Notably, when we compared PSEP levels between PT and T groups after correction for BM degree of maturation we found that PT infants had significantly higher ($p < 0.001$, for all) PSEP levels in C, Tr, and Mt fluids than their equivalent BM fluids in T infants (Figure 2).

3.3. PSEP BM and Delivery Mode

In Table 2, the PSEP levels when corrected for the delivery mode in the whole study population and for the BM sub-types are reported.

The PSEP levels in the VD PT and T infants were lower ($p < 0.01$) than in those born by CS. Conversely, higher ($p < 0.001$, for both) PSEP levels were found in PT infants delivered both by VD and CS than in T ones. No significant differences ($p > 0.05$, for all) in BM PSEP sub-types were observed among PT infants regardless of delivery mode. The same pattern ($p > 0.05$, for all) was observed in T infants. In PT VD infants, higher C PSEP than Mt was found, whilst no significant differences ($p > 0.05$, for both) between C and Tr or Tr and Mt were observed. In PT CS infants, the PSEP levels in the C fluid were significantly higher ($p < 0.05$, for both) than those in the Tr and Mt fluids, and the level of PSEP in Tr was higher ($p > 0.05$) than that in the Mt fluid.

In T VD infants, the PSEP levels were higher ($p < 0.05$) in C than Tr, whilst no differences were observed between C vs. Mt or Tr vs Mt.

After correction for CS, higher C PSEP and Tr ($p < 0.05$) than Mt levels were found ($p < 0.05$, for both). When we compared the levels of PSEP between the PT and T groups after correction for delivery mode and BM degree of maturation we found (i) higher ($p < 0.05$, for both) C and Tr PT VD PSEP levels than T ones, whilst no differences ($p > 0.05$) were detectable between Mt fluids, (ii) and higher ($p < 0.05$, for all) C, Tr and Mt PSEP levels in PT CS infants than T ones.

3.4. PSEP BM and Gender

Milk samples were corrected for gender in the whole study population and for the BM sub-types (Table 2). No significant gender differences ($p > 0.05$, for both) were observed in the PT and T total populations. Indeed, PSEP levels in the M and F PT sub-groups were higher ($p < 0.001$, for both) than M and F T male sub-groups.

In the M and F PT subgroups, we found higher ($p < 0.05$, for both) C PSEP levels than in the Tr and Mt fluids. No differences ($p > 0.05$) were found in PSEP between the Tr and Mt fluids.

In the M and F T subgroups, no differences ($p > 0.05$, for all) in PSEP levels among the C, Tr, and Mt fluids were found.

When we compared the PT and T groups after correcting for gender, we found higher ($p < 0.05$, for all) C, Tr, and MT PSEP levels in the M PT sub-groups than those of M T. Indeed, higher ($p < 0.05$, for all) C and Tr PSEP levels were observed in the F PT sub-group than the F T sub-group and no differences in Mt fluids between the sub-groups were shown. Finally, higher ($p < 0.05$) M PT Mt PSEP than F PT Mt PSEP was observed.

4. Discussion

The mother's own milk is widely accepted as a unique fluid, containing biological factors involved in the regulation of optimal newborn development and growth (including hormones, growth factors, and cytokines), through which biochemical communication between mother and child is established [1–3,24]. This especially holds true for BM's antimicrobial properties that protect particularly preterm infants from early and late infections and from major post-natal complications such as neonatal necrotizing enterocolitis [17]. The issue is of significance bearing in mind the high mortality and morbidity rates in that delicate population.

In the present study, we found that a promising biomarker for sepsis, namely PSEP, is more highly concentrated in the BM of mothers delivering a PT rather than a T infant. Notably, BM and its sub-types of maturation (colostrum, transition, mature) were delivery mode and gender dependent.

The presence of PSEP, or sCD14, and its sub-types at high levels in BM matches, in part, previous observations [28,29]. Discrepancies lie in the study population's characteristics such as ethnicity, type of disease (bacterial and fungal sepsis, HIV), monitoring time-points (1 vs 4 months), and measurement technique (ELISA, CLEIA, cytometric bead array) [30,31]. Notably, none of the mothers were complicated by any allergy and/or excess maternal weight, both of which are known to affect PSEP release in the BM [32,33].

4.1. BM PSEP

The high PSEP levels detected in BM warrant further consideration. In particular, BM PSEP levels (i) were 10–20-fold higher than others detected in different biological fluids (i.e., blood, urine, saliva) from both of healthy PT and T infants and from those complicated by early/late onset sepsis [18]. This finding is in agreement with data showing that the levels of a series of cytokines involved in immune defenses, and in brain development [17], (ii) in both PT and T groups were higher than those previously reported. The explanation for this lies in the different measurement techniques and different endpoints used [17,29], and (iii) they were significantly increased in PT than T infants both considering total BM PSEP or its sub-type levels. This finding is noteworthy and offers additional support to the notion of the release of the marker for inflammation in placenta and systemic circulation during labor, particularly in PT cases known to be mainly triggered by a perinatal infection [34]. Bearing in mind that, in the present series, we excluded all the cases in whom perinatal sepsis had occurred, it is reasonable to argue for PSEP activation through a microbial-independent pathway [35].

4.2. BM PSEP Degree of Maturation

The finding that the PSEP levels increase according to the degree of BM maturation deserves further consideration. In particular, we found that the C PSEP levels in PT infants were higher than those measured at different stages of maturation (Tr, Mt), whilst in T infants a similar pattern was observed except there were no differences between the C and Mt fluids. These findings are in agreement with previous observations aimed at measuring a series of cytokines in BM and its sub-types [17,35]. Among a series of explanations, to date still under debate, the main ones, after having excluded environmental factors, regard functional/biochemical issues. In particular, (i) considering the significant differences in PSEP between the two main districts of concentration such as systemic circulation (low) and BM (high) the high C levels support the hypothesis of a mammary gland epithelium site of PSEP production [35], (ii) BM can achieve a PSEP serum extra-aliquot through a paracellular pathway [35], and (iii) PSEP over-production by mammary glands as a compensatory mechanism to adjust immunity of PT infants [29]. Altogether, the possibility that preterm birth, in the absence of any early laboratory signs of infection, could somewhat be triggered by a cascade of inflammatory events leading to the release of PSEP into systemic maternal circulation is, therefore, reasonable. Further studies aimed at elucidating the aforementioned issues are, therefore, justified.

4.3. BM PSEP and Delivery Mode

In the present study, we also found that BM PSEP levels both in PT and T infants were delivery mode dependent. In particular, the highest PSEP levels were observed (i) in

PT infants compared to T ones regardless of delivery mode, and (ii) in C VD and CS PT sub-types both when compared to Tr and Mt PT and T BM fluids. Discrepancies with the literature data are due to the different PSEP measurement techniques, the study population (extremely PT vs. moderate and late PT infants), and monitoring time-points used [35]. The pattern of increased BM PSEP levels in PT born by VD and CS than T ones warrants further consideration. On the one hand, labor is associated with an increased immune response activation [36], whereas the increase in the immune factor in PT mother's milk after labor could be a compensatory mechanism aiming to protect the immature infant [29].

4.4. PSEP BM and Gender

In the present series, we found that BM PSEP levels are gender dependent with higher Mt protein' levels in PT males than females. To the best of our knowledge, the finding constitutes the first observation in this setting offering additional support to sex-related differences in the perinatal period [37]. Indeed, the higher impact of prematurity on male compared to female infants has also been demonstrated, as well as diversity in whole organ development [29]. The possibility that the higher Mt PSEP levels detected in PT male infants could be related to a pathophysiological cascade of events involving preterm labor, inflammation, and mammary gland PSEP over-release is, therefore, consistent. Thus, differences in the immune system will be included in a broader study aimed at investigating gender-related prenatal whole organ development.

4.5. Study Limitation

Lastly, the present study had a number of limitations such as (i) the small sample size, (ii) the lack of potential effects of maternal diseases on BM PSEP levels, and (iii) the potential bias due to maternal dietary regimen and pro-biotic supplementation on BM PSEP levels.

5. Conclusions

In conclusion, the present results showing the presence at high levels of PSEP in BM and its sub-types point to the protein's potential antimicrobial role in the perinatal protection/development of the maternal–newborn dyad. Notably, the detection of high PSEP levels in PT C suggests its potential for early diagnostic use in neonatal care settings. Future studies should investigate the longitudinal effects of PSEP levels on infant health outcomes and the potential for integrating PSEP monitoring into routine neonatal screenings.

Author Contributions: Conceptualization, E.D., C.P., M.S., R.B., A.M., A.N., V.B., A.C., E.B., F.G., A.S.A., M.C., S.P., M.D., M.L., M.T.Q. and D.G.; investigation, E.D., C.P., M.S., R.B., A.M., A.N., V.B., A.C., E.B., F.G., A.S.A., M.C., S.P., M.D., M.L., M.T.Q. and D.G.; writing—original draft preparation, E.D., C.P., M.S., R.B., A.M., A.N., V.B., A.C., E.B., F.G., A.S.A., M.C., S.P., M.D., M.L. and M.T.Q.; project administration, D.G.; supervision, D.G.; writing—review and editing, D.G. All authors have read and agreed to the published version of the manuscript.

Funding: This research was funded by I COLORI DELLA VITA FOUNDATION, grant 2/2018 and DANONE, grant 3/2019. We thank PHC Europe BV, The Netherlands, for scientific support, and Gepa S.r.l, Italy, for providing analysis kits. Authors extend their sincere appreciation to Researchers Supporting Project number (RSPD2024R750), King Saud University, Riyadh, Saudi Arabia.

Institutional Review Board Statement: The study was conducted in accordance with the Declaration of Helsinki, and approved by the Ethics Committee of ASO SS ANTONIO, BIAGIO AND C. ARRIGO, ALESSANDRIA, ITALY (Presap.ASO.Neonat.19.02/19 May 2023).

Informed Consent Statement: Informed consent was obtained from all subjects involved in the study.

Data Availability Statement: The data presented in this study are available on request from the corresponding author due to hospital privacy statement.

Conflicts of Interest: The authors declare no conflicts of interest. The funders had no role in the design of the study: in the collection: analyses, or interpretation of data; in the writing of the manuscript; or in the decision to publish the results.

References

1. Meek, J.Y.; Noble, L. Policy Statement: Breastfeeding and the Use of Human Milk. *Pediatrics* 2022, *150*, e2022057988. [CrossRef]
2. American Academy of Paediatrics. Breastfeeding and the use of human milk. *Pediatrics* 2012, *129*, e827–e841. [CrossRef] [PubMed]
3. Saadeh, M.R. A new global strategy for infant and young child feeding. *Forum. Nutr.* 2003, *56*, 236–238.
4. Lönnerdal, B. Bioactive proteins in breast milk. *J. Paediatr. Child. Health* 2013, *49* (Suppl. S1), S1–S7. [CrossRef] [PubMed]
5. Rio-Aige, K.; Azagra-Boronat, I.; Castell, M.; Selma-Royo, M.; Collado, M.C.; Rodríguez-Lagunas, M.J.; Pérez-Cano, F.J. The Breast Milk Immunoglobulinome. *Nutrients* 2021, *13*, 1810. [CrossRef] [PubMed]
6. LeMaster, C.; Pierce, S.H.; Geanes, E.S.; Khanal, S.; Elliott, S.S.; Scott, A.B.; Louiselle, D.A.; McLennan, R.; Maulik, D.; Lewis, T.; et al. The cellular and immunological dynamics of early and transitional human milk. *Commun. Biol.* 2023, *6*, 539–551. [CrossRef]
7. Gazzolo, D.; Monego, G.; Corvino, V.; Bruschettini, M.; Bruschettini, P.; Zelano, G.; Michetti, F. Human milk contains S100B protein. *Biochim. Biophys. Acta* 2003, *1619*, 209–212. [CrossRef]
8. Andreas, N.J.; Kampmann, B.; Mehring Le-Doare, K. Human breast milk: A review on its composition and bioactivity. *Early Hum. Dev.* 2015, *91*, 629–635. [CrossRef]
9. Serpero, L.D.; Frigiola, A.; Gazzolo, D. Human milk and formulae: Neurotrophic and new biological factors. *Early Hum. Dev.* 2012, *88* (Suppl. S1), S9–S12. [CrossRef]
10. Victora, C.G.; Bahl, R.; Barros, A.J.; França, G.V.; Horton, S.; Krasevec, J.; Murch, S.; Sankar, M.J.; Walker, N.; Rollins, N.C.; et al. Breastfeeding in the 21st century: Epidemiology, mechanisms, and lifelong effect. *Lancet* 2016, *387*, 475–490. [CrossRef]
11. Bauer, J.; Gerss, J. Longitudinal analysis of macronutrients and minerals in human milk produced by mothers of preterm infants. *Clin. Nutr.* 2011, *30*, 215–220. [CrossRef]
12. Kim, S.Y.; Yi, D.Y. Components of human breast milk: From macronutrient to microbiome and microRNA. *Clin. Exp. Pediatr.* 2020, *63*, 301–309. [CrossRef]
13. Gazzolo, D.; Bruschettini, M.; Lituania, M.; Serra, G.; Santini, P.; Michetti, F. Levels of S100B protein are higher in mature human milk than in colostrum and milk-formulae milks. *Clin. Nutr.* 2004, *23*, 23–26. [CrossRef]
14. Reis, F.M.; Luisi, S.; Carneiro, M.M.; Cobellis, L.; Federico, M.; Camargos, A.F.; Petraglia, F. Activin, inhibin and the human breast. *Mol. Cell Endocrinol.* 2004, *225*, 77–82. [CrossRef]
15. Blais, D.R.; Harrold, J.; Altosaar, I. Killing the Messenger in the Nick of Time: Persistence of Breast Milk sCD14 in the Neonatal Gastrointestinal Tract. *Pediatr. Res.* 2006, *59*, 371–376. [CrossRef] [PubMed]
16. Fikri, B.; Tani, Y.; Nagai, K.; Sahara, M.; Mitsuishi, C.; Togawa, Y.; Nakano, T.; Yamaide, F.; Ohno, H.; Shimojo, N. Soluble CD14 in Breast Milk and Its Relation to Atopic Manifestations in Early Infancy. *Nutrients* 2019, *11*, 2118. [CrossRef] [PubMed]
17. Vidal, K.; Labéta, M.O.; Schiffrin, E.J.; Donnet-Hughes, A. Soluble CD14 in human breast milk and its role in innate immune responses. *Acta Odontol. Scand.* 2001, *59*, 330–334. [CrossRef]
18. Botondi, V.; D'Adamo, E.; Plebani, M.; Trubiani, O.; Perrotta, M.; Di Ricco, L.; Spagnuolo, C.; De Sanctis, S.; Barbante, E.; Strozzi, M.C.; et al. Perinatal presepsin assessment: A new sepsis diagnostic tool? *Clin. Chem. Lab. Med.* 2022, *60*, 1136–1144. [CrossRef]
19. Pugni, L.; Pietrasanta, C.; Milani, S.; Vener, C.; Ronchi, A.; Falbo, M.; Arghittu, M.; Mosca, F. Presepsin (Soluble CD14 Subtype): Reference Ranges of a New Sepsis Marker in Term and Preterm Neonates. *PLoS ONE* 2015, *10*, e0146020. [CrossRef]
20. Shozushima, T.; Takahashi, G.; Matsumoto, N.; Kojima, M.; Okamura, Y.; Endo, S. Usefulness of presepsin (sCD14-ST) measurements as a marker for the diagnosis and severity of sepsis that satisfied diagnostic criteria of systemic inflammatory response syndrome. *J. Infect. Chemother.* 2011, *17*, 764–769. [CrossRef] [PubMed]
21. D'Adamo, E.; Levantini, G.; Librandi, M.; Botondi, V.; Di Ricco, L.; De Sanctis, S.; Spagnuolo, C.; Gazzolo, F.; Gavilanes, D.A.; Di Gregorio, P. Fetal chronic hypoxia does not affect urinary presepsin levels in newborns at birth. *Clin. Chem. Lab. Med.* 2024, *62*, 1643–1648. [CrossRef]
22. Bellos, I.; Fitrou, G.; Pergialiotis, V.; Thomakos, N.; Perrea, D.N.; Daskalakis, G. The diagnostic accuracy of presepsin in neonatal sepsis: A meta-analysis. *Eur. J. Pediatr.* 2018, *177*, 625–632. [CrossRef]
23. Botondi, V.; Pirra, A.; Strozzi, M.; Perrotta, M.; Gavilanes, D.A.W.; Di Ricco, L.; Spagnuolo, C.; Maconi, A.; Rocchetti, A.; Mazzucco, L.; et al. Perinatal asphyxia partly affects presepsin urine levels in non-infected term infants. *Clin. Chem. Lab. Med.* 2022, *60*, 793–799. [CrossRef]
24. D'Adamo, E.; Botondi, V.; Falconio, L.; Giardinelli, G.; Gregorio, P.D.; Caputi, S.; Sinjari, B.; Trubiani, O.; Traini, T.; Gazzolo, F. Effect of temperature on presepsin pre-analytical stability in biological fluids of preterm and term newborns. *Clin. Chem. Lab. Med.* 2024, *62*, 1011–1016. [CrossRef] [PubMed]
25. Playford, R.J.; Macdonald, C.E.; Johnson, W.S. Colostrum and milk-derived peptide growth factors for the treatment of gastrointestinal disorders. *Am. J. Clin. Nutr.* 2000, *72*, 5–14. [CrossRef] [PubMed]
26. Bertino, E.; Di Nicola, P.; Varalda, A.; Occhi, L.; Giuliani, F.; Coscia, A. Neonatal growth charts. *J. Matern. Fetal Neonatal Med.* 2012, *25* (Suppl.S1), 67–69. [CrossRef]
27. American Academy of Paediatrics. The APGAR score. *Pediatrics* 2015, *136*, 819–822. [CrossRef] [PubMed]

28. Nur Ergor, S.; Yalaz, M.; Altun Koroglu, O.; Sozmen, E.; Akisu, M.; Kultursay, N. Reference ranges of presepsin (soluble CD14 subtype) in term and preterm neonates without infection, in relation to gestational and postnatal age, in the first 28 days of life. *Clin. Biochem.* **2020**, *77*, 7–13. [CrossRef]
29. Trend, S.; Strunk, T.; Lloyd, M.L.; Kok, C.H.; Metcalfe, J.; Geddes, D.T.; Lai, T.C.; Richmond, P.; Doherty, D.A.; Simmer, K.; et al. Levels of innate immune factors in preterm and term mothers' breast milk during the 1st month postpartum. *Br. J. Nutr.* **2016**, *115*, 1178–1793. [CrossRef]
30. Holmlund, U.; Amoudruz, P.; Johansson, M.A.; Haileselassie, Y.; Ongoiba, A.; Kayentao, K.; Traorè, B.; Doumbo, S.; Schollin, J.; Montgomery, S.M.; et al. Maternal country of origin, breast milk characteristics and potential influences on immunity in offspring. *Clin. Exp. Immunol.* **2010**, *162*, 500–509. [CrossRef]
31. Okamura, Y.; Yokoi, H. Development of a point-of-care assay system for measurement of presepsin (sCD14-ST). *Clin. Chim. Acta* **2011**, *412*, 2157–2161. [CrossRef]
32. Hua, M.C.; Chen, C.C.; Yao, T.C.; Tsai, M.H.; Liao, S.L.; Lai, S.H.; Chiu, C.H.; Yeh, K.W.; Huang, J.L. Role of maternal Allergy on Immune Markers in Colostrum and Secretory Immunoglobulin A in Stools of Breastfed Infants. *J. Hum. Lact.* **2016**, *32*, 160–167. [CrossRef]
33. Collado, M.C.; Laitinen, K.; Salminen, S.; Isolauri, E. Maternal weight and excessive weight gain during pregnancy modify the immunomodulatory potential of breast milk. *Pediatr. Res.* **2012**, *72*, 77–85. [CrossRef] [PubMed]
34. Maddaloni, C.; De Rose, D.U.; Santisi, A.; Martini, L.; Caoci, S.; Bersani, I.; Ronchetti, M.P.; Auriti, C. The Emerging Role of Presepsin (P-SEP) in the Diagnosis of Sepsis in the Critically Ill Infant: A Literature Review. *Int. J. Mol. Sci.* **2021**, *22*, 12154. [CrossRef] [PubMed]
35. Labéta, M.O.; Vidal, K.; Nores, J.E.; Arias, M.; Vita, N.; Morgan, B.P.; Guillemot, J.C.; Loyaux, D.; Ferrara, P.; Schmid, D. Innate recognition of bacteria in human milk is mediated by a milk-derived highly expressed pattern recognition receptor, soluble CD14. *J. Exp. Med.* **2000**, *191*, 1807–1812. [CrossRef] [PubMed]
36. Ando, K.; Hedou, J.J.; Feyaerts, D.; Han, X.; Ganio, E.A.; Tsai, E.S.; Peterson, L.S.; Verdonk, F.; Tsai, A.S.; Maric, I.; et al. A Peripheral Immune Signature of Labor Induction. *Front. Immunol.* **2021**, *12*, 725989. [CrossRef] [PubMed]
37. O'Driscoll, D.N.; McGovern, M.; Greene, C.M.; Molloy, E.J. Gender disparities in preterm neonatal outcomes. *Acta Paediatr.* **2018**, *107*, 1494–1499. [CrossRef]

Disclaimer/Publisher's Note: The statements, opinions and data contained in all publications are solely those of the individual author(s) and contributor(s) and not of MDPI and/or the editor(s). MDPI and/or the editor(s) disclaim responsibility for any injury to people or property resulting from any ideas, methods, instructions or products referred to in the content.

MDPI AG
Grosspeteranlage 5
4052 Basel
Switzerland
Tel.: +41 61 683 77 34

Nutrients Editorial Office
E-mail: nutrients@mdpi.com
www.mdpi.com/journal/nutrients

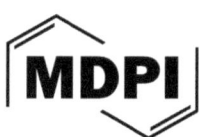

Disclaimer/Publisher's Note: The title and front matter of this reprint are at the discretion of the Guest Editor. The publisher is not responsible for their content or any associated concerns. The statements, opinions and data contained in all individual articles are solely those of the individual Editor and contributors and not of MDPI. MDPI disclaims responsibility for any injury to people or property resulting from any ideas, methods, instructions or products referred to in the content.

www.ingramcontent.com/pod-product-compliance
Lightning Source LLC
LaVergne TN
LVHW072352090526
838202LV00019B/2529